QUESTIONS ...
QUESTIONS ...
QUESTIONS ...

What physical changes can I expect during pregnancy? What should my diet be? ... What things should be bought before baby comes? ... When are fears foolish, and when is there real cause for alarm? ... What different kinds of child-birth methods are there? ... Should I breast-feed or bottle-feed? ... When should I start giving my baby solid food? ... What is a normal pattern of growth and development? ... What are common discipline problems? Health problems? Accident problems? ... Am I really being a good parent? ...

You and Your Baby has been written to help give you the confidence and authority so important for both yourself and your child. Here you will find the answers to all your questions—in a wonderful modern guide that is truly the answer to a parent's prayers.

SIGNET Titles of Special Interest

Contents

Introduction

In this book I will talk to you about your baby and how he develops before birth and grows in his first year of life. It isn't designed to be a textbook. I have written it for parents of new babies, not for other doctors. In over thirty years of practice in pediatrics I have learned a great deal from these babies and the couples to whom they were born. Now that the ten thousandth baby has come and gone through his first year, I will try to share with you some of what I have learned.

If I had written this book thirty years ago, or even twenty years ago, it would have been somewhat different. Lord Rochester once said: "Before I got married I had six theories about bringing up children. Now I have six children and no theories." That quotation is appropriate to my point, as is the following:

> Many years ago I discovered that there could be no simple formula for raising children. When I was a young psychiatrist, the father of one child, I loftily developed a lecture entitled, no less, "A Decalogue for Parents." Like a new Moses I enunciated Ten Commandments based on the successful rearing of Son Number 1. Along came Son Number 2, a nonconformist, who shattered my feelings of certainty. I changed the title of the lecture to "Ten Hints for Parents." With this change of authoritarianism I got along well until the third child was born, a girl! Then I gave up the lecture entirely.*

These comments mean that you—and I—go on learning from our children, just as they learn from you.

If you have had no previous experience with children you

*Abraham Myerson, M.D., *Speaking of Man* (New York, Alfred A. Knopf, 1951).

may have an advantage: i.e., no preconceived ideas! This gives you a chance to learn your own way. As your love for your baby and your skill in caring for him develops, you will come to know him well. His love and confidence in you grow as you care for him even if you are no expert. He is a pretty tough guy in spite of his size. He can take a lot of your learning efforts and lack of skill, as long as he gets the feel of your affection and goodwill. So take care of him happily and gain confidence. You don't have to do everything "right"—whatever that is! Don't get so involved in the techniques that you lose sight of your baby—he is the reason for all of them.

You want to do a good job as parents when your new baby arrives. The seasoned parent is no more determined in this than is the new parent. Each of you tries to give your child the best care. As veteran parents, you may find you don't need some of the details of child care I give. My goal for you, whether you are new or veteran parents, is to enable you to come up with a child-care plan of your own that makes you comfortable as parents while you help your baby get up on his own two feet during this first year.

Unfortunately, there is a continual barrage of free-of-charge advice on how to be a good parent. This showers down from newspapers, magazines, radio, and TV. The deluge can sweep you away. In the past twenty-five years there have been over seventy-five hundred volumes published on the care of the child. Without meaning to, this material often creates more problems than it solves. Authorities rush into print to argue out the bewildering intricacies of child care, often without recognizing the part that inheritance and social factors play. Everyone is confused by this. Anxious fathers and mothers come to fear that even the most innocently spoken word or careless act will harm their child and guarantee his future unhappiness. The great American preoccupation is how to succeed as a parent. I much prefer to consider the journey an individual makes from his cradle to his grave as a long sequence of different-sized steps. He starts with some basic equipment that he acquired from his parents and grandparents. Depending upon his ability to learn and use his experiences with his family, other people, and his surroundings, he makes his steps with different degrees of comfort and discomfort, success and failure. His way of going is his own. But he follows the well-worn path every human must pass along. While, as his parents, you can aid or interfere with his march to adulthood, he is ultimately responsible for his own acts and methods for gaining his goal.

Books in the field of infant care have a problem. They have to generalize in order to answer questions, but their answers may not be the answers for your child. Read if you wish, but keep your perspective. And remember that your pediatrician is the best source for specific answers to particular questions about your child.

This book was written to help you to do your job of normal day-to-day child-rearing more intelligently. An informed parent is a big advantage for your child—and your pediatrician. It is not intended to be a substitute for the regular care your pediatrician provides. Regular visits give him a chance to estimate your baby's progress, make suggestions, answer your questions. They are preferable to random visits or visits made only when your baby is ill and at his worst. Your doctor will know and understand your baby and you as time goes on. Ask him your questions as they come up. Jot them down at home so that you can ask them on your next regular visit—or use the telephone.

In reading this book, you will have to accept one basic premise. All babies are alike in that they are products of the human· race, and yet each is different, an individual. There is no great difference in the orderly way in which a baby develops, no matter what his skin color or racial derivation. What you do find is variation in babies according to the parents they have, the homes they live in, and the different backgrounds they have. As I talk about the average baby, you as his parents will have to work with the material presented here from your own backgrounds, biases, and feelings.

In giving you the facts about your baby's development, I try not to make them just a recital of statistics, but to let you see the intriguing changes that development makes in your young human beings. Examining these facts will help you to adopt a sensible program for your baby. Read the material describing each month as he reaches that age level. You need to know the facts about average development so that you have some idea of what to expect. If you know about the progress a baby makes in walking, you won't expect him to stand alone and walk at six months. You can be comfortable with your child's curiosity and not expect instant obedient response at nine months—or demand toilet training at six months.

My descriptions of the conditions for average change and development show you the wide range of differences present in normal children. Your own baby's growth furnishes his own pattern. Try to understand it. You may find this difficult if you attempt to hold too tightly to some of the guidelines and patterns of development. Don't try to make your child fit any developmental pattern but his own. He may not settle neatly into any such general group as I describe. You don't have to label him abnormal just because he decides to follow his own special pattern. Consult with your medical adviser before you imagine the worst.

In the suggestions for baby care I try to show you the flexibility that must exist in any commonsense approach. Baby care isn't just physical exercise. It has to do with management, manners, and morals, too. The "whys" and the "wherefores" are just as important as the "hows." I do try to point out the realities of child care as opposed to the theories about emotional and psychological realities that come and go. I do try to pass on to you some of the shortcuts.

If you too rigidly try to make your baby follow any plan, you're in for trouble. Don't pay too much attention to the pros and cons of any one way of doing things. There are many ways to approach the care of a child—and anything that can avoid the effort, anxiety, and worry of a full-time, overconcerned child-rearing existence is fine. Just because you don't minutely follow all my suggestions doesn't mean you will be in trouble later. If you find there is a better way for you, based on your reasonble convictions, follow it. You won't be making a horrible mistake. The whole idea is to take your cues from your baby so that your guidance can be effective and helpful, not to go against his needs or abilities.

This book is directed to both of you—mother and father. To avoid confusion, I will begin any comments especially directed to you, the father, by saying, "As a father, you . . ." You will want to read the parts addressed to your wife just as she will need to know about the material in the parts addressed to you.

Being told about your baby and what you may expect him to do, gives you understanding and knowledge, but you can't raise your child by the book. You have to experience parenthood: there is no other way to go. As you encounter parenthood you will find that you will have to make some changes in your own emotional makeup. Your ability to make a positive, constructive effort to cope with these new stresses and situations will be a plus mark for your baby's progress.

You may be surprised at some of the suggestions I make in this book. They may be different from what you have been told. I frequently indicate where you can take advantage of your baby's readiness to move ahead. This may be contrary to the latest magazine article you have read. People often have difficulty letting go of old ways of thinking and doing and taking up new ones. Discussions about babies too often pay very little attention to their demands for growth.

It would be difficult and confusing to go through the book saying "he" and "she." For my purposes assume that "he" means either a boy or a girl. If there are developmental differences, I will point them out. In general, a girl baby moves ahead a little faster for a time than a boy baby. She reaches her maturity at an earlier age as a result.

Now that all this explaining is out of the way, let's get started on this exciting journey you are to make as a family!

1.

Pregnancy

Your baby has a past before he is even conceived. The egg from which the embryo begins was in your ovary before you were born. The sperm from his father that joined the egg lay quiet in his father's testicles while he was still in his mother's uterus. The two halves of the baby's hereditary message were coded and capsuled in each of his parents years before your union occurred.

Your baby develops from his single cell gradually. His development reflects the evolutionary history his ancestors made over millions of years. He doesn't go through every step of the journey in an abbreviated form. The outlines of the path are there, but he scrambles up a lot of the sequences of the ancestral journey. He takes every shortcut he can to develop from a human egg into a full-term baby. He has only nine short months to do it in. Let us take a look at how he develops.

FOURTH WEEK (22 TO 28 DAYS)

By this time, you have missed your first period and may be wondering about the possibility. But your baby is already more than a possibility—he has a head to show it! Floating in his amniotic sac attached to the wall of your uterus, he is a fragile, gelatinous mass with almost no substance, but he has a body with a large head and at least the makings of a brain. At this stage he looks much like the embryo of any mammal. (See fig. 1.).

His blunt head end protrudes with two large upper bulges that will become his forebrain. Just below are two sets of

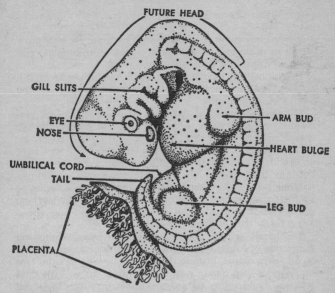

Fig. 1. Embryo at one month. Approximately three-fifths actual size. *Reprinted through the courtesy of the Johns Hopkins Press.*

bulges or folds around a central hollow place. These will become his face, with mouth, nose, upper and lower jaws, in another month. His face is only a forehead now above his future mouth and jaws. There are signs of the places where his eyes and ears will be, but no nose or outer ears as yet.

Below these is a large forward bulge, pulsating regularly and pointed to his mouth area. This is his primitive heart. It is only two millimeters long, but it is nine times as large as an adult heart in proportion to his body size. He needs this big pump to push the blood through his umbilical cord, placenta, and himself. There are three neck arches behind his big heart that resemble the gill arches in fish embryos. Behind these, down his back, are the forming vertebrae and spinal canal.

His arm buds appear on his twenty-sixth day. Two days later he will show leg buds or bulges.

There are simple kidneys, a liver, and a digestive tract. He shows signs of a rather simple umbilical cord.

FIFTH WEEK (29 TO 35 DAYS)

He reaches about a third of an inch long. He will grow a quarter of an inch in a week and look more human. You think of yourself as pregnant now.

His blunt head end with forehead and forebrain is still his most prominent feature. It is about one third to one half of his total length.

His eyes show up as dark circles where the black pigment layer of the retina is developing. You can see the eye lens forming, too, along with the future eye cover, or cornea. There is even a place showing where he will have an eyelid. A small cleft behind his eye area will be his ear, but it is quite low on his neck. He has a rather primitive mouth cavity. The wide-apart openings of his nose shape up their rims to begin the formation of the upper jaw and nose. The structures at his head end are growing ahead much faster than at the lower end.

His hands appear now, starting as rounded bumps on either side of his body, coming out of a ridge along the side of his body on his thirtieth day. The following day the arm bud divides into hand, arm, and shoulder areas. Two days later the hand shows its finger outlines through the ridged web of the hand plate. There are no finger joints yet, but the tips of the fingers push out beyond the webs. The hand part of his arm unit grows most rapidly.

His main body trunk bends forward more and more, so that his face area appears to be pushed down on his bulging heart. In fact, you can't really tell yet where his head ends and his body begins. His heart is now a two-chambered affair and quite large. The blood circulation in his body and placenta is increasing and demands hard pushing. His body circulation remains simple, with the big central aorta artery and its neck arches, a yolk sac vessel, and the two arteries to the placenta through the umbilical cord.

His skeleton is forming, but it is still cartilage. The bone outlines show. The curved-down tail will disappear as he grows. Just above this the primitive umbilical cord is forming to carry the large blood supply he needs and will be expanding as fast as it can.

SIXTH WEEK (36 TO 42 DAYS)

Now you are almost two months pregnant. The embryo is a designer this month. His body parts, arms, legs, and face take on some shape. You can see that he looks much more like a human baby at the end of this week. He measures a half to two thirds of an inch from crown to rump. He weighs less than a book of matches. His head growth continues rapidly. It is still his biggest area, about half his total length. Eyelids begin to form with ridges around the edges of his eyes. His internal hearing apparatus is being finished up, too. His face forms now as a middle piece from the forehead grows to meet the cheek parts and to shape his upper lip, nose, and cheeks. In the weeks ahead this is followed by the formation of the palate and separate nose spaces with a nose tip.

His arm buds have grown to plump webbed paws with short upper and lower arm portions. The tips of the fingers push out beyond the edge of the finger web. This week the leg buds push out to form a rounded extremity with a footplate knob on the end. This follows much the same pattern as the hands. The ridged foot nubbin pushes out in two days to show ridges in the web for the toes. Four days later it has a definite heel.

His big heart is now joined by his liver and his internal circulation. Although the bigger part of his system is still outside his body in the placenta, his whole circulatory apparatus is now quite complete and in use. The large umbilical vein returns blood with oxygen and food materials through the placenta. Now the liver is added to the system, so that some of that blood goes through it. There is now a direct connection from the umbilical vein to the heart. His trunk has not grown much, so that his umbilical cord originates almost between the leg buds. His head end is still way ahead of the rest of him. But he has his vital organs, some of them already at work.

His soft skeleton of cartilage is quite well along in its formation. No bone yet, but the ribs are coming around to meet in front of his chest. His muscles are connecting up his skeletal parts. Also, his nervous system is increasing its tie-up to his muscles. Muscles and nerves now begin to work together. Lip stroking at this time would give a body reaction. He would bend his upper body to one side and throw his arms back.

His body covering is thin and translucent. Beneath this covering the skin is forming. The outer skin cells start to make hair, sweat, and oil glands. He continues to float in his amniotic sac, well anchored by his umbilical cord. He is almost weightless as he floats, well protected from shock.

No work is required in this indoor swimming pool. It is filled with a salt solution that wets his body cells. His body recycles this fluid. Some is swallowed, some is absorbed through his digestive tract, some is expelled with waste material, and he makes more of it all the time.

SEVENTH WEEK (43 TO 49 DAYS)

He weighs in at one thirtieth of an ounce, but he has stretched up to just under an inch. His interior structures are all there, but not functioning yet. He is sturdier now, with less chance of serious damage from outside influences.

His brain is starting its job of control to coordinate some of the functioning of his other organs. He has the complex structure of a mature brain, but in miniature. His brain develops more connections with muscles to control movement, but these are whole-body movements. His first movements—not felt by you—come this week or began last week. He can pull back, throw his arms back, or he can twist his whole body.

His eyes are well formed and begin to show the bluish color that he will have as a newborn. His eyelids and his external ears are forming delicately. Internal ear structures are quite well completed. He has good upper and lower jaws with a formed mouth, lips, and beginning tongue. The buds of his twenty first teeth are in the ridges of his gums.

His arms and legs have lengthened so that he has not only hands with fingers and feet with toes, but elbows, wrists, knees, and ankles. His hands show separate fingers, and thumbs with finger parts. The touch pads in the fingertips are very prominent.

His digestive tract is trying to produce some digestive secretions. His liver starts to produce young red blood cells with a nucleus in them. His kidneys start to filter blood as it comes through them. His genitals are beginning to sprout.

His umbilical cord is now a substantial structure with its two arteries and a single vein bulging with blood. He curls up more in his salt fluid-containing sac. His head is folded down on his chest.

His completed cartilage skeleton of last week is now due for a change. The first true bone cells appear in the bones of his upper arms. They will develop in all the long bones and eventually replace his cartilage cells. This marks the end of his first period of living—his time as an embryo.

With the appearance of bone cells, he ceases to be an embryo and becomes a fetus, or young unborn person.

EIGHTH WEEK (50 TO 56 DAYS)

Now he is over 1 inch in length (See fig. 2.) He will get to weigh one fifteenth of an ounce this month. After this week his physical structure is essentially complete. Every-

Fig. 2. Embryo at two months. Approximately three-fifths actual size. *Reprinted through the courtesy of the Johns Hopkins Press.*

thing is present in his body that will be found in a full-term baby. His job now is to perfect the equipment and get it to function properly.

His brain continues to improve its ability to coordinate his functioning. Covering membranes begin to develop over the delicate brain, in addition to its thin skin covering. These membranes start at the base and grow toward his crown to form a protective shell. His brain is furnished with a fluid bath to float in. The supporting structures are strengthened as the future flat bones of his skull start to form bone. They shape up like the petals of a flower to surround and protect the brain. They will not join at the top, but remain free for later shaping and molding during his journey down the birth canal. They must allow room for the brain to grow for some time to come. The junction areas are covered by strong membranes.

His eyes look partly closed, as if he is half asleep. He has formed nostrils, filled with protective material. His face is still forming. The features are present but not complete. There is more face now below his eyes, but the lower part of it still looks missing. This makes his ears appear lower set than they really are. From now on his lower face will grow more rapidly.

He can make some slight head and trunk movements. His arms have grown enough to touch his face. He may even get his fingers in his mouth and suck. He can move his fingers and arms about enough to grip something when his palm is touched. His legs may even do some gentle kicks, just enough to stir up his surrounding salt fluid. You won't feel them yet. He shows the distinct parts of his arms and legs now—arms, elbows, forearms, wrists, hands, and fingers, thighs, knees, lower legs, ankles, feet and toes. His fingertips are shaping up but still show the touch pads.

In case you've been wondering how we know all this, it should be said that as a result of very painstaking observations by patient investigators, working with aborted fetuses or making observations with the fetus still in the abdomen, a great deal has been learned about fetal behavior. Some of these findings are summarized in this section.

During this same period long bones are replacing cartilage bone cells, but the fetus doesn't have much of a body skeleton yet. His growing muscles and an increasing body give him a more rounded-out appearance. Connective tissues are also moving out from in back of his body to strengthen his trunk. His internal organs continue to develop into functioning units.

During previous weeks the genitals have been rudimentary, a mere slit-like opening with a bud in between a swelling on either side. Now the external genitals show some change, but still not enough to determine the baby's sex.

The magnificent root system of the placenta is working at top speed to carry out its multiple functions.

NINTH-TENTH WEEKS (57 TO 70 DAYS)

In his ninth and tenth weeks he reaches 1½ inches, weighs half an ounce, and his face becomes formed in all its parts.

His well-developed eyelids close over his eyes to seal them until the seventh month. His tenth week shows greater and more skillful use of his nervous system. His nerve-muscle communication improves and he increases these connections about threefold in these two weeks. This means a great surge ahead. He moves on his own without any stimulation. He can weave his body back and forth in his fluid bath. He can turn his head, bend his elbow, wrist, or knee, or straighten out his leg. He can't make a fist yet.

He develops sensitivity to touch. First his eyelids and palms react to stroking by squinting or closing. Later he will swallow if you stroke his lip. His whole body develops this touch awareness except for the sides, top, and back of his head. These remain insensitive, probably as a protection against pain when he is born head downward.

PLACENTA. In the past four weeks the placenta has appeared as a rapidly increasing, importantly functioning organ as the demands of your fetus increase so fast for food and oxygen.

The placenta is attached to the uterine wall, and the fetus is connected to the placenta by the umbilical cord. The umbilical cord and placenta make it possible for the baby to be a self-contained unit. He is a separate individual, although he is a parasite since he is completely dependent on his mother.

What he gets in the way of nourishment is delivered from his mother's reserves. This is one reason that his mother's diet is so important. The fetus receives only what she has to share. Whatever the mother takes and absorbs into her bloodstream travels to the placenta and is picked up through the placenta by the baby in one and a half to two hours.

The blood systems in fetus and mother are separate. Your mother's blood comes in contact with a placental membrane, then goes back into your circulation. It does not mix with the fetal blood. In the same way your fetus has his own closed circulation system. One set of blood vessels belongs to you and another set to your baby. There is a wall of cells between you. The blood-vessel walls are permeable. Oxygen, dissolved food, waste matter, carbon dioxide, and other chemicals pass through the cell walls. The blood from the fetus goes to the placenta from the two umbilical arteries in the lower part of his body to pick up material and lose some. It returns to the fetus through the big umbilical vein in the umbilical cord.

The umbilical cord, the link between baby and placenta, forms along with the placenta in the embryo. It extends from his navel and grows with him. At term it probably reaches 2 feet in length, although it may be as short as 5 inches and as long as 4 feet. It is an excellent piece of equipment designed to carry large amounts of blood.

I have called your baby a parasite—and he is! He is a foreigner inside your body. If his blood system were connected directly with yours, your body would reject him as a foreign substance. But with the placenta protecting him, he lives for nine months as a foreign parasite, your body acting as a host.

ELEVENTH WEEK (71 TO 77 DAYS)

By his eleventh week your fetus is 2 to 2½ inches long and weighs three quarters of an ounce to one ounce. His bones have been forming rapidly. His body is shaped and closed up in front so that everything is inside. The front of his body has grown from behind forward. Many of his organs lay outside of his body before this time. His nervous system is developed to the point where the nerves control his muscles to move his bones and produce movement. His teeth are forming. He now has hair on his scalp. His short, clumsy fingers still show touch pads that are quite large, but the nail beds are forming.

TWELFTH WEEK (78 TO 84 DAYS)

In this first trimester your baby has grown to 3 inches or more in length and weighs two ounces or more. (See fig. 3.) He shows a whole set of new responses. He is an individual in the way he acts and looks. This is the end of the period of formation of his body systems. The cartilage skeleton that was changing at eight weeks to solid bone is now serving as a form for the bone cells to lay down solid layers of bone. His cartilage is literally dissolved. It is replaced by these busy cells working from the middle of his bones outward. He now has bony ribs and vertebrae. He is becoming more solid. His head is still big for the rest of his body. His face is losing that fetal look and he is becoming more attractive by adult standards. He begins to show his family patterns. His eyes are almost fully developed and are moving closer to his nose. His ears are moving up. His outer ear is now more fully formed. Tooth sockets and buds are more complete in his jaws. He squints, frowns, and opens his mouth. His fingers and toes are well formed. The prominent touch pads are going away. His hand now looks like a finished product. The development of his feet is about two weeks behind that of his hands. His first hair appears

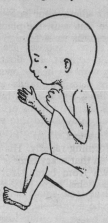

Fig. 3. Embryo at three months. Approximately three-fifths actual size. *Reprinted through the courtesy of the Johns Hopkins Press.*

as early as the beginning of his third month. It looks like little stiff whiskers on his upper lip, eyebrows, and on his palms and soles.

He rehearses breathing, eating, and movement. He continues to swallow considerable amounts of amniotic fluid. As yet he has no breathing-control center in his brain, and his lung tissues are not ready for breathing. He begins to practice inhaling and exhaling movements. He sends amniotic fluid in and out of his lungs, even though they are primitive lungs, in order to form their air sacs. He has vocal cords but no air to make a voice. With his new sucking muscles he presses his lips together in a grimace that is the first step of his sucking reflex. He has no definite rooting or sucking reflex as yet. His palate closes. He has salivary glands and tongue taste buds in his mouth.

This first trimester marks the end of an important period for your baby. His nervous-system muscle responses are changing. They lose their mechanical pattern and show a more coordinated rhythmic quality. He is very active, and his reflexes are appearing. He can kick or pull up his legs, turn his feet, grasp with his feet, curl or fan his fingers, make a fist, curl or fan his toes, bend his wrist, turn his

head, press his lips tightly together, pull his lips up into a
sneer, open and close his mouth. With a lip stroke he
grimaces. With a foot stroke he kicks one leg and draws up
the other. All of these responses are designed to avoid
rather than to seek contact. He floats about lazily. He
doesn't always stay with his head downward in the pelvis.

By this time, his digestive glands are working. As he
swallows amniotic fluid, it is used by his body. He urinates
the waste fluid. His sex cell organs are now quite definite.
The genital folds have developed into either labia for girls
or a penis for boys. There are also primitive egg or sperm
cells present in the internal genital organs. The testes have
descended into the well of the pelvis and stop there until
about the seventh month.

You won't be feeling him yet, since he is still well down
in your pelvis, and he is so small that his motions are not
vigorous enough to be noticeable. If you are quite thin you
may show a little bulge in your lower abdomen. Your
uterus has increased in size and has changed into a somewhat globular shape.

FOURTH MONTH

During this month he shows tremendous growth, increasing from three inches at twelve weeks to 5½-6½ inches by
the end of this month. (See fig. 4.) His weight increases
four to six ounces by the end of this time. All of his organs
are formed and functioning. The main thing he does from
now on is grow.

By the end of this fourth month his increase in size
brings your enlarged uterus out of your pelvis to show as
a low bulge in your abdomen. Since he is growing and
getting stronger you will begin to feel him moving against
your abdominal wall. This is called quickening, and may
not be experienced by some women until sometime next
month. During the fourth month a dense, fine growth of
hair, known as the lanugo hair, develops. The primitive
whiskers on the upper lip, eyebrows, palms, and soles disappear as this softer lanugo hair develops all over the body
like a downy covering. It is mainly gone by the time birth
occurs, so that only a faintly noticeable downy covering
remains on the face and perhaps on some other parts of the
body. Eyebrows and scalp hair begin to appear as coarser
terminal hair. The scalp hair appears in the bright pink

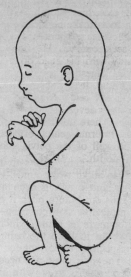

Fig. 4. Embryo at four months. Approximately three-fifths actual size. *Reprinted through the courtesy of the Johns Hopkins Press.*

skin, which still is quite transparent and very thin. It is replacing the protective membrane present before. The surface vessels are very clearly seen through the thin skin.

FIFTH MONTH

During this month he grows to about 10-12 inches and increases in weight to about one pound. His skin is covered with the fine lanugo, especially over his legs and back. His eyebrows and scalp hair are more definite. He is growing a fringe of eyelashes. Nipples and mammary glands appear in both girl and boy babies. He has a hard skeleton now, with stronger muscles so that he is more rounded out. Because of this you will be aware of more activity on his part. He does more kicking and turning. There is still enough room in the sac for him to do this. His fetal calisthenics answer his need to practice everything he has to do later. He may practice sucking his thumb as soon as his hand gets close to his mouth and the thumb slips into it. This is to get him ready for sucking and nursing as soon as he is born. His nails are about to reach his fingertips, so that he may scratch himself. He makes the motions of crying, and may react to loud outside noises. By now his arms and legs move vigorously when he is not asleep. And he has begun to develop a sleep-awake pattern.

SIXTH MONTH

During this month the fetus grows to 11-15 inches and increases in weight to about two pounds. He has quite long head hair now. His lanugo hair is even more definite. Before most of this falls out before birth it is involved in the formation of the protective skin covering—vernix. Next to each hair are one or more oil glands which provide an oily substance called sebum to keep the hair lustrous and the skin soft. This is especially important for the unborn baby floating in water. The skin must not become sodden.

His eyelids have eyelashes to go with his eyebrows. The tooth buds for his second teeth come into his jaws at about this time.

He spends his time in growing bigger, laying down muscle, and starting a fat layer. He can grip with his hands strongly enough to support his hanging weight. His grip is stronger now than it will be shortly after his birth. He is starting his reflex movements.

His sleep habits are shifting to those of a newborn baby. Periods of rest alternate with periods of activity. He exercises his arms and legs with great persistence. He bends and stretches his body, sucks, swallows, kicks, makes a fist, and makes breathing movements now and then. The space around him is smaller and smaller, so that your baby feels every motion that you make. He falls asleep when rocked by your movements and wakes up when everything is quiet again. Expectant parents will soon learn what sort of temperament their child has. Some babies are calm and reasonable in the uterus and react only occasionally with the movement of a hand or foot to remind the outside world of their existence. Others are easily upset. They protest with vigorous kicks if they are not softly rocked by mother or if absolute quietness does not prevail. This little character in your womb is no longer anonymous, he has a personality.

His breathing is regular, but his breathing and digestion are not yet good enough to help him survive outside your uterus. The youngest surviving premature has been about twenty-three to twenty-five weeks in utero and about one pound in weight.

SEVENTH MONTH

By the end of this month he will average three pounds and measure about 15 inches. His development is virtually complete. The extra time from now on gives him added strength and health. If he was born now he would have a chance to survive, but he needs the protection of a heat-insulating fat layer, which he doesn't yet have. He would have difficulty with respiration, as his lung tissue is not well formed. Also his immune substances are not yet present.

He floats in less fluid now since the amnion adjusts to hold less fluid to permit a bigger baby to reside inside the sac. His skin is quite red and deeply wrinkled. It will smooth out as he lays down a fat layer. He is losing some of his hair, but his scalp hair is growing longer.

His eyelids are opening, and he is able now to turn his eyes in all directions. Thumb-sucking may be his favorite pastime. This may be so continual that he is born with a callous on his thumb.

If he was born now his testicles would still be inside his body and the scrotal sac would be empty. The testes started on the back of the abdominal cavity and moved downward along the walls, so by the third month they were in the pelvis, to remain there until this month. In the seventh month they move downward out of the well of the pelvis into the inguinal canals to reach the scrotum by the end of the eighth month. The ovaries remain in the abdominal cavity and do not move out of the pelvis.

EIGHTH MONTH

In this month he reaches an average of four and a third pounds and increases to about 16½ inches. His chance for survival is much greater if he is born now. He is beginning to lay down his heat-insulating layer of fat, which is the source of his weight gain. He is more confined now, and can't flip about much. This doesn't stop him from moving and stretching.

NINTH MONTH

During this ninth month he gains several more pounds and becomes even more prepared to be born. He now averages seven and a quarter pounds and 18½ inches. He settles down to a preferred position, most often the head-down position, which is best for the shape of your uterus. When he moves now he makes the surface of your abdomen move. This is an important month for him to make his final additions to his body and to store away his reserve materials. During his eighth and ninth months he grows to be more and more a typical, fully matured human baby. His skin is smoother and less pink. His lanugo hair is disappearing as hair grows on his scalp. This scalp hair can be light and sparse or quite abundant. He sheds both lanugo hair and vernix into the amniotic fluid, which he swallows. This helps to form his first bowel movements. He has a good heavy insulating layer of fat now, which serves as a food source and a protective coat after he is born. His ears and nose now have cartilage in them. His paper-thin nails have grown out beyond his fingertips. His skull bones are firmer and closer together to form a protective cap. The fontanelles are open, but smaller in size. His eyes are the slate-blue color of the new baby's.

In these last weeks your baby stops growing by about the 260th day, the week before his birth at 266 days or thirty-eight weeks. About three out of every four babies will be born within 11 days of the 266th-day figure. In these 266 days one cell has mutiplied to 2 billion cells and weighs 6 billion times the original cell weight by dividing through 30 generations. Does this give you some idea of that remarkable human success story, a human baby?

THE MOTHER

Think back to the time before you were pregnant. Perhaps you and your husband had not even gotten around to thinking about children. Or you may be one of those well-organized couples whose family addition was planned. In either case, now your lives are changed. You'll be in for much discussion and planning ahead.

DETERMINING PREGNANCY

You can suspect pregnancy—and you probably did—if you go ten days or more past your regular menstrual date. When you miss a second period you can usually be quite certain that you are pregnant, although it must be cautioned that severe stress may cause you to miss a period or two or to become irregular.

If you can't wait for the natural symptoms of pregnancy to convince you, there are tests that are 95 percent to 100 percent accurate for an early diagnosis. This may give you a chance to start making your plans sooner.

You may first realize you are pregnant because certain changes are taking place in your body. It is more than just your missed period. Your nipples show a change in size. The color of the areola deepens. Enlarged veins appear as blue lines. Your breasts may feel tingly and swollen. You may urinate more frequently and even have to get up at night. Nausea or just not feeling well in the morning may occur. The pigmented areas of your body may grow darker. Since such changes raise the likelihood of pregnancy, you need to seek professional advice.

CHOICE OF DOCTOR

If you don't already have or know of an obstetrician-gynecologist, get in touch with your local medical society or large hospital center. They can advise you.

Make your choice of a doctor as early in your pregnancy as you can. You have a choice of a single doctor, a group of doctors associated in practice, a clinic group, or a large institutional maternity clinic. Base your decision on which seems most comfortable for you and which credentials or performance are most acceptable. Finances will have some influence in your decision, too. After you and your husband have talked about it together and made a decision, make an appointment with the obstetrician. If your husband can possibly go with you, he should. He should meet the people who will be taking care of you during your pregnancy. On your first office visit you are given a thorough examination. You give your family histories and any other information necessary. Don't forget to be as accurate as you can in remembering previous illnesses, problems, and menstrual history. You receive your preliminary instructions. Ask your questions. Your husband can ask his, too. You will also receive directions about future appointments. Ask your medical adviser when you can expect the baby. He will give you a date that can be either two weeks early or two weeks late. The length of your pregnancy can vary from this date and be perfectly normal.

CALCULATING YOUR DELIVERY DATE

You can calculate the date, too. Count back three calendar months from the first day of your last menstrual period, then add seven days to get your expected date of confinement. For example, say that June 1 was the first day of your last menstrual period. Count back three months to March 1, then add seven days. Your due date will be March 8 of the following year. However, your calculations may be all wrong if you run an irregular menstrual cycle.

FINANCES

At your obstetrician's office make your arrangements with his bookkeeper. What is the basic fee? Are there any extras? What doesn't it cover? What if you have twins? What about a caesarean section? Can you pay in installments? When is it all due? Arrangements will differ from one office to another, but get a clear picture of what is involved. Discuss fees and charges at once so that you know how to plan.

HOSPITAL

Talk with your obstetrician about hospital arrangements. His office can make your reservations early. What are the identifying numbers of your medical plan? You need these for the hospital and your doctor.

Call the business office of the hospital you're scheduled to go to. They will give you information about the cost of room and board, delivery-room charges, laboratory fees, nursery fees, and drugs.

Make a trip from your home to the hospital, to determine the most easily traveled route. At the hospital, get some of your questions answered in advance. Check on the locations of the admitting office and parking area, and on any other details that can be time-consuming later on. Be ready when labor starts to go to the proper place with the least delay.

CLASSES

Try to attend classes on parent education in your area or town. These classes help to prepare you for parenthood by giving you factual information about pregnancy, labor, and delivery, and by teaching you some of the techniques for the physical care of your baby and giving you a chance to practice them a little. Classes for both parents are more valuable than just for mother alone. Of course, some aspects of instruction are just for mother-to-be. Prepared childbirth classes that teach exercises and breathing techniques are good instruction for any pregnant girl. She is taught what to expect during labor, how to relax, how to cooperate with the obstetrician. Look in your newspaper, call your local Y or other community agencies, check with your doctor, hospital, or the local medical society for information about such classes.

REGULAR MEDICAL CARE

Your care of your baby starts the day you realize you are pregnant, not the day he is born. As discussed earlier, regular visits to your medical adviser give you the best chance for a normal pregnancy, safe delivery, and healthy, normal baby. The basic part of your prenatal care is the careful attention given to keeping you in good health through diet, hygiene, exercise, and prevention of complications.

Here are some suggestions for sound health care to follow throughout your pregnancy.

INFECTIOUS DISEASES

Avoid contagious diseases. Such infections may cause you no great distress but may be dangerous to your baby. This risk is greatest in the first three months but may be present to some degree during your entire pregnancy. Report any possible exposure to your doctor, and check with him if you have any questions.

HYGIENE

A daily bath is a good idea. Tub bathing is permissible in early pregnancy. In late pregnancy take showers. But don't chill—and don't slip!

Every morning and night clean the genital areas with soap and wåter. Careful cleansing after a visit to the toilet is necessary, too. Don't douche late in your pregnancy unless you check with your doctor. Some thin, whitish-to-pale-yellowish vaginal discharge is common during pregnancy. As long as it isn't thick and doesn't itch, burn, or cause discomfort, no treatment is needed. But check with your obstetrician if there is any question.

Continue sexual intercourse in your normal pattern until the last six weeks. Both partners should follow the rules for cleanliness. Avoid the introduction of bacteria or foreign materials into the vagina after the baby's head drops down into the birth canal.

BREAST CARE

Examine your breasts regularly during your pregnancy. (You should do this whether you are pregnant or not.) Learn your own breast anatomy so that you can pick up any changes in the breast tissue. If you notice that one breast is different from the other, have this checked at your next regular office visit.

If you intend to nurse, have your breasts inspected to reveal any possible anatomic problem that may interfere with nursing. Contrary to what you may have heard, small or flat breasts are often the best milk producers. Large breasts may be mostly fat and not glandular tissue.

Wear a well-made, nonconstricting, wide-strapped brassiere with a supporting under band—a good uplift type. This should push your breasts up with no pressure on the nipples. Proper support helps to keep the breast tissue intact. A maternity brassiere is adjustable to allow for expansion and later nursing.

Condition your nipples for the job of nursing if you wish to breast-feed. In early pregnancy don't do anything but wash them well with soap and water at the time of your daily shower or bath.

After the fourth month your breasts produce a slight amount of liquid called colostrum. This is normal, but may be enough to require a little pad in your brassiere to protect your clothes. Wash this fluid off regularly so that the nipples won't become irritated and sore. Before touching your breasts be sure your hands are well washed. Avoid any possibility of infection. With your right hand grasp the dark ring, the areola, surrounding your right nipple, so that the nipple protrudes. With your left hand use a rough, clean washcloth and soap and water to wash the breast and nipple with a rotary motion. Then hold your left breast in the same way and wash it with your right hand. Rinse the nipples and the breasts with clear water. Dry with a rough towel. Don't be too rough in your toweling. You may take off the superficial layer of skin. Cold water dashed over tender nipples may help to toughen them. There is no advantage in the use of so-called hardening processes designed to toughen the nipples. Such procedures may increase the likelihood of cracking or fissuring later. Now cover the nipples with a lubricant to keep the skin in good condition. This may be cold cream, Vaseline, lanolin, mineral oil, or cocoa butter. In the last three months you start regular nipple exercises, particularly if you have nipples that are stiff, hard, or flattened. You are getting them ready so that your baby won't have a difficult time getting hold of the nipple to nurse. The first of these exercises is to start the daily milking out or hand expression of the colostrum. It is easier to learn and practice before your breasts are engorged in early nursing. Learn something about the structure of your breast. (See figs. 5 and 6.) Deep in the breast there are small grape-like clusters of milk glands (alveoli) whose linings manufacture milk. These sacs open into large passageways, which

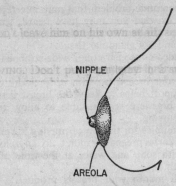

Fig. 5. The external structure of the breast.

end up in the fifteen or twenty sinuses under the areola. These are reservoirs, each of which drains a different part of the breast. They empty out through a small duct or canal, which goes out through the nipple. Try to stimulate the nipples so that the ducts are open and empty. Here is how to do it.

Wash your hands. There are two parts to hand empty-ing the breast. The first is to circle your breast with your

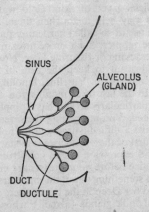

Fig. 6. The internal structure of the breast.

hands at its base and stroke toward the areola. (See fig. 7.)
Do this several times to urge any secretion in the breast
tissue toward the nipple. (After your baby is born, when

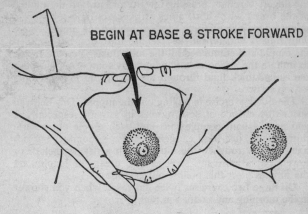

BEGIN AT BASE & STROKE FORWARD

Fig. 7. Milking the breast. Part I.

your breasts contain milk, you will do it ten to twelve
times.) The second part is the actual milking out of the
breast sinuses. (See figs. 8, 9 and 10). Put your thumb

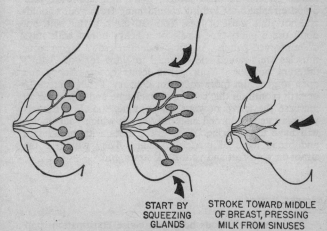

START BY
SQUEEZING
GLANDS

STROKE TOWARD MIDDLE
OF BREAST, PRESSING
MILK FROM SINUSES

Figs. 8, 9, 10. Milking the breast. Part II.

above and your index finger below the nipple at the edge of the areola, using the opposite hand for each breast. The bulk of the breast should rest in your hand. Gently squeeze the fingers together, pressing inward and toward the middle of the breast with short, quick strokes, six times or more a minute. Don't bring them forward toward the nipple. Move your fingers and repeat the exercise until you have circled the nipple and stimulated all the milk ducts. You are trying to imitate the action of a nursing baby's jaws. As you push the rather thick fluid through the ducts, you may get only a drop or two.

The other exercise is pulling out the nipple. This helps to lessen the chance of sore nipples in nursing, especially if you have a light complexion. Pull each nipple out several times firmly, just hard enough to cause discomfort but not pain. Gently roughen the nipples with a dry washcloth or towel. Put a lubricant, such as cold cream or lanolin, on the nipples after this pulling-out exercise.

Do these two exercises twice daily, say when you shower in the morning and undress at night.

DRESSING CORRECTLY

Don't wear tight clothes, tight brassieres, tight girdles, or round garters. In other words, don't interfere with your blood circulation. Clothing should hang from your shoulders, not your waist or legs. You can use a garter belt, but don't use a panty-type girdle or a heavy corset with stays or reinforced panels. As your abdomen grows bigger your muscles are strained and changed to allow for your baby's different positions. Your pelvic joints become loose and open to give him more room for delivery. From the fourth or fifth month on this can cause backache and fatigue. You increase the curve of your lower spine, too. For support you may need a special maternity corset which your doctor will have to prescribe. Wear good shoes with broad toes and broad heels of moderate height. They will ease the strain on your feet and your back strain, too.

BOWEL ROUTINE

The changes in your body can cause constipation, particularly in the last three months. Regularity with a relaxed

approach is your aim. An important part of bowel care is
proper diet. Eat three meals a day. Try to drink a glass of
water or fruit juice as soon as you get up in the morning,
and drink several glasses of fruit juice daily. At breakfast
eat a cooked heavy cereal like oatmeal or a bran cereal,
and stewed or fresh fruits like figs, dates, prunes, oranges,
or baked apples. Use raw leafy green vegetables during the
other meals of the day. Don't forget exercise, too. Enemas
and harsh laxatives are out. Consult your doctor if you
need further help.

HOUSEWORK AND EXERCISE

Keep on with ordinary household duties as long as you
remember how to lift, bend over, and reach properly. No
furniture moving or heavy scrubbing. And don't get too
tired.

You need exercise—but in moderation. What you do now
in the way of exercise depends on what you did before
pregnancy. If you drove, played golf, swam, or rode horse-
back, keep it up, but stop before you get overtired. When
you are pregnant you tire more easily and recover more
slowly from strenuous activity. If you have any questions,
ask your doctor. Begin daily morning and evening walks
outdoors. (Your housework doesn't count as walking.)

SLEEP

Sleepy and lazy may well describe you in your first
months as your body adjusts to its changing function.
Throughout your pregnancy you must arrange to sleep
eight hours a night, with one or two rest or nap times during the day. Take more rest than this if you feel tired. Don't
fight your sleepiness.

SOCIAL LIFE: DRINKING AND SMOKING

Continue your outside interests. See your friends as much
as possible. Your concern should be that a cocktail has 80

to 160 calories. You can't tolerate a one- or two-cocktail occasion or a bottle of beer in the evening if you are having to watch your weight.

Heavy smoking combined with a poor diet definitely puts your baby in danger of prematurity or poor weight gain. You do a better job in your pregnancy if you eliminate smoking completely. Limit your smoking to one-half pack a day if you can't stop altogether.

SELF-MEDICATION

Don't prescribe medicines for yourself. Medicines can affect your baby. A good rule to follow is that no drugs or medications are to be used unless they are prescribed or approved by your doctor.

THE WORKING MOTHER-TO-BE

If you want to work during your pregnancy, this is a decision that you, your husband, and your obstetrician should make together. Staying active can be a good thing for your morale and give added zest to this new adventure. Use a simple rule of thumb for this. Keep working as long as you can function as a homemaker, wife, and companion to your husband. Financial necessity may make you continue up until the last week or two of your pregnancy—but take care and be prepared. You may have to make a sudden run for the hospital. Some of the larger organizations set definite rules as to how late in pregnancy an expectant mother may work; in part these limitations are for their legal protection in the event of accident.

TRAVELING

You may travel during pregnancy if you have had no bleeding during your first four months, if you have had no complicating physical condition during this time, and if your trip will not burden your body more than your usual day does. The main problem is fatigue.

CARE OF TEETH

Don't forget the care of your teeth. Keep them in good shape with after-meal brushing, restriction of sweets, and regular dental examinations. You do not furnish calcium for your baby from your own teeth and bones, contrary to popular belief. "A tooth for every child" has never been true. The needed calcium comes from your own diet.

NUTRITION

Daily adequate, nourishing foods eaten by a pregnant mother decrease the chance of prematurity and inadequate nutrition in her baby. The basic food groups from which you should eat each day to give yourself high-quality diet-building blocks are meat–meat substitutes, milk–milk solids, fruits, vegetables, bread–cereal, and fats–oils.

MEAT–MEAT SUBSTITUTES. In this group are meat, fish, fowl, seafood, eggs, and occasional meat substitutes like dried beans, peas, or nuts. The cheaper cuts of meat are just as nutritious as the more expensive. Animal protein should make up about two thirds of the total daily protein intake. Organ meats are excellent. Heart, liver, and tongue especially should be eaten often because of their high iron and mineral content. At least two liberal servings a day totaling eight to ten ounces of lean meat, fish, chicken, turkey, or organ meats is the requirement. Eat one or two eggs daily.

MILK–MILK SOLIDS. One quart of milk or the equivalent milk solids should be included in your daily diet. Dried powdered skim milk may be added to many foods without dilution to give straight milk-protein solids. Cheese in its many forms can be used in place of milk. Cottage cheese is better than creamed cheese or cheese spread.

FRUITS. Use two or three servings daily of the whole fruit or juice, of which at least two servings should be Vitamin C-containing fruit or tomato juices. Use Vitamin C-containing fruits like oranges, grapefruits, and melons, as well as other, noncitrus fruits, like stewed prunes, bananas, apricots, peaches, applesauce, or prune juice.

VEGETABLES. Use two or more servings daily of this group

with one or more dark-green or deep-yellow vegetables. Use raw vegetables often. Don't emphasize the white starchy vegetables, such as potatoes.

BREAD–CEREAL. Use three to four servings daily. Use any of the whole-grain cereals, either cooked or prepared, once daily. Use whole-wheat bread at the other two meals. Always use whole-grain or enriched cereals and breads. One serving can be replaced with noodles, macaroni, corn, lima beans, rice, spaghetti, or white potato. Cut down on size of servings if you are gaining too much weight.

FAT–OIL. Use one teaspoon of margarine or butter three times daily. As substitutes use cream, lard, fat, olive oil, cottonseed, peanut, and fish oils.

Avoid foods such as white bread, cake, pie, cookies, sugars, jams, syrups, soft drinks, gravy, candy, and highly processed cereals and grains. For desserts use cheese, Jell-o, junket, custard, fruit, and fruit whips. Make your between-meal snacks nutritious and not just something to fill up on. Use proteins whenever possible.

Avoid excess salting.

Drink six to eight glasses of water or clear fluids daily. (Milk is not a clear fluid.)

Use an all-purpose vitamin containing calcium and iron throughout your pregnancy and during your nursing period afterward.

If you gain weight too fast, cut down on the fats–oils group as well as on the bread–cereal group. Keep your total weight gain fifteen to twenty pounds above your desirable nonpregnant weight. If you were underweight to start with, gain more. If you were too heavy before, gain less. To help you in thinking about your weight, here are some rough indicators. A nonpregnant twenty-five-year-old woman 64 inches in height and weighing a desirable 128 pounds maintains her active life on 2300 calories a day. In the second half of her pregnancy she will require 300 calories more a day.

A caution! Don't diet unwisely! If you eliminate essential foods in trying to lose weight, your baby is deprived of needed elements for his growth. He needs all the basic food items he can get. Don't play the crash diet game with him.

DANGER SIGNS

If any one of the following occurs, get in touch with your doctor immediately. Don't take any medicine until you have checked with him. Lie down and keep quiet until you have had specific directions.

1. Vaginal bleeding
2. Swelling of the face, hands, or feet
3. Severe, continuous headache which doesn't yield to the ordinary remedies
4. Dimness or blurring of vision
5. Pain in the abdomen
6. Persistent vomiting
7. Chills and fever
8. Sudden escape of water from the vagina
9. Hard fall

FIRST THREE MONTHS

In these early days of pregnancy you may feel as if you are going to have your period at any time. You feel heaviness in your lower abdomen because of the increased blood supply. Your uterus is growing larger, too. One of your earliest complaints may be the urinary frequency mentioned earlier. This common symptom disappears after this period. You will get it again some weeks before your delivery, when your baby's head starts down into your pelvis and presses on your bladder.

Your eating habits may be in for a change, too. At this stage many a mother-to-be will eat less. You may lose your ability to keep food down. Nausea or morning sickness is experienced by at least half of mothers-to-be. No definitive cause for this condition is known. It may be the result of some of the physical changes occurring in your body. Your anxieties and tensions will aggravate the underlying condition. Your obstetrician will be able to help you a great deal with this unpleasant symptom. Normally it is gone after the first three months.

As a father-to-be, you can play a helpful role here. You can give your wife sympathy and show a philosophical acceptance of the situation. Your lack of understanding can create trouble for the two of you if you believe that the problem "is all in her head." She needs to know that she is still charming and loved by you even when she feels very unattractive. And this period of upset is usually brief. An occasional dinner by candlelight or a night-on-the-town will help.

As you probably know, there are emotional changes during your pregnancy, too, as your baby creates changes in your hormone balance, which is closely connected to your nervous system. You are likely to experience sudden shifts in mood and may stop feeling very comfortable with yourself. Expect this to happen and you won't punish yourself when it does. Even the healthiest, happiest mothers-to-be go through these mood swings.

It may be hard for you to separate your feelings of uncertainty about your new baby from your feelings of concern about yourself. These two major fears are common during pregnancy. Your concern about yourself is more prominent during these early months. Your reaction to physical symptoms, your discomfort, your mixed feelings of happiness and sadness, your changing moods, your wish to be taken care of—these feelings are all part of this period.

Your other big worry is your baby. You may fret as to whether he will be normal. Even if you are getting good medical care and supervision, your fears about your baby's fitness and your own safety linger.

Try to talk about these worries with your husband, your doctor, or an understanding friend. You can face them better when you can bring them out into the open to be looked at. Usually they are not as serious as you imagine.

As a father-to-be, you can do a great deal about your wife's fears. Be aware of her moods and concerns. Encourage her to talk to you about them. Explore them as to their source and truth. Reassure her with facts, but present them in acceptable ways. Above all, treat her feelings seriously. This is no time for indifference or teasing.

Each man comes into this business of becoming a father in his own way. It is of no help to say, "Do what comes naturally" (you may feel like running away), or "Just be yourself" (you may not know exactly who "yourself" is in this new situation). No matter how prepared and accepting of your new role you are, you will have some mild anxieties and reservations about the whole business. Talk to your doctor or to some wise friend. Don't unload your fears on your wife at this time. She's asking you to hear her and help keep her in emotional balance.

MIDDLE THREE MONTHS

This middle period may be the most tedious of all for you. The months may seem to drag along without much happening. But this is the time you will get your first thrill. Your baby moves and stirs about. You feel life. This occurs anywhere from the fourth to the sixth month. He may give you little rest once he starts, or he may be lazy and quiet. Whichever, this movement is a confirmation that your baby is really there.

You may still have difficulty thinking about your baby as a person, even if you feel him moving about. Don't worry about it. Your active participation in baby care will come along soon enough. Then your center of attention will shift from yourself to the new baby.

This is the time for those do-it-yourself classes in baby care. You aren't too unwieldy to get around easily and you have plenty of energy. Your early pregnancy slowdown is over and you feel like doing something.

This is also a good time to begin assembling the clothing and equipment your baby will need, and to organize your home for his arrival. (For suggestions, look ahead to *Preparing for the Baby*.) You can do a lot, but do it wisely. Don't push too hard.

Begin to think about your choice for a pediatrician. Also conside whether you will breast- or bottle-feed. Discuss this with your husband. A nursing mother needs the support of father-to-be to do as well as she can. You can feed your baby equally well by either method. (Look ahead to the section on *Breast-Feeding and Bottle-Feeding*.)

No matter what you do or plan, don't forget your eight-hours-a-night sleep time plus adequate rest or nap times during the day. Keep up your social life, but slow it down to a more sedate speed. Travel comes under this same heading.

It is during this period that you discover you have difficulty controlling your appetite. You will be beyond your first three months and your morning nausea. Heartburn may be an unpleasant sensation now. It is a sour, burning sensation in your throat or under your breastbone. As the size of your uterus increases and it comes up into your abdomen, its bulk can cause pressure and trouble. (Don't use baking soda to treat this. Your obstetrician can give you something for it.) You may crave food. Your tendency to self-indulgence must not result in an inadequate diet or excessive weight gain. Nibble occasionally on exotic foods if you like, but keep to your good three-meal diet. Your doctor will decide when you need to restrict or substitute in your diet.

LAST THREE MONTHS

This is the time for patience. The days seem to grow longer as you near termination and you feel increasingly heavy and unwieldy. There is a change in your equilibrium. Your walk has to adjust itself to your changes in contour and posture.

Sitting down and getting up need a little thinking about. When you sit, choose a chair with a straight back, not a deep, overstuffed chair or sofa that you sink deeply into and need help to get hoisted out of. When you sit, sit up straight, with your hands in your lap or on the chair arms, one foot a little ahead of the other, or with your ankles crossed. Forget about trying to cross your legs. When getting up, put your hands beside you on the chair arms or seat to support yourself, and then give a push up and out. If one foot is forward you can put your weight on this leg.

When standing, you will have to come to terms with your changing center of balance and size. Stand so that you reduce the increased curve of your back. Hold your head up, chin back. Walk this way, too. But don't stand for any length of time. If you have to, don't stand solidly on both feet—stand straight but shift your weight from one foot to the other.

And then there is bending over—that makes you laugh? Until you got so large you didn't realize how much bending over and picking up you did during the day. Squatting is the proper method now. Stand with your feet apart and flat on the floor. Hold onto something solid, then squat down. You'll have to practice a little, but it is a good exercise to condition and limber up your pelvic muscles. You avoid extra strain on your back muscles, which are already straining, and you remain a lady by not exposing too much of a rear view.

Gymnastic exercises help to strengthen your back and abdominal muscles. Maybe you'll even get an extra feeling of well-being. But don't get fooled into thinking that gymnastics guarantee a painless delivery. They are a help but not a cure-all. Here are a few good exercises.

Pinch or squeeze your vaginal muscles as if you were trying to keep from urinating, then relax and squeeze again. This maneuver exercises the muscles of your pelvic floor.

Sit cross-legged on the floor. Alternately place one hand on your head and the other straight out, turning your head toward the side. (See fig. 11.)

Sit cross-legged on the floor. Clasp your arms as if you were hugging yourself, then rock backward and forward. (See fig. 12.)

Stand on the outsides of your feet with your toes pointed in, then curl your toes. (See fig. 13.)

Lie on your back with your arms flat on the floor along your sides. Raise your legs and pump them as if you were riding a bicycle. (See fig. 14.)

Figs. 11-19. **PRENATAL EXERCISES**

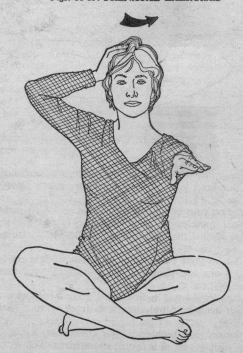

Fig. 11. Exercise I

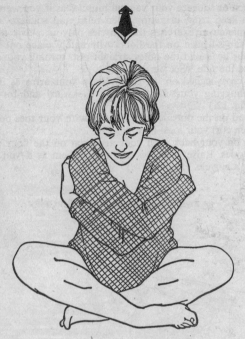

Fig. 12. Exercise II

Lie on your back with your arms at your sides, bend your knees, but keep your feet on the floor as you raise your hips. (See fig. 15.)

Lie flat on your back with your knees bent. Contract your abdominal muscles, tense your buttocks, and press your back flat against the floor. Then relax and sway from side to side. (See fig. 16.)

Lie flat on your back with your arms straight up in the air. Raise one leg, then the other, touching your hand to the knee as it comes up. (See fig. 17.)

Sit cross-legged on the floor, and make a scissors motion with your arms held out straight in front of you. (See fig. 18.)

Lie flat on your back with your knees bent. Relax. Then breathe deeply. Be sure your abdomen moves with the breathing. (See fig. 19.)

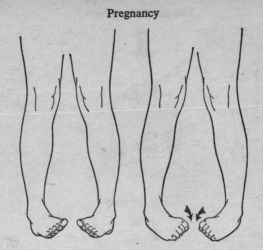

Fig. 13. Exercise III (A) (B)

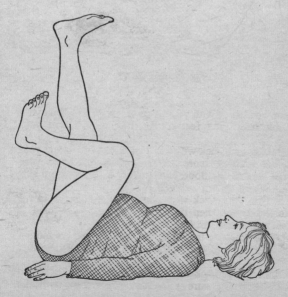

Fig. 14. Exercise IV

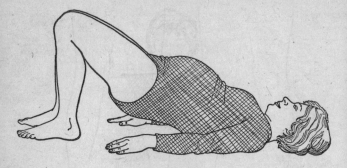

Fig. 15. Exercise **V**

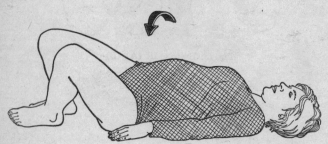

Fig. 16. Exercise **VI**

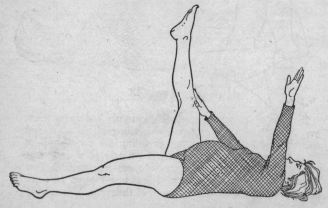

Fig. 17. Exercise **VII**

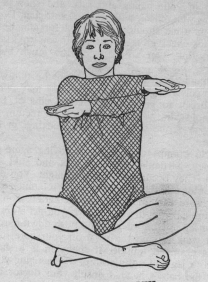

Fig. 18. Exercise VIII

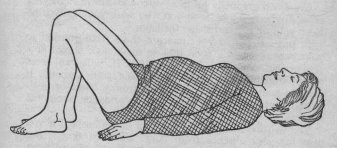

Fig. 19. Exercise IX

Because of the increased pressure in your lower abdomen, you may show quite noticeable swelling of the feet and ankles. Try to avoid standing or sitting for any length of time. If you notice swelling, lie down and raise your legs up with pillows. Turn to one side or the other. Larger shoes help with swollen feet. Also, never wear circular garters or roll your stockings to hold them up. If you have swelling of your hands and face and show a change in weight as well, check with your obstetrician. Don't put this off! Your urine should be checked for albumin. You can do a quick check on this yourself: If you can't take off your wedding ring, you are carrying too much fluid in your body.

Pregnancy increases the strain on the thin-walled veins of your pelvis, rectum, and legs. They may dilate and the valves break to give you varicose veins of the legs, or hemorrhoids, the varicose veins of the rectum. Your doctor may prescribe special support stockings or some other measure.

Muscle cramps can be an annoying symptom in late pregnancy, particularly if your feet and ankles are swelling, too. They occur most often at night. You may be putting your leg and thigh muscles under too much strain. Strain and pressure can impede your circulation. Sometimes you need more calcium in your diet. If you get a cramp, stretch out your leg in front of you and push down hard with your heel, or walk around the room in your bare feet, or massage the cramped muscle. If the pain is a shooting pain down your leg and not a cramp, try changing your position to shift the baby's head. Consult your doctor if cramping is frequent.

Cut down gradually on more strenuous activities as your unwieldy body indicates to you. But walk your daily stint. Keep yourself in good shape for labor.

In this last period your concern shifts from yourself to your baby. Now is a good time to make your choice of a pediatrician. Make a visit to his office. He will want some background information about you and your husband. If you are going to use pediatric care from a clinic or institution, contact the clinic to obtain information about the services.

You will have a more relaxed stay in the hospital if you plan for your absence from home ahead of time. Your husband may be quite familiar with the details of your household management—or he may be like a lost soul in the kitchen. Make your plans with his present capabilities in mind—although he may surprise you with his speed in learning. Give him details and instructions.

Make a list of essential telephone numbers and tape it near the phone or some other place where he can find it. Then make another list, this one of people he should call after your new production is an accomplishment.

If you have a freezer lay in a supply of frozen dinners

and foods you have cooked yourself. Stock up on canned and packaged foods, too. Buying food in advance is especially important if there are other children at home.

If you do have other children, try to keep them in the familiar home surroundings. In this way your absence is less bothersome to them. If you can afford to have a housekeeper, try to have her start a little before your due date. (Look ahead to *Your Other Children and the Baby*.)

Now decide what you need to take with you to the hospital. Pack these articles in a small overnight case that you can carry yourself—you may need to! Do this several weeks before your expected date of confinement. Your new baby may decide to arrive sooner than you expect, or at the last minute you may be excited enough to forget everything. Here is a suggested list:

Nightgowns (1 or 2, washable, lightweight, with front openings if you will be nursing) or
Pajamas (1 or 2 pairs)
Bed jackets or negligees (1 or 2)
Robe (washable)
Brassieres (2 or 3, nursing or regular)
Sanitary belt (napkins are usually supplied by hospital)
Shower cap
Slippers
Cosmetics
Comb and brush
Bobby pins
Hand mirror
Cleansing tissues
Bath powder and lotion
Toothbrush
Toothpaste
Hair curlers
Manicuring set
Watch or clock
Reading material
Money (including small change)
Stationery
Birth announcements
Stamps
Pen and pencil

A word of caution. Don't expect to fit into all your pre-pregnancy clothes as soon as your baby is born. Remember this when you choose what you will wear in the hospital and what you will wear to go home.

Pack baby's going-home things separately from the items listed above. You can take them with you, or your husband can bring them along with your going-home outfit. The baby's case should contain:

    Diapers and pins
    Nightgown
    Cotton receiving blanket
    Lightweight sweater
    Quilted pad or plastic pants
    Lightweight (heavy, if winter) blanket or shawl

2.

Preparing
for the Baby

CLOTHING AND BEDDING

Your baby's needs are modest in the first few months. It is wise to plan for three complete changes of clothing—one for wearing while another set is in the wash, and a third set tucked away for emergency use. Buy the bare essentials now and wait to see what you need later. Your baby grows rapidly in his first month. In wardrobe planning you will also consider the climate you live in, the season of the year, your facilities for laundering.

There is one basic fact about your baby that is important to keep in mind: He is a throbbing, going, growing, red-hot energy machine. When you are cold, he is quite comfortable. When you are comfortable, he is too hot. His metabolic rate is greater than an adult's. He just produces more heat. He feels warmer with less clothing. You don't prevent colds by overdressing any more than you give him a cold by underdressing. He gets an infection through some other human being. Colds come from people—not climate. At first, you will usually make the mistake of overdressing him because he seems so little. He *is* little, but he is functioning at top speed unless he has had some definite problem. A good rule: Dress your baby the way you think you should—then take half of it off. Indoor dressing is much the same across the country. His outdoor clothing is what you vary according to the weather.

What are the basics? His clothing should be simple in

51

design and cut, lightweight, easily laundered, made of soft, color-fast material that will stand up under frequent washings, require no ironing, show minimal shrinkage, have smoothly finished seams to avoid irritation, and be large enough to allow for easy dressing and his freedom of movement. Their design must allow them to be put on and taken off with the least possible effort on your part and the least discomfort on his. Raglan sleeves are better than the set-in type. Avoid irritating embroidery or edging along sleeve and neck margins. Avoid anything that has to be dry-cleaned.

For items like diapers, nightgowns, shirts, blankets, towels, and washcloths, cotton is the best all-around material. You can get it in light- and heavy-weight weaves. Some of the new synthetic materials are excellent, but be certain that they are nonflammable or flame-resistant. Don't use inner garments of flannel or wool. They are too hot in the modern-day house or apartment. Use them only for outer heavy-weather clothing. Allow for growth change. Start with the small-size garment but don't get too many. If you do not overbuy your next purchase can be for the next growth period. In garments for children there is a shift away from sizes given in age levels to sizes designed for weight differences. Check on the garment to see what weights the small, medium, and large sizes are intended for. Extra-small often means under 12 pounds while small may be indicated as 12 to 18 pounds, and so on.

In buying clothes, consider types of fasteners. Snap fasteners are best for inner garments. Ties, strings, ribbons, hooks, are all cumbersome to use and can be risky if your baby gets tied up in them. Overalls that zip down both sides, pajamas that unsnap at the waist, and snowsuits that zip open from top to bottom can save a lot of time.

Remember: *Avoid overbuying and overdressing.*

Below is a minimum list of the things you should have on hand before you go to the hospital. You will find the minimum list quite adequate for the first weeks, although you may want to add items from the material on the pages following it.

Diapers (4-6 dozen)
1 box Disposable diapers
4-6 Nightgowns
4-6 Shirts
4-6 Crib sheets
4-6 Mattress pads

4-6 Receiving blankets
2-3 Light blankets

CLOTHING

DIAPERS (4-6 dozen). These are useful in many ways. You can use them for wipe cloths, burp rags, extra sheeting, towels. Two to three dozen may be enough if you use a diaper service.

Although you may buy printed or colored ones, the material is the important element. Heavy-woven gauze diapers are more absorbent, less bulky, and dry more quickly than the cheaper lighterweight gauze ones which lose their shape and get sleazy with washing. Diaper sizes vary a great deal but 27″ x 27″, 21″ x 34″, and 13″ x 22″ are common sizes. You may find other sizes but in folding modify them according to your baby's specifications.

You can use the larger sizes for a longer time. Some of these are available with fold lines woven into the fabric. There are also prefolded diapers on the market.

For a first diaper, I recommend the cotton birdseye; it has a distinctive geometric woven pattern, is less expensive than others, heavier, stronger, soft, warm, quite absorbent, and usually hemmed. There are some with pinked edges, which are less bulky and quicker drying.

There are knitted diapers in tubular and contour shapes adjustable to fit the body. These are not as absorbent as others and dry more slowly.

Fitted diapers are more expensive than others. They are more suitable for the older infant than the very young one.

SAFETY PINS. Use regular safety pins of good size or get some special diaper pins. Clips and snaps are available, too.

DISPOSABLE DIAPERS (1 box). Keep disposable paper diapers on hand for emergencies and for traveling or visiting. They are expensive for day-to-day use. They come in sizes designed for weight differences so check on the carton for the proper size.

DIAPER LINERS. Diaper liners are disposable panels made of coated paper. They are used inside a regular diaper or a diaper holder to reduce diaper soiling. Liners are good in the early weeks when your baby has quite messy stools.

You just lift up your baby, fold up the soiled liner, and throw it away.

DIAPER SERVICE. If you are planning to use a diaper service, arrange for it before you go into the hospital so that you will have a supply on hand when you return home. It is a little more expensive overall than home laundering, assuming that you have an automatic washer and dryer available, but you may feel it is well worth the cost. You get a continuing supply of freshly laundered, sterilized diapers, the number depending on your arrangement with the company. Every-other-day service to start will allow you to find out how many diapers you will require at each delivery.

DIAPER PANTS (3-4). These are waterproof pants made of plastic-coated, or rubber-coated material, worn over the diaper. The edges of the openings should be properly bound to avoid skin irritation. There is a pull-on type and a type with side snap fasteners, which opens out flat for putting on.

If the pants are airtight, they act like an incubator and cook the skin of the diaper area. If you use pull-on pants get pants that have snap closings and allow some ventilation through the sides, and check for air holes that allow evaporation of moisture in the diaper area. Don't use diaper pants for more than a few hours at a time. They keep your baby too warm and wet—a bad combination for his skin health. Use two diapers or a folded diaper inside his outer diaper instead.

Don't use a knitted wool pant called a wool pilcher or soaker. It is too tight and hot.

NIGHTGOWNS (4-6). Get nightgowns made of lightweight knit, seersucker, terry cloth, cotton jersey, or synthetic material. These launder easily and dry quickly. The length should be enough so the baby can stretch out and kick easily. Start with the small size for the new baby and increase the size as he grows. Dress him in a nightgown and diaper both day and night until he gets to moving about more. Drawstrings at sleeve ends and at the hem will help at first. *No drawstrings at the neck.* Pull the sleeves down over his hands if he waves his hands about his face and scratches his skin. Later, you can turn the sleeves back so the baby can use his hands. Turn the neck opening so it goes in back. Then he can't catch his hand or arm in the

opening. Don't use the button or zipper-in nightgown unless he can kick freely. Cotton stretch-cloth or terry-cloth
pajamas or sleepers with pull-back mitten cuffs and attached booties are good after the first weeks. They have a
zipper or snap fastener down the front or back and inner leg
for easy access. They require minimum care in laundering.

For the very young baby his nightgown and double diaper
are enough clothing at night, with the sheet and blanket
well tucked in at the sides. Add more bed clothing if the
room really chills down.

For older babies and toddlers, you can use two-piece
sleepers with legs. Two rows of snaps at the waist let you
adjust the fit as the baby grows. Another style has a deep
tuck at the waist for letting out. Sleepers usually have
booties attached, sometimes detachable for simpler laundering. Booties with plastic soles give longer wear. For sum-
mertime, cotton-pelisse, cotton-seersucker, or cotton-mesh
nightgowns or pajamas are good. None of these fabrics requires ironing. For winter, fabrics made entirely of man-
made fibers and those with a good portion of a hardy synthetic hold warmth well, dry quickly, and are not apt to
shrink. And don't forget the stretch ones.

SHIRTS (4-6). You don't need shirts in the early weeks since
you will be using nightgowns. Don't use both the shirt and
the gown. Get the small size, for the baby under fourteen
pounds, to start with. Shirts come in basic styles like slip-
overs and those with snap closings, side ties, or side zippers.
They can be sleeveless, short-sleeved, or long-sleeved. Some
have tabs for fastening to the diaper.

The sleeveless or short-sleeved slipover type, of porous-
like cotton fabric, is best for year-round use. The head
opening must be large enough to stretch over the baby's
head easily. You drive him wild if you put anything over
his face and then have to struggle to get his head through
the opening. The arm holes must be large enough, too.

If more clothing is needed for outdoors, use a sweater or
heavier outer clothing. Dress your baby as you do yourself
—you don't wear an extra undershirt just because you're
going outside.

SUITS (OR DRESSES). When your infant begins to try to
crawl, pull up, and move about, he will need a garment
other than his nightgown. For everyday use you will find
rompers, one-piece stretch suits, creepers, sunsuits, over-

alls, or similar garments handiest for both boys and girls. These clothes should be of cotton, such as poplin, broadcloth, gingham, corduroy, or of any of the easy-to-wash blends. The important feature is how easy they are to remove, so that you can change diapers with the least effort.

Garments should not have trimmings that will irritate the skin. Be sure that buttons or snaps are well anchored. Don't use pins in your baby's clothing where he can reach them. He explores and learns all too quickly how to remove pins.

Overalls or long pants are helpful since they protect the baby's legs.

Tights, or half-leotards like old-fashioned drawers, are popular. Both little girls and boys can use these in the early months for outdoor wear during chilly weather.

FOOT COVERINGS. Don't put stockings on your baby unless you are in the Arctic. His hands and feet normally feel cool. No foot covering is necessary for indoor use, but for outdoor use, socks and booties are fine to start with.

SWEATERS (2). Choose a cardigan. A slipover is too bothersome. The sweater must be large enough to fit comfortably over the other garments. Acrilan, nylon, Orlon, or other synthetic fabrics wash and dry easily and don't shrink. Wool shrinks, is hard to dry, and can irritate the skin.

OUTER CLOTHING. A sweater, coat, snowsuit, or similar garment is used when the baby is taken outdoors, depending on the temperature. For the first few months cover him with a lightweight blanket or shawl when he is outdoors, just as he is covered during the cool part of the night. A wool bunting or similar covering can be used when he has to travel outdoors in truly cold weather. Add a snug cap or hood when you dress him in a snowsuit—if he will leave it on! Never leave your small baby in his crib or carriage with a cap on if he can push it around or get it pulled over his face.

BIBS. You will need these when your infant starts to be fed sitting up. You may need them earlier when he is drinking. A bib should be large enough to cover his whole front, with closures at neck and waist to keep it in place. Don't leave him alone with his bib on. He may choke himself. Bibs can be rubberized, plastic-covered, or of terry cloth. They should be easy to wash. If necessary, you can use a diaper.

BEDDING

MATTRESS PADS (4-6). A quilted pad 18″ x 18″, rubberized pad, flannel-coated waterproofed cotton pad, or lightweight rubber Kleinert-style pad is best over the mattress and under the sheeting. (No heavy red or black rubber sheeting—too hot!) The pad catches moisture and does not hold odors. It must be washable with soap or detergent. Change it daily or oftener. You may buy material for pads by the yard and cut it to the size you wish. Small pieces may be used to slip under the diaper area or between the nightgown and diaper to absorb moisture.

CRIB SHEETS (4-6). Ordinary cotton crib sheets or knitted crib sheets are used over the pad. Fitted contour bottom sheets are more expensive, but they are easier to put on and give a smoother surface. Unfitted sheets should be long enough to tuck under the mattress generously so that they don't pull out easily. (The same is true for blankets.) Don't ever use a pillow—it's unsafe. Put a diaper or small pad under your baby's head to catch any drooling or spit-up food, firmly pinned at the sides so that it can't be dislodged or wadded up. This may save changing all his bedclothes every time he spits or drools. A folded diaper or pad under his diaper area will also spare the bedclothes. Always make certain that such bedclothing is carefully secured in place. Don't use thin plastic bags or sheets like those used by dry cleaners anyplace around your baby. They are dangerous!

BLANKETS (2-3). Warm, lightweight crib blankets are best for your baby. A heavy blanket is not usually necessary unless the sleeping-room temperature drops quite low. Washable, dryer-safe fabrics are preferable (cotton, Orlon, Dacron, nylon, and some types of rayon and wool). The baby is placed between the sheets, and this blanket is used over the top sheet. Always tuck his bedclothing in well under the mattress so that it is snug and not lying free. The same is true for comforters and quilts. A stroller blanket or pram robe is useful to have.

Wrapping, carrying, or receiving blankets (4-6) made of cotton or cotton and synthetics are lightweight, washable, and about a yard square. These are used for loose wrapping, papoose style, but not for tight swaddling. Use these

when you pick up your baby to feed him or move him about
the house.

Never use sleeping bags or blanket sleepers that tie to
the sides of the crib, or any other type of restraint arrangement. *No restraints. No harnesses.* Use blanket clips instead.

Zippered sleeping bags with sleeves, where baby has free
use of his hands and arms, and can turn or roll, are safe
to use. But if you are given any other kind as a gift trade
it in for some other layette article you need. It is always
dangerous to harness or tie your baby down. If you deny
him freedom of movement, you take away some of his
natural protective defenses.

Give your baby's bed and bedclothes a thorough daily
airing. Make his bed up fresh each day, throwing the covers
back to air beforehand. Wash the mattress surface weekly
or oftener to keep it clean and germ-free.

Check on the things you put in his bed. Any danger from
loose objects that he can get tangled up with, like toys or
extra blankets?

LIVING ARRANGEMENTS

Whether you will be raising your new baby in your own
home, an apartment, or a mobile home, the same rule applies: Live by yourselves, not with your parents. If young
parents are to make mistakes (and you will!), it is better
to do it out of sight of the ever-watchful eyes of grandparents. Even a good relationship between parents and
grandparents can be badly strained by the older couple's
well-meaning attempts to teach. (Look ahead to the section
on *Grandparents* for a fuller discussion of grandparent-
parent relationships.)

BABY'S ROOM

Try to manage so that your baby has a room for himself right from the start. It doesn't have to be large. You
will find it is important to have your infant out of your
bedroom at night. He will sleep better. More importantly,
you will sleep better. He will let you know if he needs
you. You will quickly find out that "sleeping like a baby"

is a monstrous joke. He will make noise every few minutes all night long. He grunts, he sucks and sighs, he passes gas, stretches, squirms, and so on. You may get used to it. But why put yourself through this? Later he needs a room of his own anyway. Why not start now? If a separate room is not possible, sleep your baby in a room with another small child or in any quiet place in your home. Ordinary household noise is all right, but screen him off adequately.

If you have the space to supply your baby with a real bedroom of his own, here is what it should be like ideally. You may not be able to meet all the specifications, but they will give you some idea of what to strive for.

Your baby's room should be light, airy—and childproof. It must have a door that can be closed. There should be no lock on the inside or he may lock himself in later.

Cover the lower four feet of the wall with a hard-surfaced hardboard-type material that washes easily but is difficult to mar. Cover the floor with a non-slippery, mar-proof, easily cleaned vinyl-type material.

A ceiling painted off-white diminishes shadows and light glare. Lighting is distributed evenly and with the least glare from fluorescent sources. Cover all electrical outlets so that curious fingers are safe from harm.

Windows should be adequately screened. Curtains or draperies should be washable. The windows should have roller shades that can be pulled down to cut out light sufficiently at any time and to keep the room cooler in hot weather. They cost less than venetian blinds.

Your very new baby can be left in a room with a 70°F. temperature day and night. After the first few weeks, 65°– 68° is better. A minimum temperature of 45°–50° is allowable. Your baby should be warm but not perspiring. His hands and feet are normally cool to the touch. A wall thermometer is a good investment as a guard against your inclination to keep his room too warm.

Room ventilation must be adequate. Fresh air is important, even at night and on rainy days. A high relative humidity is an excellent environmental help. Cross ventilation is good, but keep baby's crib out of the direct line of the cross draft. In very hot weather, get air circulation by using an electric fan (one with a protective grille) directed away from the baby, or an air conditioner.

Room heat can be furnished by central heating or a room unit. Keep in mind the possible danger if you heat his room with an oil or gas heater or portable electric heater. An oil heater can be knocked over. A gas heater may leak gas or be blown out unless all connections are metal and solid. Some portable electric heaters are possible electrocution machines when wet hands are used on the switch. Avoid any open flame. In a room with a fireplace, solid, well-fitted, and immovable fire screens must be in place. Don't put his crib near any of these units. A fire extinguisher in good working order should be in every home in a convenient spot.

Furniture should be simple, rugged, and free of dust-catching decorations. It must be easy to clean, have smooth varnished, waxed, non-lead painted or enameled surfaces. Cabinets and open shelves for storage are useful. Anchor furniture so that it will not fall over on him when he climbs on it later.

When you have completed the room, step back and check. If you have prepared his room adequately, he can have complete freedom and safety there in the years to come. Look and see. In roaming, crawling, walking along the wall, looking out of the window, pulling the drawers out of the dresser, will he run any hazard? Fix the windows so they can't be opened widely. This will prevent him from falling out. The windows may need to be protected on the inside with heavy mesh or screening so he cannot break the glass.

FURNITURE AND EQUIPMENT

You won't need all of these items right away, but you need to plan for them in your buying budget. You may be able to borrow some of these things from friends and relatives. Don't forget that many of these pieces of equipment can be found in second-hand shops.

BASSINET. You can use a bassinet or basket for a maximum of about three months. One on legs with casters is convenient. A large, flat rectangular clothes basket, wooden box, or bureau drawer with straight sides may be a substitute. It must be big enough and wide enough. A 30-inch length is about right. You can make a mattress of several thicknesses of heavy cotton matting or cotton blankets. It must fit snugly at the sides so that the baby can't get caught in a crack. A fitted Airfoam mattress or pad is better and safer. Any pad you use must be smooth and firm. As noted before, do not use a pillow, either as a mattress or a pillow. Such a carrier is convenient if you take your baby in an automobile or sleep him away from home. Make certain that it has adequate handles. Place the carrier on the back seat of the car, never on the floor of your car or on the floor at home. Always anchor it securely. Everything in your baby's bed must be firmly anchored.

CRIB. You can start with a one-year-old crib. This is equipped with casters or rollers, and can be pushed easily from room to room. You may find a six-year-old crib, 54" x 27" or larger, more practical from the first. Select it for its ease in cleaning, safety, durability, and stability. This piece of furniture will take a great deal of punishment from your growing baby. Check that the sides are high enough to prevent his climbing or falling over them later. They must lock in place securely. Look for sliding mechanisms that are as sturdy and foolproof as possible. The slats or bars on the sides must be placed closely enough so that your baby is not able to get his head through the spaces or catch his arm or leg between them. Smooth sides are better than posts. No exposed sharp points, please! Flat springs are all right, coil springs are not essential. The finish may be shellac, varnish, wax, enamel, or non-lead paint. It is a help if you can raise or lower the level of the bed. You should be able to screen it for insect control.

You need crib bumpers or padding to go around the lower sides of the crib inside. Even a young baby moves surprisingly well and may end up banging his head.

A mobile for his crib is an extra, but he may enjoy it quite early. A cradle gym is a good alternative to this.

MATTRESS. Get a mattress made of any stuffing that holds its shape well and lies flat. Innerspring or foam-rubber mattresses are best but most expensive. No tufts—they are too easily pulled out later and the mattress insides ruined by urine or water. The covering should be water-repellent or, even better, waterproof. The fabric must be tough. An Airfoam plastic-covered mattress is probably best.

CHEST OF DRAWERS OR WARDROBE. This holds all his needed items, including bed linen and diapers. Bath articles and medications can be put on top of it. Centralizing things saves steps for you.

DRYING RACK AND SCREEN. A drying rack is very handy to have nearby when you are dressing, bathing, or changing your active infant. A folding screen heavy enough not to be knocked over easily has many uses in a nursery.

CAR BED (see under *Bassinet*).

INFANT SEAT. This is a molded plastic shell with a mattress pad. In it your baby can half sit, look around, and go to sleep. It permits him to be portable. Don't leave him in the infant seat for feedings. Don't use it after the third or fourth month except for transporting him from one place to another, as in the car, well anchored. He needs to be free to move and may struggle to get out. Be sure to anchor it wherever you put it. This is essential as your baby becomes more active.

HIGH CHAIR. Many models are now available. There are certain requirements that they should all meet. The high chair should have an adjustable foot rest that can be raised or lowered. Pick one with a tray that can lock in place and that slides backward and forward for adjustment. Don't get the kind that swings up over his head. A plastic tray with smooth corners cleans most easily. A chair pad can be included. Widely spaced legs will avoid easy tipping over. The finish should be durable and able to withstand frequent washings. Check for sharp edges. A safety waist strap is a must.

There are specific feeding tables available on the market under various trade names. These platform multiple-purpose feeding table-chairs have sold extensively. They are expensive. The objection to them is that your baby is expected to eat, play, and exercise in the same equipment. His high chair should be identified in your baby's mind with eating and not playing or discipline. This means that he will be kept there only during feeding times—not for long periods of recreation or just to keep him out of the way.

WASHBASIN. This is not used for bathing. It can be useful for small cleaning chores.

BATHTUB. Almost any container can be used as long as it is large enough to allow your baby room to splash and move about. Any 28-inch enamel, plastic, or metal basin or tub is satisfactory. Always place it on a sturdy table or ledge of sufficient height to allow you to work comfortably without stooping. A very good substitute for this is the kitchen sink. It is a good height for you, but remember that the hot-water faucet can be manipulated by infant hands as well as adult ones. Never leave an infant or child in a tub while hot water is being added. Don't use the family bathtub until your child becomes sufficiently developed to handle himself in the water to some extent. Never have the depth of water too great.

BATH TABLE. One type is called Bathinette. It is a widely used piece of apparatus with the advantage of folding up for storage when not in use. It is at a good height for the work top and appliances. Don't leave your baby strapped on the bath table for any period of time. Never leave him *alone* strapped on the top.

You will find a sturdy folding or stationary table useful for dressing and changing your baby if you don't have a bath table. *Never leave your infant alone on any table*. You may not think he can crawl or roll, but you may find that he has developed these abilities when you leave the room—and he's on the floor when you return!

BABY CARRIAGE OR STROLLER. If you use a carriage it must be large enough to permit your baby to lie down comfortably or to sit up. There must be a firm full-length mattress that lies flat with no gaping spaces at the sides or ends. You can use the carriage for his outdoor sleeping in his first months.

More popular today is the lightweight collapsible stroller with an adjustable back, in which your baby can sit, recline, or stretch out. The cushions are firm with washable plastic covers. Sturdy construction will insure use for a long time. Pick a stroller with a wide wheel base, one of the low-silhouette types, to avoid tipping over. A restraining crotch strap, foot rest, canopy cover, adjustable front bar or tray, adjustable handle, brake, and a basket for holding bundles should be included. It is good for shopping. You will use it longer than a carriage.

Don't leave your baby unattended in his carriage or

stroller or without his restraining safety harness for any long period of time. If he can climb, stand, and pull up, don't leave him on his own at all.

SWING. Don't put your baby in a swing when his playpen would give him more exercise and a chance to find himself and explore. A swing is fine for short periods. It will teach your baby to bounce, but not to stand or pull up.

WALKER. A walker does let your baby push around as he sits in his sling seat, but he misses out on learning to pull up and down and to crawl.

CAR SAFETY BELT OR HARNESS. This is a must after the first months to hold your baby in a safe position. A similar harness can be used to control him when you are out walking and he is walking too. An auto seat is a convenience, but it must always be safely anchored. The adult-type lap seat belt should never be used for a child weighing less than 40 pounds.

CANVAS SLING SEAT. You can use this for baby carrying after the first weeks. Your baby is draped across your hip with the strap over your shoulder to take his weight. You are free to use your arms for other things. For long periods of carrying there is the knapsack type of carrier that goes on your back. Get the kind that allows your baby to face forward, his legs going through openings on either side of the seat. Make certain the holes are big enough for him.

CHAIR (FOR MOTHER). You need a low, comfortable chair, especially at feeding time. You may like this during the last weeks of your pregnancy, too.

PLAYPEN. The most suitable type is one that can be easily folded up and moved about. It must be sturdy, as it will have to take a lot of fancy gymnastics later on. The bars or slats must be close enough together so that your baby can't get his head caught between them. The finish should be smooth and nontoxic—he will chew on it later. Its floor requires reinforcement to prevent sagging. It should be several inches from the floor to avoid drafts or damp ground. Small wheels or casters are a help in moving it about. Get it as large as space permits to allow the baby to practice crawling, rolling, standing, and even walking. Net playpens are not as satisfactory for later use.

A washable, plastic-covered, easily cleaned pad makes a good bottom cover. Ties for the four corners are needed unless the pad is extra heavy. A soft blanket may be used over this at first to make it more comfortable. Unless the floor is unusually drafty, it is best not to use side bumper pads. They obstruct baby's view when he is too little to sit up. When he is bigger, they restrict his fun in putting toys outside and fishing them in again.

The playpen has been called "mother's helper." She can go about her chores knowing that her baby is contented and safe, not crawling dangerously about underfoot. You can use the playpen a good part of the time for many months. Just remember three simple rules: Start your baby in his playpen at an early age. Make it an interesting place for him to be. Don't confuse him as to why he's there.

You must make an early start. Use the playpen as soon as he begins to raise up, look around, or push himself about. If you put him in no later than two or three months of age, his little fenced-in place won't seem like a jail at all.

You don't need to stay near him all the time, but do look in on him often. Give him a cheery "hello" or a short conversation and smile. A lot of his playpen pleasure in his early learning comes from being where he can hear and watch some of the household activities.

Think of his playpen as his school. He may learn to turn over there for the very first time. The bars and the solid flat surface help him. Then he will figure out how to sit up. With much effort he will pull himself up to his knees and then onto his feet to hang onto those bars. While he is still holding on he will take his first wobbly steps. During all this, you will have the pleasure of watching him without the bother of chasing after him every minute.

By the time your baby is getting around by rolling or crawling, don't make the mistake of turning him loose in the house just because he fusses at you when he is in the playpen. If he fusses, turn him loose in his childproof room —and close the door so he stays put—or move the playpen to another room where he can't nag at you. Don't forget that a change of scene often works wonders with a baby.

3.

Having
the Baby

LABOR AND DELIVERY

ADVANCE SIGNS OF LABOR

Toward the end of your pregnancy, your body begins to make its preparations for the big event. Following are some of the signs that serve as advance notice that you are almost ready for labor.

"Lightening" occurs anytime from several weeks to a few days before labor sets in. This doesn't mean that your baby is any lighter, only that his position has shifted forward and lower down into your pelvis, his head settling down into the birth canal. (Ninety-five percent of babies are born head down.) This may happen quite suddenly. You feel less pressure in your abdomen. You can breathe better. Your ribs don't feel so pushed on. You climb stairs without as much trouble or puffing. But you find that the pressure has merely shifted downward. Now the pressure on your bladder makes you urinate more often. You may have some trouble having a bowel movement. If you have had a baby before, lightening may not come until you actually start labor.

Another sign you may have is a sudden burst of energy. This happens just when you seem to be dragging around at your worst. Or you may not have it at all.

Another indication of preparation for labor are the false

pains that come and go. Such pains always make you wonder if this is the real thing. But they are short and irregular and not too severe before they peter out. You don't want to go to the hospital too early and have the embarrassment and nuisance of going home to wait all over again. You can test the pains yourself a little when they come. They are across your lower abdomen or lower back. Change your position or activity. See if they continue. If they go away you are probably not in labor yet. If they keep on, clock them. How frequently do they come? How long do they last? Are they getting more intense? You may be starting the real thing!

START OF LABOR

When your labor begins, there are three important cues. They may not show up in the order indicated here. They are not always proof positive that labor has started.

"SHOW." One cue is "show." A small amount of bloodtinged mucus is discharged from your vagina. This thick, sticky mucus has served as a plug closing the opening of the cervix of your uterus and protecting it against infection. Now the way is clear for your baby. If this show is followed or accompanied by a cramping pain, it is a good sign that your labor is beginning.

RUPTURE OF MEMBRANES. Another cue is the breaking of the bag of waters. The pressure in the amniotic sac increases when the muscles of your uterus tighten. The baby-containing sac finally bursts to release a flow of colorless fluid. This may come as a sudden gush of water or may be only a trickle if the tear in the membrane is small. By itself this doesn't necessarily mean that labor is actually beginning. The sac can rupture a couple of days or more before labor really starts.

If the sac breaks before your pains start, you should let your doctor know at once. Stay off your feet until you get directions. If your baby's head is not yet down in your pelvis, there is some risk of infection. Induced labor may be necessary. (Induced labor may have to be used for other reasons, too, as when medical problems in the mother re-

quire that the pregnancy be terminated prematurely, or
when it is necessary to prevent postmaturity.)

Often with your first baby the membranes may not break
until you are in the hospital in labor. If this doesn't happen
spontaneously during labor, your doctor ruptures them.

CONTRACTIONS. Labor may start as an ache at the lower
part of your back that spreads out around and across your
abdomen, or as a cramplike sensation much like the cramping at the beginning of a menstrual period. Although contractions may only feel like a backache at first, these muscle
tightenings are slowly pushing your baby down against and
through your cervix. Your abdomen becomes hard and soft
again as your uterus contracts. The contractions last ten to
forty seconds and come about ten to thirty minutes apart.
The increase in their regularity, force, and duration tells
you that your labor has started. Your husband can keep
track of these contractions and time the intervals between
them. When the pains begin to come regularly at eight-to-
ten-minute intervals, call your obstetrician. Don't head for
the hospital before you talk with him. Be able to tell him
where you can feel the pains, if they are coming at regular
intervals and increasing in severity, and if walking changes
them. And don't eat or drink anything once the pains have
started: The OB man commonly says, "Well, it sounds like
you're ready for the hospital." You grab your prepacked
overnight bag and head for the door.

AT THE HOSPITAL

If, as advised earlier in this book, you have made a tour
of the hospital before now, you will know its layout and
you won't waste any time getting to the admitting office.
Someone there checks your reservation, confirms pertinent
identification, fills out forms. Be sure you have your medi-
cal-insurance registration card with you. It seems like a
very long time before you get to the elevator, go to the
obstetrical floor, and are introduced to a hospital bed in
the labor room. When you look at your watch, you realize
that it really hasn't been very many minutes.

You are separated at this point from your husband for a
time while you are checked in medically. The nurse or

doctor will perform a rectal examination to determine the position of your baby's head and the condition of your cervix. This determines how far labor has progressed. If you are definitely in labor, you will be shaved in the pubic area. In hospital talk this is called prepping. Most likely, you will be given an enema. Other parts of the examination include such things as taking your pulse, temperature, blood pressure. These details must be watched to determine the well-being of you and your baby. As the estimation of your condition is made, your obstetrician checks and advises. The anesthetist comes to do his part to aid you in your labor. Finally your obstetrician directs the nurses to get you into the delivery room.

At this point, let's back up a little and talk about the stages of labor. The following descriptions are based on the assumption that you will be awake during labor and delivery.

FIRST STAGE

The first stage of labor consists of the time between the beginning of labor and the full opening of the cervix. If your bag of waters has not broken, you may get up and walk about. This may help. If your bag of waters has ruptured, stay in bed, or you may get yourself into difficulty. As mentioned before, these first pains are like a dull backache, or a cramplike feeling as the intensity and duration of the pains increase. With the contractions your baby is pushed down against your cervix. The cervix has softened to be ready for stretching. It gradually stretches and thins out to be pulled down over his head as he is pushed deeper into the birth canal. (See figs. 20 and 21.)

This first stage is the longest and most tiring. It takes about six to eighteen hours for a first baby and about two to eight hours in subsequent pregnancies. There is no way to determine the exact duration of this stage ahead of time.

You may start out with quite strong pains or contractions, which taper off for a time. Use this time for a nap or some quiet rest. The contractions will start again, perhaps with some stimulation given by your doctor. Between contractions you may want to read, or chat with your husband if he is with you in the labor room. As your contractions become more frequent, there will be moments when you feel you are being swept along by forces bigger than yourself. That's when you want some real help, someone to hold onto, like your husband, the nurse, or the doctor. During this time the members of your hospital team will be doing

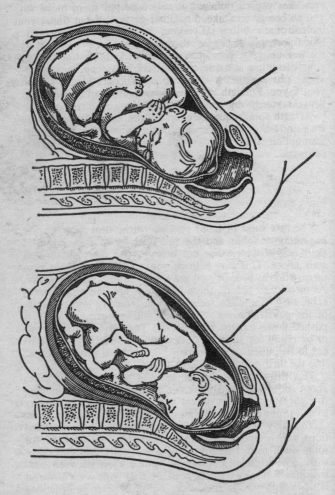

Figs. 20-21. The first stage of labor. Reprinted from *Education for Sexuality*, John J. Burt and Linda Brower (W. B. Saunders Co.).

all they can to make you comfortable. You may be given some medication now to help you relax. During this first stage you relax with the contractions. Don't strain. Bend, curve your back, breathe with your whole abdomen. This relaxes your abdominal muscles and lets them move with each breath you take. The contractions are not under your control at this time. If you push and grunt at this point you will just wear yourself out without doing any good. If you tense up and fight the pain you will only make it worse and lengthen the time of labor. If you take it easy during this phase of your labor, resting while you can, you will save your strength for the time when you will need it.

As your baby gets further down your birth canal, the strength and frequency of your contractions increase. You begin to aid in the pushing in spite of yourself. With a local anesthesia the strong muscle contractions of your uterus continue to force your baby along the birth canal, but you don't feel pain—you feel the hardening of your abdomen with the contractions. Your doctor or the delivery-room nurse checks you at intervals during this first stage to determine the progress you are making in your labor. Other checks are done to make certain that both you and your baby are in good shape. When your cervix is fully dilated and your baby's head has moved far enough down the birth canal, you have entered the second stage of labor.

SECOND STAGE

The second stage starts when your cervix is open to its fullest, and ends with the delivery of your baby. (See figs. 22-26.) It can last as long as two hours if this is your first birth. If your membranes have not yet ruptured, they will be opened now to speed the descent of your baby's head into the birth canal. The bag of waters has helped to prepare your vagina for delivery, serving as a cushion over your baby's head. This is the point when the contractions make you feel like bearing down with your abdominal muscles. You may be surprised to find that the hard pushing pains when they come are a great relief. At last you are doing something to help your baby along. Your doctor or nurse will let you know when to push and when to relax. As you continue to push your baby down the birth canal, you will feel pressure but no alarming pain because of the action of the local anesthetic. Between contractions and pushing, relax and let your drowsiness take over. As your baby's head moves into position, you will be prepared for the delivery and moved to the delivery room.

The delivery room looks like an operating room. There is the table in the center of the room with a great deal of bright light about it. There stands the gowned nurse, already busy with the instrument table. To the side is a warm bassinet waiting to receive the baby. Here comes the obstetrician from his surgical scrub, ready to get into a sterile gown, followed closely by his assistant. Then you are busy getting on the table. The delivery-room nurse shifts you about. Your legs are put up on supporting stirrups. You are scrubbed, draped with sterile sheets, and all is ready. The anesthetist stands by to watch over you. Your hands and wrists are placed loosely in wristlets to remind you to keep your hands where they belong. They serve as a grip if you need one. Your husband is ushered in now if he is to be present, looking very strange with a surgical cap, mask, and gown.

From this point on you listen to your obstetrician as he tells you what is happening and what you can do to help. If there is an overhead mirror you can watch so that you aren't ignorant of what he is talking about. As you look you can see, with each contraction, something appear in the birth-canal opening. Can it be? Yes, it is! Your baby's head. (See fig. 22.) More of it appears as you push him

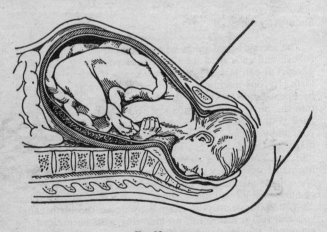

Fig. 22

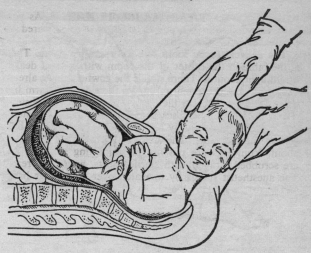

Fig. 23

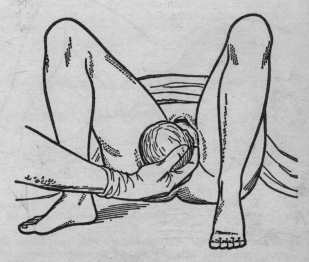

Fig. 24

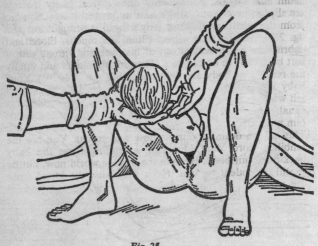

Fig. 25

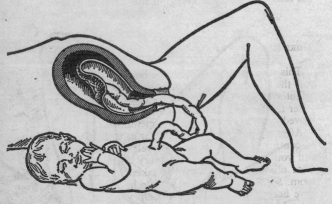

Fig. 26

Figs. 22-26. The second stage of labor. Reprinted from *Education for Sexuality,* John J. Burt and Linda Brower (W. B. Saunders Co.).

down the birth canal. You push hard with your whole abdomen, then relax between pushes. But something has to give—and it does. An episiotomy, a surgical incision made at the opening of the vagina to avoid tearing of the perineum and vagina, is frequently done. Most likely, forceps are slipped over your baby's head to protect it as it emerges from the birth canal. Your baby's head is brought out (see fig. 23), and his face wiped. Fluid and mucus, blood and debris, are gently sucked out of his nose and throat with a soft bulb syringe or catheter. Then his shoulders and finally the rest of his body are delivered. (See figs. 24–26.) Your baby is usually born face down and head first. You can't tell whether he is a boy or girl until he is out of the birth canal. Then the obstetrician announces his sex and holds him with his head downward below the level of your hips. This aids in draining out his nose and throat. You see the umbilical cord, dark blue, still extending from the baby back into your body. He is in the outside world now, but he is still dependent on you. He is still using the blood from the placenta. Then the cord is clamped and cut, usually after the pulsations have stopped and your baby is no longer getting any blood from it. Cutting the cord doesn't hurt him since there are no nerves in it. About 2 inches of a stump are left. The cord is tied or clamped to prevent bleeding. The baby is now on his own. He is held up for you to see before he is put in a warm blanket that the nurse has ready. At last, you and your husband are parents!

THIRD STAGE

This stage consists of the time between the baby's arrival and the delivery of the placenta. It can last from a few minutes to several minutes, sometimes as much as an hour. After the placenta has separated from your uterus, it is removed with the now useless sac membranes.

After the delivery of the afterbirth, your uterus contracts to control the blood flow. The relaxing incision is closed and you are taken to the recovery room. After a time of close observation, you will be taken to a regular hospital room. Some details may be a little hazy at this point. You have been given a sedative to help you rest and relax for several hours. People are there, but they blur together. All you can think of is, "I am a mother!" You will do a good deal of resting, sleeping, eating, and enjoying yourself from this point on. The resting part is the most important for the first few days.

4.

The
Newborn Baby

GENERAL APPEARANCE

Perhaps you have seen newborn infants before the arrival of your own, but even so you may feel a pang of anxiety as you gaze at this messy-looking creature with the gray-blue color that your doctor is holding aloft for you to see. He doesn't look like the picture-babies that you had in mind. Is he all right? How can he be and look like that? Well, he probably is. Most new babies look this way until they are cleaned up and begin to use their lungs in the approved fashion when they take on a pink-to-red look.

But you need to take a closer look at this small, squirming object—your newborn. (He is designated a newborn for the next month and then he is called an infant.) You are struck by the fact that he looks so totally helpless. Of all the creatures in the world, the human baby is the most completely dependent. His helplessness lasts for a much longer period than any other animal's, although his ability to cry gets him a good deal of attention.

INDIVIDUALITY

Although he may look a good deal like any other newborn, your baby is unique. He is more than a combination of you and your husband; he is a brand-new article. Not only does he differ, if only slightly, in size and weight from all the other babies in the nursery, even his manner of acting and responding is different. He doesn't have too many ways to express himself, but the signs are there for you to see. Your baby may cry sooner or less quickly than another baby. He may keep his body moving continually, or he may be quiet with only slow or little movement. Already he is an individual!

While your baby is not actually thinking yet—his brain isn't very mature and he has no memories to use in associating one thing with another—he is experiencing and feeling. Whatever goes on about him or happens to him, he records and stores away. Whatever is uncomfortable he protests about, at first with no idea that such a protest will bring assistance. Eventually he will make associations: he is hungry—he cries—you come—he is fed—he is comfortable. I suppose that you could say that this is his first glimmer of a thought.

PHYSICAL CHARACTERISTICS

WEIGHT

From past experience I would say that the first question you will ask, after asking if the baby is all right, is, "How much does he weigh?" You may feel just a little glow of superiority if you have a big baby. But before you puff out your chest too much, let me talk about this weight business.

Ranges: Boys 5.8–10.1 lbs.   Average 7.5 lbs.
Girls 5.8– 9.4 lbs.   Average 7.4 lbs.

As you can see from these figures, the normal newborn can vary almost two pounds in either direction from the average weight. First children are usually somewhat smaller than subsequent ones. It is not always true that big parents have big babies. It is more often true that parents who have been big babies will have big babies themselves. Older mothers are more likely to have big babies than young mothers, but this can vary, too. A baby's weight at birth is influenced by several factors: heredity, his mother's general health and nutritional status, the placement of the placenta in her uterus during pregnancy, her glandular condition, and the length of gestation.

INITIAL WEIGHT LOSS. Your baby weighs in heavier at birth than he really is, because of his water-logged tissues. He will lose weight during his first few days. His initial fluid loss is usually about 5 to 7 percent of his birth weight.

WEIGHT INCREASE. His weight loss stops about his third or fourth day. Then he will begin to gain. If he continues to lose weight he is not getting enough to eat, or, less commonly, he may be sick. His weight gain from now on is not a steady one, it will vary from one period to another. He will usually be back to his birth weight or even exceed it by ten to fourteen days, if he is fed with formula. If he is adequately breast-fed, he may regain his birth weight sooner.

There is no great difference in weight increase between babies fed by breast and those on formula. If he gets enough to eat by either method, he will gain weight. How satisfactory his nutrition is will be demonstrated by the character and rate of his growth. You will find considerable variation in weight increase among normal babies.

HEIGHT

The height ranges below show how much variation there can be from the average. It is difficult to get an accurate measurement on your young baby. He wants to curl himself up into the position he has used for nine months.

Ranges: Boys 18.2–21.5 in. Average 19.9 in.
          Girls 18.5–21.1 in. Average 19.8 in.

The newborn's length depends mostly on his heredity and on constitutional factors. If he doesn't get enough to eat for a considerable period of time, his increase in length may begin to lag, but not as rapidly as his weight does.

SKIN

If your newborn is a well-nourished, full-term baby, you will see a moist, somewhat wrinkled skin with a bluish-gray color immediately after his birth. His color become more normal as he breathes and increases the amount of oxygen taken into his lungs. His hands and feet often remain bluish for some days.

Vernix, the prenatal skin covering discussed in "The Unborn Baby" section, makes your newborn look as if he has been dipped in thick buttermilk. The amount can vary a great deal, but is most abundant in the body folds and creases.

OIL-FILLED GLANDS. The skin of the newborn's face may show some "white heads," small oil-filled glands or pores. These empty spontaneously as his face is washed.

JAUNDICE. The yellowish tinge that may come to his skin about the third day is jaundice, or icterus. This is physiological or newborn jaundice and is not a disease. Extra blood cells that your baby no longer needs are broken down at this time. The yellow bile pigment from the blood breakdown piles up in his blood faster than his immature liver can handle it temporarily. His skin loses this yellow color and returns to normal after a week or so as his liver behaves more efficiently. Jaundice that isn't normal is the kind that goes with Rh disease or prematurity.

FAT LAYER. The fat layer of your baby's skin is normally a thick, protective, insulating layer. Exceptions are the premature baby, who hasn't had time to put this fat on, and the postmature baby, who is using his up. You can appreciate this layer best by pinching a fold of skin between your fingers. It is a good indicator of the state of his nutrition at birth.

BIRTHMARKS. Birthmarks are so common that you should almost expect your baby to have one. Contrary to various superstitions and misconceptions about birthmarks, there is no connection between them and any mental or physical act or injury on a mother's part. You didn't mark your baby. Don't overemphasize the importance of birthmarks. The most common types fade out over the years.

There are several kinds of birthmarks, not all of which are present at birth. Medically, they are called vascular or pigmented nevi, meaning that they are discolored spots on the skin made up of either extra blood vessels or extra pigment deposits.

Birthmarks related to blood-vessel change differ from each other only in the type of blood vessels that make them and the extent of the skin involved. Girls are more often found to have them.

Your baby, like many if not most babies, will show blotchy pale pink to light red or purplish marks at the back of his neck, perhaps around his eyelids, forehead, nose, or upper lip. These are called stork marks or stork's beak marks. These tiny blood-vessel blotches shrink so that the marks fade gradually during his first year. The mark on the back of his neck often remains. Many of you parents will still show this mark.

If the port wine stain type is present, it is usually present at birth. The extra capillaries make it red to purple in color. It isn't a raised mark and can vary considerably in size, shape, and location. These marks don't fade out when you press them and they usually don't disappear spontaneously. Camouflage with cosmetics is the best treatment later.

The strawberry mark, or *capillary hemangioma,* is a deep red, raised, rough surfaced area with extra capillaries in the whole skin layer. It can come anywhere on the body. Most appear in the first month and are in the head region. Prematures frequently have one or more. Such marks often grow rapidly in size during the first six months, then remain about the same until they gradually shrink over a three-to-six-year period. Small pale areas appear and join together at the center and move outward. They are completely gone by seven years, leaving only an area of whitish skin. Watchful waiting is best, as scarring is greater when treatment is carried out. If their location and size cause problems, some treatment may be required.

Cavernous hemangiomas are strawberry marks with large veins and vascular sinuses in them. They involve not only skin but the tissue under the skin. They may occur without the strawberry mark on the skin surface. They are soft, deep, bluish masses from which you can squeeze the blood on pressure. They enlarge before they start to shrink. Again, watchful waiting is the best treatment unless they are so large they create problems that make removal necessary.

Moles, or pigmented nevi, are not common in the newborn but appear in later years. They are collections of pigment-bearing cells. Pigmented nevi are important primarily for cosmetic reasons. They rarely undergo malignant change, particularly in infants and children.

Mongolian spots are dark blue or purple blotchy spots. The blue color is caused by the changes in the cells and pigment layer of the skin. Usually located over the lower back, they may extend up over the mid-back or even onto the back of the arms or legs. Such staining has also been found on the inside of the cheeks. They are a common finding in infants with darker complexions of all races. They disappear spontaneously during the first four years. They are not the result of injury or pressure.

Accessory or supernumerary nipples occur as a single spot or multiple flat tan or brown spots along the front of the chest in a line below the true nipples in both boys and girls. They often darken in color at puberty. These evolutionary remnants may look like pigmented nevi. If you stretch the skin around one, it goes in. Their location and dimpling make their identification possible.

TEMPERATURE REGULATION. Your baby's skin is a temperature regulator as well as a protective covering. Just as the newborn's skin is not too protective at first, so his temperature regulation is not too accurate to begin with. After a few days his temperature apparatus begins to function more efficiently. He develops the ability to regulate his internal body temperature by adjustments in his skin activity.

His circulation, especially at the skin surface, is not sufficient to keep his extremities as warm as the rest of his body. Your hands and feet are several degrees cooler than your trunk temperature. It is the same with him. The skin of your baby will respond to change in temperature by a purplish mottling. This indicates the pattern of the blood vessels in his skin.

HAIR

Hair color and texture can change. Blonds may become brunettes, brunettes redheads. Curly hair may become straight. Many new babies are almost bald, while others have enough hair to braid it into little pigtails. At the start, boy babies often have more hair than girl babies. Don't expect a heavy head of hair to stay. Much of the hair present at birth may be brittle and break off easily. This may produce a period when scalp hair is sparse. New hair comes, often quite light in texture.

Over his body there may still be some of the downy fuzz called lanugo hair, discussed earlier in more detail in "The Unborn Baby" section. Most of it is on his back, shoulders, forehead, and cheeks. It disappears fairly rapidly as it falls out or is rubbed away in his early weeks. There are some dark-skinned babies who come from dark-skinned families who keep a fairly heavy growth of body hair. This is a family or inherited characteristic.

NAILS

While his fingernails are developed enough so that they extend out beyond his fingertips, his toenails don't reach anywhere near the end of his toes as yet. Infant nails are layered and very soft. They flake off and tear easily.

HEAD

Your newborn's head will look remarkably large to you. The length of his head, top to chin, is about one fourth of his entire length. By the time he is a grown man this will change to one eighth to one tenth of his body length. Most of the growth in the size of a human's head occurs during his first year of life.

The soft spots in the head, or fontanelles, are the openings where the bones of the skull have not yet grown together. (See fig. 27.) You will be able to identify only two of the six soft spots present at birth. His rear, or posterior, fontanelle will admit only the tip of your little finger. His frontal, or anterior, fontanelle, on top of his head, will measure 1 to 2 inches. The fontanelles are covered by heavy membranes, which are ample protection. These open areas are obliterated as the bones grow together. The big anterior soft spot, the last one to close, usually does so between the fifteenth and eighteenth months.

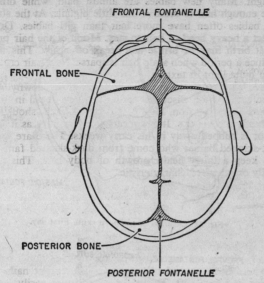

Fig. 27. The fontanelles.

Your baby's head may show any one of various minor departures from the average. Most of these variations result from the position of and pressures on the fetus in the uterus, or from the stresses of delivery. The baby's head circumference at birth is between 12 and 13 inches. This is usually larger than the circumference of your birth canal through which it has to pass. This means, as mentioned earlier, that his head will have to be shaped to fit. All babies coming through the birth canal show some shaping, but sometimes it may produce quite an irregularly shaped head. (See plate 1.) His brain is not damaged by these changes in shape.

This shaping process makes his head seem longer, with his forehead flattened, and the point of his head almost looks like a dunce's cap if the shaping is extreme. The skull bones are often overlapped to form ridges on his scalp. By the end of the first week much of this is gone. By a month he has a normally long head. (See plate 2.)

The following diagram (see fig. 28) shows a newborn's skull in the first day of life. It shows the molding of the

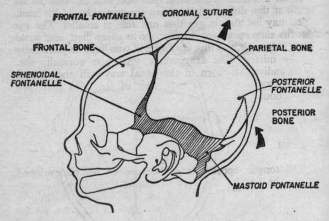

Fig. 28. Diagram of newborn skull. First day.

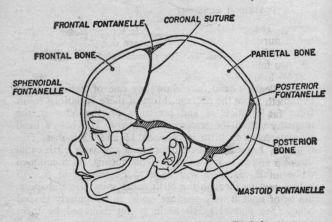

Fig. 29. Diagram of newborn skull. Third day.

bones of his skull, with overlapped edges and narrowed sutures caused by the normal process of squeezing during his passage through the birth canal. The other diagram (see fig. 29) is of his skull on the third day of life, and shows the reexpansion of his cranium and widening of the sutures and fontanelles. The parietal, occipital, and temporal bones have returned to their normal positions.

Even a month after birth you will still be able to see some of the differences between the two sides of his head. You may be able to see that one side is smaller. The eye on this side may look smaller, go to sleep first, and wake last. You may pick this up faster if you look at your baby in the mirror. This exaggerates what you normally see. Most individuals born in the usual way will show some asymmetry between the two sides of the head and face throughout their lives.

MOUTH

His tongue appears large because of his undeveloped chin. The frenum, the cord under his tongue, may appear too short or too tight. Usually this can be left alone. Tongue-tie rarely causes speech defects in children. As his jaw grows his tongue appears more normal. The tongue-tie disappears. If your baby can bring the tip of his tongue to his lower gum line or further, he has no trouble. I don't feel that this short cord should be blamed for ineffective nursing. The action of the tip of the tongue is not important in nursing as milking motions are done with the middle part of the tongue.

If you find teeth in your new baby, they will usually be the two lower central incisors. You do not need to have them pulled unless they are loose. Sometimes a baby will erupt teeth in his first two weeks as well.

The fat bulges in his cheeks are sucking pads. A small, thin baby will show these prominently. They disappear in about six weeks. His lips may show something blisterlike or calluslike. Look closely. These are sucking pads, on his upper lip and two on his lower. They help him to close his lips about the nipple tightly for good suction. They may peel several times before they disappear by two or three months of age.

THYMUS

The thymus is a mass of tissue in the chest behind the breastbone. It is normally large at birth. The thymus has never been implicated as a cause of respiratory difficulty, although formerly it was often blamed for this. It is an important organ in your baby's immunity system. It is not talked about so often nowadays, but some parents are still needlessly concerned about stories they have heard concerning an "enlarged thymus."

HEART

The baby's heart lies in a horizontal position in his chest. The apex beat at the tip of his heart can be felt at, or just outside, his left nipple in the space between his third and fourth ribs in front. His pulse varies from 90 in sleep to 180 when he is active or crying. You may not be able to feel any pulse in his legs for several weeks. He may show a heart murmur for a time until his heart and circulatory system have made the changes from that of a non-air breather to an air-breathing baby. These are called functional murmurs. The murmur that is heard after he is five or six months old is often significant, but the presence of a heart murmur doesn't have to mean any organic disease. This is the reason a diagnosis of congenital heart disease is made with great caution and some reservations.

LUNGS

After the first forceful cries that start a baby's regular breathing, he may settle down to very quiet breathing in his newborn shock period. After that he may cry vigorously and start a very irregular breathing pattern for his next weeks. His lungs need several days to expand to full capacity. You will find a wide variation in the rates and rhythms of your baby's breathing. He may breathe twenty to one hundred times a minute, although the average is forty-five. This depends on whether he is physically active, awake, asleep, or crying. His breathing is done almost entirely with his diaphragm. This makes him pull in his chest and stick out his abdomen when he takes a breath. His rhythm of breathing changes, too. He is a periodic breather—shallow and rapid for a time, then some big, irregular ones, then back to shallow. He may be a slow and deep breather, or he may show a very irregular pattern.

ABDOMEN

Your child's pot-bellied look lasts for the first few years and is actually what gives him that "baby" look. His abdomen is protuberant because of his weak abdominal muscles, large internal abdominal organs, and sometimes a considerable layer of fat. This size fits in with what is required of your infant. He is going to have to take in, absorb, and transform a tremendous amount of food in order to attain his quite remarkable increase in size. For this reason the stomach and intestinal system has to be a prominent feature in your new baby. It has an important role.

UMBILICUS

His umbilicus, or navel, shows a 2-inch to 3-inch stump left from the umbilical cord. The stump dries to a brown or black, gradually to mummify and drop off cleanly at the junction of the cord and skin, usually between five to nine days.

STOMACH

The size of the stomach is subject to wide variations in individual infants. Any infant is capable of taking much more fluid than his anatomical capacity would lead you to believe. His physiological capacity, in other words, is greater than his anatomical capacity. This is due to the fact that food leaves the stomach while more is being taken in. It is possible to distend the stomach considerably without any difficulty. The amount your baby's stomach will hold varies with how often you feed him and how much he has to take in order to be satisfied. A dilute feeding with not many calories to satisfy him will require larger amounts for him to maintain good nutrition. More concentrated feedings mean that his hunger is satisfied for a much longer period of time. Larger amounts, which distend his stomach, may increase the actual time it takes for food to leave his stomach. Your infant can take phenomenal amounts if you compare him with an adult relative to his size.

The stomach of the newborn lies across his upper abdomen. As he begins to get into an upright position, his stomach begins to change to a more up-and-down position.

SPINE

Your newborn infant's spine is essentially in the shape of a curve. (See plate 3.) It is rubbery and mobile. This curve is gradually replaced by the adult set of curves as your child comes to an erect position and learns how to walk by developing adequate equilibrium.

You may notice a deep dimple at the end of his spine, sometimes with a little tuft of hair in it. It is like the stem spot on an apple. This point is the part of his spine that was closed last. Keep it well cleansed so that material won't collect and irritate.

His legs are most often seen doubled up against his abdomen, in his prebirth position. If you stretch his legs out straight, it will surprise you to find how short they are in comparison with his arms. His knees stay slightly bent. The bowing of his legs is usually temporary. As the hardening of his long bones occurs, they straighten out.

His hands and feet may look too large for his skinny arms and legs. His feet look more complete than they really are. X rays would show you only one real bone in his heel. His other foot bones are still in the cartilage stage. The skin is loose and wrinkled. Abnormal positions of the feet will be a special matter to take up with your pediatrician. Overlapping toes are a family characteristic and don't need treatment.

Your baby holds his hand in a fist with the thumb inside. He may suddenly swing his arm out and bring his hand around, clutching at the air. If he hits his face, he claws it. If he hits his mouth, he sucks.

If you open his hands out flat from their characteristic fist position, you will see that they have finely lined palms, tissue-paper-thin nails, dry, loose-fitting skin, and deep bracelet creases at the wrists. Both feet and hands have skin-line patterns that are individually characteristic and may have been used by the hospital for identification purposes.

GENITALS

The swollen, puffy genitals of both boy and girl babies will appear large in comparison to later size; this is a response to the hormone effect of the mother's blood. In the baby boy, fluid sometimes accumulates before birth in the scrotum or the sac about the testicle. Pressure during birth causes a certain amount, too. This condition is called hydrocele (water in the sac). The testicle may look like a water-filled balloon. Such fluid is gradually absorbed. No special treatment is required.

Erection of the penis is common in newborn boys. This does not indicate abnormality. The prepuce or foreskin is always sticking fast to the glans or head of his penis and may be quite full and long. If there is an opening in his prepuce sufficient to allow unobstructed urination, circumcision is not a must-do procedure.

Your baby girl may have a white vaginal secretion for a few weeks, or even a bloody vaginal discharge. This is not menstruation. Her mother's hormones are responsible for it. The hormonal effect wears off by four to six weeks.

BREASTS

In both boys and girls the breasts may be swollen and tense for the first few weeks of life. Again this is a physiological reaction from the hormones in the mother's bloodstream. It gradually subsides as the hormone effect diminishes. There is sometimes a small amount of secretion. This has been called "witch's milk." No attempt should be made to squeeze out this "milk." The breasts are not to be manipulated, massaged, rubbed, or touched, except for gentle washing.

POSTURE

At first your baby's muscles are limp. He has pliable joints. (See plate 4.) He loses his excessive joint flexibility at about six or eight weeks.

Your baby tries to stay in the curled-up fetal position for some weeks after birth. His legs are pulled up and his arms held close to his body. His hands are closed in tight fists.

Your newborn can usually raise his head when lying on his stomach. He can turn his head from side to side, but not with good control.

Bowel Movements

Your baby may have his first bowel movement soon after birth, or in the first day or two. The lower part of his large intestine is filled with meconium at birth. His first bowel movement is made up of this meconium, a very thick, greenish-black, sticky material consisting of what he swallowed during the time he was in the uterus plus debris from the lining of his intestines. This matter must be eliminated from his bowel before his normal bowel movement will appear—in two or three days time. The first stools after meconium, whether you breast-feed or formula-feed, will be loose and pale white to yellowish brown, with milk curds present. These will be replaced in the breast-fed baby by a soft, granular yellow-orange stool with a not-unpleasant odor. The color doesn't mean too much. The number of movements varies with the number of feedings and the amount of food your baby receives. He may have a great many a day or only one every four or five days. The stool of a formula-fed baby has a pasty, thick consistency, varying from yellow to greenish-yellow in color with a fairly strong odor. His movements are usually fewer than those of the breast-fed baby at this time.

Urination

Your newborn usually urinates soon after birth. This event may be delayed even to the second day without causing concern. His early urine may contain uric-acid crystals, which stain his diapers pink. This should not be confused with bleeding. The amount of urine that your infant makes depends entirely upon his fluid intake. This may be quite scanty during his early days of life. By the end of a few days, when he is starting to take increasing amounts of food, his urine production equals his fluid intake, unless there is excessive fluid loss from his skin. This can happen if he is kept too warm.

REFLEXES

The newborn's most obvious tools for living that you can see at birth are his reflexes. He doesn't have conscious control over his movements as yet. His behavior is almost entirely automatic in nature.

Although he spends most of his time sleeping, he does do other things. He lies on his side with his arms and legs drawn up. He lies on his abdomen with his knees drawn up, his buttocks high, his head turned to one side. He starts, yawns, quivers, coughs, sneezes, hiccups, stretches, salivates, and cries on the slightest provocation. He can see, smell, taste, hear, and feel. His breathing and temperature are irregular. He can suck and swallow, but he may swallow in the wrong direction.

Most of these acts are involuntary. They follow after specific stimulation. They are reflexes, unlearned and inborn. They are not behavior patterns. They are not learned or the result of coordination of his growing nerves and muscles.

These reflexes may be defensive or protective or may serve as the framework on which your baby gets his start in the complicated business of learning how to control his body parts.

STARTLE REFLEX

This is also called the Moro reflex. A loud noise or quick movement, a rapid shift in the baby's position, or a sudden bright light can produce this response. (See plate 5.) The baby can cause it himself if he jumps suddenly. His body stiffens. His arms shoot out from his body with his hands open, then come together as if to hug or surround something. His head may extend and his shoulders rise. He may open his eyes wide as if he is looking far off, and his breathing may speed up. His legs may make jerking motions. Finally, there may be a cry—or he may quiet down without making a noise. Not all babies show this response to the same degree. It's sometimes hard to believe that your baby can get into such a state over practically nothing as far as you can see. This reflex gradually diminishes in strength by the third month, to be gone by five or six months. Remnants of it are still seen in a grown-up when he is startled by a loud noise.

TONIC-NECK REFLEX (TNR)

You will see the classic fencing position of this reflex when your baby is lying quietly on his back. (See plate 6.) He may be asleep. His head is turned to one side. The arm and leg on that side are stretched out. The arm and leg on the other side are flexed. If you turn his head to the other side, his arms and legs reverse their positions. The flexed limbs will stretch out, and the stretched-out limbs will flex. This response disappears gradually by six to seven months.

SPINAL REFLEXES

These are reflexes that have to do with his trunk. (See plates 7–12.)

TRUNK INCURVATION REFLEX. This is also called Galant's reflex. Put your baby on his stomach, and run your fingers or a pin lightly down one side of his trunk between his ribs and hip. He will bend his back and swing his bottom toward your stroking fingers. (See plates 7 and 8.)

MAGNET REFLEX. Put your baby on his back, half bend both his legs, and put pressure with your fingers on the soles of his feet. His legs will straighten out to push him away from you. (See plates 9 and 10.)

CROSSED-EXTENSION REFLEX. Put your baby on his back. Stretch one leg out by pressing his knee down, and stroke the sole of the foot. His other leg will bend at the knee, then stretch out. This reflex is usually gone after his first month. (See plates 11 and 12.)

ORAL REFLEXES

ROOTING REFLEX. This is also known as the search reflex. It occurs when his cheek is touched. He turns that way and roots or nuzzles for something. This reflex helps him find the nipple. It is followed by sucking if he finds something he can grasp with his mouth. He may turn toward the smell of milk and start rooting. If you touch the corner of his mouth, he lowers the lip on that side and his tongue moves that way. His head turns to follow if you slide your finger away from the corner of his mouth. If you stroke the middle of his lower lip, he lowers the lip and his tongue heads for that point. If you move your finger down on his chin, he will open his jaw and bend his head down. If you touch the center of his upper lip, he lifts his lip to bare his gums, and his tongue points that way. If you touch the tip of his nose with a light upward sweep, he throws his head back, stretches backward with his trunk, turns his arms backward, pushes out with his forearms, turns his hands palm downward, and pushes out with his legs. Most of these mouthing-type reflexes described strengthen during his first weeks after birth to gradually fade out after mid-year.

SUCKING REFLEX. You can provoke this by putting your fingertip or a nipple in his mouth. This produces vigorous sucking at once. You can do the same with lip stroking to get him to purse his lips and get him to suck. He is perfectly capable of sucking when he isn't a bit hungry. He may get a certain amount of pleasure just from the muscular actions involved in sucking. He practices sucking before he is born, perhaps with his finger or thumb, but sucking is not fully developed until after he is born. By twenty-four to forty-eight hours the sucking reflex is usually mature enough. Your baby may not suck well immediately after he is born—maybe not for two or three days. Later he may get interested. Until he gets well coordinated in sucking and swallowing he may choke, gag, or dribble while he eats.

In sucking there are two distinct rhythms. The nonnutritive or nonfeeding way is broken into alternating bursts of sucking and rest with a frequency of two sucks per second. It can occur at any time except during deep sleep or extreme excitement. When he is feeding, the pattern depends on the flow of food. It is organized as a continuous sequence of sucks with one suck per second. In your newborn, sucking involves no looking. If his eye catches something, his sucking stops. His sucking at this time is a mass movement of his mouth parts. It isn't differentiated yet. It is combined with the swallowing reflex.

SWALLOWING REFLEX. Your baby can swallow, but he does it by reflex action. It lacks the voluntary cheek or mouth phase of mature swallowing. His swallowing is a separate reflex from the sucking reflex, but it is closely associated with it. If you stroke his lips, you will cause a set of muscles in his throat to contract in consequence. This produces sucking, then swallowing. His mature suck-swallow pattern will be a burst of thirty sucks with a two-suck-per-second speed, then a rest before a sucking sequence again. His swallows come frequently during his sucking bursts.

GRASP REFLEX

Usually he holds his hands closed. If you touch the palm of his hand his fingers will grasp your fingers and hold on firmly. (See plate 13.) This is the grasp reflex. It may surprise you how much strength there is in his grasp. Now, with his fingers on one side and his thumb on the other side of your finger, if you pull your finger gently upward you get his traction response. You feel the reaction spread to his upper arm. This grasp can be strong enough so that you can lift him right off the table to let him hang suspended by your grasped finger.

If you touch the back of his hand you get the opposite reflex as his hand opens. It is usually gone between the second and third month. True voluntary grasping comes later.

PLANTAR RESPONSE

If you press the bottom of his foot at the base of his toes you will provoke his plantar response reflex. His foot acts like a hand. His toes turn down to grasp when you stimulate the sole of his foot. This is like the grasp reflex of his hand, but doesn't disappear until the end of his first year.

If you stroke the outside of his foot toward his toes, his toes spread out and his big toe points up in the air. This is the Babinski reflex.

WALKING REFLEX

If you hold your baby in a standing position on a hard surface and move him forward, he does alternate bending and pushing with his legs to imitate walking. (See plate 14A.)

This kind of stepping disappears after a month. You can see it after this time if you push him up under his chin as he is held upright. If you press the soles of his feet on the table, his legs and body straighten.

His *placing reaction* occurs when you bring the front of his lower leg or forearm against the edge of a table. He will lift his leg to step up on the table or bring his arm up to put his hand on the table. This disappears after a month also.

OTHER REFLEXES

There are other reflexes but these are harder to demonstrate in a newborn. His seeing and hearing reflexes are discussed below under "Senses."

SENSES

The newborn baby receives countless messages through his sense organs and his skin, which are sent on to his brain for sorting, labeling, associating, remembering, and responding. The equipment is all there, but experience and memory are lacking. The messages he gets from his sense organs don't mean much to him at first. He has to get some experience to learn what they mean. He has to develop his ability to take in messages from his sense organs and interpret, relay, and associate them with his past experiences or memories. And he has to learn how to act with discrimination and purpose after absorbing this information. But he will learn rapidly from the messages he is sent. He grows through his sense organs—his sensations.

SIGHT

In his first days of life the newborn keeps his eyes shut more often than open. He may open first one eye and then the other, or keep one closed. If you hold him up straight and pivot around with him, he will open his eyes. He isn't accustomed to light yet. It makes him blink and frown and screw up his face.

The whites of his eyes have a bluish tint because they are still quite thin coverings. He is farsighted, and his pupils are contracted. The irises of the eyes are at first a grayish-blue in light-skinned babies and grayish-brown or brown in dark-skinned babies. Pigment is gradually deposited to produce a final eye color at about six to twelve months.

His tear glands don't function this early. But by one month eighty percent of babies will produce tears.

The tear ducts leading from the inner corners of his eyes down into his nose are tiny and easily plugged. This causes any tears or other discharge to collect. Massage the ducts if this continues.

If you see a red spot on the white area of the eye, don't let it alarm you. It is one of the effects of his trip down your birth canal. It may look like a bright red crescent on one side of his iris or may extend entirely around it. The blood absorbs in seven to ten days with no aftereffects.

His eyelids may be quite puffy for a few days and show some discharge, the result of drops put in his eyes at birth to prevent infection. These drops are silver nitrate, or one of the potent antibiotic solutions. State laws require that these be given to all newborns to prevent gonorrheal infection. Warm-water irrigation is all that you should do if this condition continues, unless your doctor directs otherwise.

His upper eyelids often show extra skin and an extra skin fold—the epicanthal fold—running down parallel to his nose to cover the inner corner of his eye. With his wide nose bridge, this wide stretch of skin creates the illusion that his eyes are turned inward. This is most noticeable when he looks off to one side, especially in photographs. As his face grows this disappears.

All parts of his eyes are fully developed at birth except the center of his retina, the light-sensitive ending of his optic nerve. This is the macula, or central spot, which provides acute central vision. This specialized area of his retina begins to separate out during his first month to be organized at four months with full growth by eight months of age. It isn't entirely perfected in use until he is five or six years of age. At birth he has fully developed peripheral vision around this area. This doesn't get much better as he grows older. So his newborn eyes are far advanced in the assembling of parts, but they don't function yet to give him complete vision.

He can tell the difference between light and dark. He has the ability to fix on an image and follow it with both eyes momentarily. This shows he has eye movement with both eyes working together even this early. He adjusts his eye movements to bring an object into his range of vision. He is born with the ability to perceive the form or shape of objects. His color vision has not quite arrived. He develops this gradually in his next few months. By six weeks he will be responding to bright colors. Clearness of vision comes when his macula goes into action. Before this you see temporary eye wandering. With increasing control of his eye muscles and improving central sight, he gains consistent coordination of his eye movements, usually by four months on. From a newborn you can expect random movements, jerky, uneven following movements, off and on turning, or jerking of one or both eyes. Like the quivery chin or the jumpy arm or leg these are signs of the immaturity of the nervous system.

BLINK REFLEXES. A sudden noise, a bright light, a painful touch, can cause blinking or eyelid tensing, as can tapping the bridge of his nose, stroking his eyelashes, or stroking over his eye on his forehead. Protective blinking doesn't come for seven to eight weeks. True blinking doesn't appear until about six months.

HEARING

At birth your baby's hearing equipment is more complete than his sight. When he is born his outer ear canal, his middle ear, and the Eustachian tube leading to the back of his throat are filled with fluid in the spaces where there should be air. As soon as these are clear and air-filled his hearing is acute. An indication that he can hear loud noises is that he may react with a startle reflex, blink, jump, cry, stop what he is doing, or turn his eyes or his head. But this is not an infallible test. He may not seem to be aware of a piano or radio playing in another room. He can certainly hear clearly his own hi-fidelity crying. The vibrations of his crying in his voice box down in his throat are conducted readily through his body as well as to you on the outside.

Hearing and equilibrium centers are both located in the ear structures. They are closely associated. When either center is stimulated enough, a fear or startle reaction is the response. You may wonder how much noise control you should have in your home. By and large your family may continue the amount and type of noise that they usually make. Your baby won't be bothered. He accepts it as background noise. Later he will imitate these same noises. What he hears becomes natural to him.

Your baby's outer ear may be found curled over on itself. His position in the uterus is the usual cause of this. This curling or folding gradually smooths out with the normal growth of his ear.

TASTE

Of your baby's five senses his taste perception is the best developed at birth. The delicate papillae of his tongue are highly sensitive. He may react to sweet, sour, salt, and bitter. It is possible that taste can guide him to proper foods later if this sense isn't interfered with.

SMELL

Taste is so closely associated with the ability to smell that it is difficult to know which sense is operating. His sensitivity to smell seems quite acute. It may be that when he begins to identify you in a few months he may do it primarily by the way you smell. Just as soon as he can he will get things to his mouth. His first best guide to discovery is the taste-smell-touch combination.

TOUCH

The first sensations he receives probably have to do with his sense of touch. The process of being born involved a whole group of pressures, proddings, pains, and an abrupt drop in the temperature of his surroundings. He cries from pain, exposure, or discomfort. Contrary to an adult, it is not his fingertips but his skin surface that is sensitive. When he begins to explore the world about him, he will begin by feeling things with the palms of his hands, not with his fingertips.

Sensation such as pain is received in different ways by your baby. Although his skin can feel pain, he will not give a quick response. If he is stuck with a pin, there may be a lag of some seconds before he cries. On the other hand, sensation in his intestinal tract is particularly acute. As a result, he reacts to even the smallest discomfort in his abdomen quickly and even violently. This will gradually change in three or four months. Then the reverse will be true. But internal sensations will be important in his months and years ahead in training and control. Sensation coming from his bones and muscles are part of his learning how to stand and walk upright.

HOSPITAL STAY

NURSERY DAYS

Your baby sleeps through this first period following his birth. He may actually go on sleeping pretty continuously into his second day if he feels tired enough. On the other hand, you may find you have the other kind of fellow, who wakes after his birth binge and insists on something to eat in spite of his headache. He is given glucose water, usually between six and twelve hours of age.

When he holds his temperature level, has a good skin color, breathes without any problem, and begins to show he has joined the human race by his noise level, he is given his first bath.

Sooner or later, he gets around to that important subject —food! He sounds off to let someone know he wants to fill the empty space in his middle. If you are to breast-feed him, he will have to put up with the glucose water in the nursery, but will be getting colostrum from your breasts before the milk comes in; if on a bottle, he will be fed formula. He may not need much to start with, but he does want even that small amount. When he gets it, he settles back down for more sleep.

But even this very new baby does more than just sleep and demonstrate reflex activity. You will see him show his first recognition of pleasure in these first few days when someone pats him, cuddles him, and talks to him. When he is hungry and you feed him, he stops crying. Later he will show his pleasure by spreading out his toes or opening and closing his hands and making contented sounds. You will begin to see his signs of displeasure, too, and learn more about the kind of baby he is.

Your baby takes his first shot before he takes his first meal. This is an injection of Vitamin K to prevent a bleeding tendency called hemorrhagic disease of the newborn. Also, a drop of blood must be taken from your baby's heel to rule out the presence of a rare metabolic disease called phenylketonuria (the PKU test).

Liquid vitamins are started about the third day. Pediatricians usually prescribe a multiple vitamin drop, which contains vitamins A, C, D, and some of the B vitamins. You will be given a prescription for this. Fluoride is added if it is not in the water supply.

CIRCUMCISION

If your baby is a boy, the question of circumcision will come up. This is something you and your husband will have to decide. Most families will wish to have this done, whether for reasons of hygiene, cosmetic appearance, or religious teachings. It is a very common procedure in the United States, and is practiced by about one sixth of the world's population. It is probably the oldest surgical procedure known.

Circumcision is the removal of the collar of skin—the foreskin or prepuce—that covers the end of the penis. The foreskin is still adherent to the head of the penis at birth. This gradually separates, so that by three years 90 percent of boys have a foreskin that retracts easily. Retraction of the foreskin is necessary for the removal of excess smegma—the cheesy substance secreted for protective lubrication under the foreskin. Gradual easy retraction can be carried out over the early months and years so that the foreskin is adequately stretched. But in the circumcised child the cleansing process is more easily taken care of. You won't know by his actions that your young man has had his first surgical procedure. Circumcision is momentarily painful but there is no particular afterpain for your baby.

GETTING ACQUAINTED WITH YOUR BABY. After the period of recovery for you and the baby, he will be brought to you. You will try to feed him, first with glucose water and later with breast or formula. His first feeding period usually occurs in the first twelve hours after birth. You will undoubtedly feel very strange as you first begin to handle your baby, and you may find the first feedings of glucose water a little trying. He often refuses any part of it. When he does take some, he spits it out. This is the usual process, so don't be concerned! It will give you some experience in handling your baby when he is trying to spit up. Just sit him upright —wipe his face—talk to him—put him back and try again. Your baby's sleepy period may persist for several days. Don't feel that you are not doing a good job if your baby follows this pattern.

FIRST DAY. Now that your day of delivery is past, you find that you feel proud and wonderful, even if you are still a bit groggy. You may have some uncomfortable spots in your body, but you will find that surprisingly enough you can manage to get about quite well. In most instances the sooner a mother gets out of bed and resumes normal activity the better she feels. If you are an exception, your obstetrician will tell you.

Most mothers leave the hospital on the third to the fifth day after delivery, although some obstetricians allow a mother to leave as early as the second day. The average baby requires about three days to reach a satisfactory balance in his adjustment to outside living. The nursing baby may not handle his nursing adequately, or the breast produce sufficiently, until the fourth or fifth day. As a result your departure day will be determined by your obstetrician, and your pediatrician, with several factors in mind.

Yesterday your pediatrician came in as soon as he saw your baby to tell you that he was fine. Today he will be around again to report on his progress. Your baby's nurses will also stop by to check with you. Your obstetrician is in and out, too.

SECOND DAY. By this time you will have been back and forth to the nursery, looking at and comparing this new baby of yours. If your baby is to be breast-fed, he will receive glucose water freely after and between your nursings if he will take it. If he is formula-fed, he will be given formula as he announces his need. You will be the one to give many of his daytime formula feedings. The formula feedings in the middle of the night you will skip. On breast, your baby will not be brought out in the middle of the night until your milk comes in. Your rest is more important in the first few days. You may worry if your baby regurgitates or spits up. This is not uncommon at first, possibly because his stomach just isn't ready yet to accept much. It doesn't mean you are doing anything wrong in your feeding or handling of him.

Either today or tomorrow you will find your breasts engorged. This occurs before your milk flow really starts. After this becomes established, your breasts will be less hard. Your baby will have less trouble getting hold of the nipple. At feeding times, gently stroke or press the nipple to stand out, bringing down a little liquid on the end of it so that your baby can get an adequate grip. Expect him to be hungry at every other feeding only.

I hope that you don't start pressuring to go home at this point. You may feel wonderful today, but tomorrow you may have the "weeps" or "blues." Your baby needs at least another day of watchful care, even if he is the biggest, huskiest thing you ever saw. If you are breast-feeding, even another two days is not too much.

THIRD DAY. You may find that by today you feel almost ready to assume your normal routine, except that you have a little hitch in your walk from the stitches. If you are an old hand at breast-feeding and your milk is well started, you may be ready to go home. If not, give yourself at least another day to practice. Also, don't underestimate the physical and emotional adjustments you are undergoing. You may not be ready yet to assume full maternal responsibility. As for your baby, it takes him seventy-two hours or even longer to stabilize himself. He is a sitting duck for any infection that comes along, whether from family or visitors.

Your baby has now become more wakeful. He will usually take every other feeding quite well. He may be quite vigorous about his wants.

This is the day that you will attend the class for going-home mothers. You will be shown methods of handling, bathing, diapering, and feeding. You may learn something new even if you are not a first-time mother.

Rooming-in. Rooming-in is the name given to a plan of care in which your new baby is kept in your room with you instead of in the nursery. In some rooming-in systems, the baby stays with you twenty-four hours a day. In the more moderate rooming-in setup, the baby spends nights in the nursery. If you start rooming-in during the first twenty-four hours after delivery, you should have a special nurse in attendance. It is important for you to get your rest at night. You don't want to go home tired out before you even get there. You will be on "night duty" soon enough.

Rooming-in is not a new idea, but one adapted from old-fashioned home care. It gives you a chance to get acquainted with your new baby by handling, feeding, and changing him. It helps you to get to know him and to discover the meanings of his strange activities and noises. Supervision on the part of the nursery staff will help you learn your chores and will answer your questions. Rooming-in also gives your husband a chance to see and handle his new heir.

Rooming-in is a matter of choice. If a mother welcomes it, then she should by all means enjoy it. The nursery method would be wrong for her. But for anyone to take the attitude that rooming-in is in itself better, because in some mystical way it is more natural, is romantic nonsense.

As a mother who does not room-in, you can rest as much as you want to. Your only obligations are to feed your baby and tend to your own grooming and eating. On the surface this may sound selfish. In reality it probably is not. Following the difficulty of labor, many a mother needs a psychological rest as well as a physical one. You may need some time to restore your own sense of identity and to ease into your new arrangement.

Physically your body is undergoing drastic changes. Hormones are flooding your system, preparing your breasts for nursing, contracting your uterus, and generally getting your body ready for its brand-new role. This can give you a tremendous sensation of well-being. It also can be quite fatiguing. When you feel tired, you need uninterrupted sleep. Rooming-in denies you this.

Another factor is your emotions. As a new mother you are quite emotional. The cry of your new baby may produce these feelings in a headlong rush. You can feel overwhelmed by the whole affair. You need a chance to adjust to these new emotions, to learn to hear your newborn baby cry and accept it with a little smile, to learn that it is his way of talking and not directed at you.

What about the baby's feeling in all this? What does he lose in the nursery method by not rooming-in? I'm not sure he loses anything. Mothers might like to think that their babies gain a sense of intimacy and closeness to them. Actually a baby couldn't care less. A newborn has no sense of who he is or who his mother is. The important thing to him is when and how he gets fed and cuddled, not who does it.

There are some limitations to the rooming-in system. You must be up and about and able to take care of yourself. Rooming-in is done in a private or two-bed semiprivate room. Rooming-in in larger wards can be too disturbing for the other mothers. Visitors are strictly limited to husband and grandparents, no more than three people at a time. This is done to lessen the chance of contact with infection. No flowers are allowed in a room where a child is rooming-in. No smoking is allowed, either. If grandparents or husband have an infection they should stay away from the baby. The baby cannot be taken out of the room or left unattended at any time.

FATHER AND THE NEWBORN

A word about father's reactions to his new baby during your hospital stay. The father is rare who can fall deeply in love with a newborn baby seen only for a minute through a pane of glass. When you are chatting ecstatically about your "wonder child," you may notice your husband looking bored and obviously wanting to talk about something else. Don't be hurt! Wait until you have the two of them home together. The baby isn't your exclusive property. His heart and mind belong to his dad, too. It is your job to build up a fine companionship between them. To do this you must let them be together from the first. Show your husband how to hold the baby so his head is supported. If he forgets once or twice the baby's head won't snap off, so don't snap his head off either! Try listening to his fatherly suggestions, and follow all of them you can. Help him understand the reasons for doing things a different way. A cooperative method of family life is the most beneficial to all concerned, particularly for Junior. It is well to start this whole process early.

THE PROBLEM BABY

If your baby weighs five and a half pounds or less, he is called a premature baby or low birth-weight baby. If he arrives ahead of your estimated date of confinement, he is premature. If he is not too early but he is small, he is a low birth-weight baby. Either way he requires more careful handling and watching during his early days than the average baby.

If your baby arrives two weeks or more after his normal 266 days of internal living, he is postmature. The longer he waits, the more he has to live on his own tissue. His placenta ages and slows down its normal nourishing activity so that he begins a process of starvation. The baby who has been through this kind of undernourishment will have to be treated carefully for a time until his internal balance returns and he can benefit from the food he takes.

His incompleteness is the cause of the premature baby's problems. If he can be helped through his maturing period in the outside world, then he catches up and later maintains a quite adequate and normal pattern of growth.

Your pre-term baby is developmentally behind to the extent that he is premature. If he is two months early, he will act like a three-month-old baby at five months, but he will follow a normal development pattern at this behind-schedule rate. At birth the premature baby in no way corresponds to a full-term baby. The low birth-weight baby and the postmature baby look and act like full-term babies but have more adjustment problems.

How does the premature baby look? (See plate 15.) His head is the first feature you notice. It looks much too big for his body. He isn't as long as a full-term baby, although he may appear longer because he is slender. His body isn't rounded, due to lack of fat. You can see the vein pattern in his thin, delicate skin. He shows more lanugo hair at birth than does the full-term baby. His eyes seem large. He has no eyebrows. For a time his ears lie pressed close to his head. He has very short, soft fingernails and toenails. The yellow tinge to the skin caused by newborn jaundice may be deeper in color and last longer in the premature.

The bigger the premature baby is, the more he will look like a full-term baby, and the faster he will catch up.

How does the pre-term baby act? He shows rapid, uncontrolled movements of his arms and legs. He twists and turns his body. The full-term baby's movements are better coordinated.

The premature baby is a much more "floppy" infant than the full-term baby, due to his poor muscle tone. (See plate 16.) Harmony between his muscles and his nervous system just hasn't come far enough yet.

Reflexes in the premature baby are less well developed than in the full-term baby.

The premature baby is put in a special intensive-care or premature nursery, which contains equipment designed for this type of baby. Several days in the incubator after a few hours in protective oxygen, and they are ready for a regular bassinet in the regular nursery group.

The problem premature, however, needs special care in several areas. He reacts very easily to changes in temperature about him. He has no insulating layer of fat. He can't warm himself up by shivering (not enough muscle). His built-in temperature regulator doesn't function well for a time. His incubator keeps the air around him at an adequate temperature level so he doesn't chill or overheat.

His immaturity is shown by the way he breathes. His nerve centers are not too well developed. His breathing can be quite irregular. Besides keeping him on his abdomen with his head down (to drain out secretions), some special equipment may be used to aid him in his breathing efforts.

The premature baby needs as much rest as he can get. He tires very quickly, and sleeps most of the time. It is really like a half doze or a half-conscious condition. He seldom cries because crying is hard work for him. No effort is made to bathe him until he has settled down in some of his important functions.

The pre-term baby will lose more weight after birth than the full-term baby, and will regain it more slowly. Glucose water is all that is given at first. Since he can't be depended on to demand food, he will be urged frequently at first to take small amounts. He will determine the amounts he will take himself. No set amount is scheduled. If a baby is too small or weak to suck a small, soft nipple, then cup, pitcher, or a small gavage feeding will be used. In gavage feeding, a small plastic tube is inserted through the baby's nose into his stomach. It can be kept in place several days or re-inserted at the time of each feeding. You may be concerned when you see this unfamiliar object in your baby's nose, but the premature baby scarcely seems to be aware of its presence.

The pre-term baby has not developed his sucking or swallowing reflexes. This takes time. Sometimes a fairly strong small baby sucks poorly, but will cup-feed quite well. He is able to swallow easily, but doesn't make adequate motions for sucking.

After the initial use of glucose water, a very dilute formula is started and gradually strengthened as the premature's needs change. As you can see, breast-feeding is not possible at first. You can pump your breasts to keep your milk supply going and after you leave send the milk to the nursery for him.

At this point let me talk a little about your feelings as the mother of a baby born prematurely. In the hospital you will have little chance to do much for your baby. It is frustrating to want to help but find that you cannot. You really see very little of your baby, even if you do go down to gaze through the nursery window. This waiting will be difficult for both you and your husband. You will agonize until some news is announced. It will be wonderful when he gains half an ounce.

You will go home at the normal time, leaving your premature baby in the nursery. You can check on his day-to-day progress by calling your pediatrician's office or visiting the hospital. The nursery staff will be able to give you only limited information. Your pediatrician is ready to explain any detail to you. Eventually there will be a day when your baby can be shifted to the regular nursery. He is on his own now and will be treated just like any normal full-term baby. At last you will have a chance to hold and cuddle and feed him. Soon you may take him home.

Your first few days at home may be rather confused and frantic but try to relax and enjoy him in spite of your earlier concern. He takes more time to do with and for than the full-term baby. He eats more slowly and tires more quickly. This means more frequent feedings and a longer feeding time. He fills more diapers. He will be making up for lost time. You can expect him to gain more rapidly than the usual baby for a time.

Visitors coming into the house can cause infection problems for your premature during these early weeks. *Keep people away from him.*

His prematurity hasn't slowed down your baby's great urge to grow and develop. His push to catch up is tremendous. He will follow his own individual pattern, but most prematures catch up by a year or so. He will sit, stand, and walk at a little older age. By the time he is two years old you probably won't be too aware of any differences.

Before then, don't try to compare him with the neighbor's child who is full-term.

Your greatest concern, made greater by all the scare stories you hear and read, probably centers about his future mental progress. Most prematures weighing three pounds or more at birth develop quite normally, as do many who weigh less. Your pediatrician will discuss his physical and mental development with you at his regular checkups.

From the emotional standpoint, your youngster's progress will depend in large part on you. If you are able to allow him freedom and responsibility as he grows, he will mature emotionally in healthy fashion. Overprotecting and overcontrolling will make it difficult for him to grow up. His self-reliance comes and is learned by exploring and by meeting frustrations. Like any other child, he needs affection and acceptance as well as your firm support and guidance.

Every minute there are eight new babies born in the United States. One out of twelve is born ahead of time. Perhaps it may reassure you to know that Sir Isaac Newton, Charles Darwin, Julius Caesar, Rosseau, Voltaire, Victor Hugo, and Sir Winston Churchill were all premature babies.

5.

Breast-Feeding
and Bottle-Feeding

FEEDING YOUR BABY

Whether he is on breast or bottle, your baby's first pleasure in life is eating and getting full—his first unhappiness is being hungry. What a picture he presents when his stomach tells him its needs—a red face with a wide-open mouth and a rigid body straining with anger and discomfort. All of which changes after a few moments of eating as, blissfully, he begins to settle down.

Your baby wants what he wants instantly. In the early weeks you should feed him when he is hungry and give him as much as he can take—and then feed him again when he lets you know he is ready. If this happens too often, he is telling you that he isn't getting enough to eat at each feeding. If he cries very soon after a feeding, he needs a great deal more than he is getting. Take his word for it. He is hungry. There is no reason to let him cry it out. Feed him until you're certain he isn't hungry any longer. In these early weeks always assume first that he is hungry when he cries. Usually he is not sick. As he gets older you have to distinguish between social crying and hunger crying. But in these early days he cries most often because he is hungry.

His eating can be a very active process. He may act almost savage in attacking his food. He works so hard that he breaks out in a sweat. When he is full he falls deeply asleep, perhaps not without some complaining first. He may even finish eating after he has fallen asleep!

In these first weeks you satisfy both his physical hunger and his emotional hunger, his need for food and love, in his feeding experience. Feeding is his first taste of life, his earliest contact with the world. His early ideas of life are set up by his feeding experiences. If they go well, the world appears as a satisfying place to him. You appear when he is hungry and make him happy by feeding and holding him. He needs you to cuddle him gently, talk to him, hum to him, stroke his skin. These needs are no less essential than an adequate food supply.

It isn't long before he starts to reach out into the world. He smiles at you and pays attention to his surroundings. His feeding time becomes a social experience between the two of you. This relationship can involve satisfaction or frustration, security or insecurity, love or hate. His early idea of people starts with the person who feeds and cares for him. You are forming the first basis for all his future relationships. He is learning to adjust his own actions to someone else's behavior—you are teaching him to trust you, to wait a little for food, to adapt himself to changes in routine. Thus as a parent you contribute a great deal to his developing personality. This should make you feel important and valuable—not frightened and worried.

Your ability to feed your baby is not automatic. You won't be an expert at once. Both you and baby will have to do some trial-and-error practicing, whether you bottle-feed, breast-feed, or spoon-feed.

These early weeks can be a time of great emotional tension and physical fatigue. Recognize that it may be hard for you to give much of yourself to your baby at first. If you are anxious about his feedings or involved in a domestic struggle, your tenseness may be sensed by your baby. He hears it in your voice, the feel of your body as you hold him, the suddenness and jerkiness of your movements. You can have a bad time starting out if you and your baby are both high-strung types who catch fire from each other. Your confidence in your ability to take care of him can be badly shaken. But you can gradually come to a happier, more relaxed way of feeding and handling him as you practice.

BREAST VERSUS BOTTLE

There is no scientific support for the idea that breast-feeding is the best method for every mother and every baby. The accumulated evidence doesn't show that breast-feeding your baby gives him a better medical or psychological background for growth and development, nor has the theory that emotional instability results from bottle-feeding been confirmed in any way. The fact is that it doesn't matter which method is used, so long as the proper attitude toward your baby is present during the feeding. Over the years I have seen babies fed by breast, bottle, spoon, and cup from the early weeks on. Their physical health and psychological growth depend not on the technique of feeding but on the relationship and communication between mother and child. A good mother is someone who takes care of her baby's needs, whether she breast-feeds or bottle-feeds. The most important thing about feeding, whether by breast or bottle, is that you feed your baby lovingly. He needs to be cuddled and talked to. Loving handling is what is important, not the type of milk container.

Try to keep this matter of feeding methods in perspective. It is not a life-and-death issue. A diet of milk alone, whether from breast or bottle, is in any case satisfactory only for a short while. And breast-feeding, while it can be rewarding for both mother and child, is not an insurance policy that comes to you neatly designed to avoid all the emotional ills of childhood.

Your choice as to feeding method should be based on what you see as best for you and your baby—not on what someone else tells you. The best way for you both is the method that fits in with your feelings and your way of doing things, coupled with your awareness of your baby's personality and the best approach for him.

Which method fits in with your ideas of motherhood, with your work and social patterns? Are you being pressured into choosing one way over the other? Are you comparing yourself with other women you know? Would you feel more confident and natural feeding by one method rather than the other? Do you feel you would be closer to your baby one way than the other? Consider the answers to these questions in making your choice. And once you have made it, stick to it—don't try to shift back and forth between the two.

BREAST-FEEDING

Try to make your decision about breast-feeding in the last months of your pregnancy—the earlier the better. The time to decide is not as you come out of the delivery room. An early decision gives you time to develop a positive approach toward nursing, which can later aid in your ability to produce milk.

HUMAN MILK

Milk from a healthy mother whose diet is nutritionally adequate contains sufficient amounts of most of the nutritional factors necessary for her infant in the early weeks of his life. The exceptions may be iron, vitamins D, C, and B_1. The full-term baby should have put aside adequate iron stores to compensate for this. Missing vitamins are supplied by the vitamin drops you give your baby. Human milk is an excellent balance of the needed ingredients in its curds and whey for a full-term normal baby, with 20 to 22 calories per ounce. It is easily and quite completely digested. In appearance it is bluish-white and watery. It looks like watered-down cow's milk.

Basically there are few important variations in the quality of human milk between individuals. There will be some differences in amounts depending on the size and structure of your breasts, your emotional makeup, the amount of rest and exercise you get, the extent to which your breasts are emptied, your diet, the time of day you nurse, and the duration of milk production.

Colostrum comes first to accommodate your baby's first needs. This is high in protein. Somewhere between the second and sixth day after delivery, it is replaced by milk that is also fairly high in protein. As the milk supply comes, milk with less protein and more carbohydrate is produced. The last part of a nursing contains more calories. Colostrum and your first milk are released slowly. When the baby begins to swallow and suck better, he gets the milk faster. The shorter his sucking time, the more often he will have to eat. As he gets stronger and sucks longer, he gets more milk and goes longer between feedings. Also your milk supply increases. But you must not be impatient. Even with a good baby who nurses well on filling breasts, there is a lag of seven to ten days before the normal nursing letdown reflex occurs. The smaller amounts of milk in these first days are adequate for him.

ABILITY TO BREAST-FEED

Can you breast-feed your baby? All breast-feeding requires is a relaxed, healthy mother who really wants to breast-feed, a hungry baby, and a bit of practice to learn how. The most successful breast-feeder is nearly always an emotionally calm, emotionally secure individual who has a normal desire to enjoy to the fullest degree the achievement of motherhood by nursing her infant. The success of breast-feeding depends on the basic psychosomatic breast-feeding mechanisms—the let-down and milk-ejection reflexes. A mother's tension and worry can interfere with these reflexes, and the result will be an inadequate milk flow, a hungry baby, and an anxious mother whose concern further depresses her milk-producing apparatus.

You need a happy, unworried state of mind. This doesn't mean you won't have concern and that you won't be shaky during your first attempts to learn. But it does mean that you won't feel needless worry about things that are really quite usual. Remember that the minor difficulties at the beginning are temporary. Don't enlarge them. It may be difficult for you not to feel rejected and inadequate if your baby refuses your breast, cries, and acts hungry. Don't let him hurt your feelings. He does not know any better. And he does need help in learning how to eat at the breast.

In most instances your supply of breast milk becomes adequate after you leave the hospital. If it has not been established beforehand no serious problem arises, nor is a drastic remedy needed. Give yourself a chance. Most mothers come too quickly to the conclusion that their breast milk is inadequate.

There really is nothing worse for adequate milk production than worrying and thinking about your nursing constantly. If you find this happening, indulge yourself and get away from it all. Use a baby-sitter while you shop, or visit the girls, or step out with your husband. Probably your baby will be the better for it too. You should get away from your baby and house completely at least once a week, anyway.

You need to recognize that motherhood is a growth process for you. I've tried to say this before. You become a mother in a physical sense with the birth of your baby, but emotional or psychological motherhood takes more time. Mothering has to be learned step by step as you leave your pregnancy behind and move into your relationship with your baby. Your love as a mother doesn't strike you like a bolt from the blue when you first see your new child. It is only as you take care of him over and over again that you learn to love him deeply. You can't stay unresponsive to any young fellow who depends on you so completely for food and care. This provides a stepping-stone into genuine mothering. In the first weeks of our getting-acquainted process you are learning how to give. If you are successful in your growth into motherhood, you discover that your attitude toward breast-feeding helps your breast-feeding performance. You relax with your baby, cuddle and feed him comfortably. You enjoy his closeness and your ability to answer his needs.

Your husband can be a big help to you during your early adjustment period when your baby is starting to nurse. His calm, reassuring cooperation can influence your ability to produce milk.

NURSING DIET

The production and quality of your milk are influenced by the number and kinds of calories eaten, by alcohol, smoking, and drugs. Your diet directly affects the chemical composition of your milk, and your food protein directly influences your milk protein. The same is true of fat.

Unlike the period of your pregnancy, when you are nursing you are really eating for two. You need the extra calories that it takes to make milk plus what the milk contains. Your milk production comes first when food is portioned out. You must supply strategic storage materials similar to those substances going out in the breast milk. You increase your diet by 60 calories a day per pound of baby weight the first month, 50 calories per pound in the second and third months. This is about a 20 percent to 25 percent increase over your pregnancy diet and 40 percent to 50 percent increase over your regular diet.

Look back at the diet recommended in the section on *Pregnancy*, and add extra proteins like lean meat, milk solids, eggs, and cheese. Include an extra serving of whole-grain cereals or enriched cereals each day, as well as extra servings of raw or fresh vegetables and fruits. Additional milk solids for additional protein can be gained by adding dry powdered skim milk to soups, vegetables, cereals, puddings, and cheese dishes. Try to drink two, even three, quarts of fluid a day. Don't count milk as a fluid. Remember that drinking milk doesn't produce milk. You can substitute milk solids for liquid milk if you don't want to drink the quart or more a day usually recommended. A vitamin supplement is needed to insure adequate amounts of vitamins in your breast milk.

Certain foods like garlic and onion may make some difference in the odor and taste of your milk. Your baby isn't bothered by this after he gets accustomed to it. If a food seems to upset your baby, leave it alone for a time or use it in moderation. Large amounts of fats in your diet, such as chocolate, may cut down on your milk supply.

You may use small amounts of alcoholic beverages and smoke moderately if a drink and a cigarette truly contribute to your peace of mind or sense of well-being. Heavy smoking or drinking does your breast supply no good.

Drugs are excreted in your milk, but most types won't bother the baby unless the doses you are taking are quite large. The laxatives you take may bother your baby. Control constipation by diet, with raw fruits and vegetables, whole-wheat bread, bran cereal, and adequate amounts of water.

You may have to pay attention to weight control during your nursing period. Take a good look and use some common sense. If you are ten pounds overweight, you should aim at losing a pound a week. Use your basic protein foods but decrease the starches and fats. No crash diets. Your baby and the whole family suffer if you are tired out from skipping breakfast or eating too little.

BREAST CARE

DAILY ROUTINE. Thorough daily washing of the breasts and nipples with soap and water should be done at bath time. Don't use lotions on your nipples unless your doctor tells you to. If he has recommended a nonmedicated lubricating material, be sure to remove it before nursing. You don't need to sterilize the nipples with alcohol or soap at nursing time. Drying agents irritate them and interfere with the normal healing process between nursings. Just use normal cleanliness. When you are to touch your nipples at nursing time, wash your hands well with soap and water. Before and after each nursing, wash your nipples and the surrounding breast area with clear water or a solution of one teaspoon of salt to one pint of water. Use a clean washcloth or sterile cotton for this. Dry thoroughly. Exposing your nipples to the air for a time after nursing can be helpful. It is important to keep the nipples dry. Most nursing brassieres have soft removable pads that absorb leaking milk. You can also cover the nipples with pads made of sterile gauze, tissues, a square piece of a sanitary napkin, or clean cotton cloth. There should be enough space inside your nursing brassiere so that the pads fit over the nipples without pressure. The free circulation of air is important in helping to keep the nipples dry. Change the pads as often as necessary, since milk may leak from the breasts between feeding. Don't use plastic cups or pads made of a rough material inside your brassiere.

Your nursing brassiere must give good support to your breasts. It should be worn at all times. Have enough brassieres so that you can change at least once daily. Don't wear soiled or stained ones.

HAND-EMPTYING. The importance of manual expression of milk from the breasts has been mentioned. (Look back to "The Mother" in the section on *Pregnancy* for the proper technique.) Use hand-emptying when your nipples are sore, your breasts engorged or not emptied, or when you need milk for some reason. If it is necessary for you to discontinue breast-feeding temporarily, continue to hand-empty your breasts so that they will be ready to be used again.

You may get only a few drops at first, but after a few strokes, a squirting stream should be obtained. If this doesn't happen, you aren't grasping far enough back on the breasts to let the milk down into the nipple area. Don't touch the nipple. Don't let the fingers slip forward on the breast. The thumb and forefinger should stay on the same piece of skin and not slide over it.

You can collect this milk in a sterile container for use later in cereal or for a substitute feeding within the next 24 hours if it is kept refrigerated. Milk enough out so that the spray actually decreases to drops. You will always be able to get some milk, even from an apparently empty breast. Avoid damaging the skin by milking too hard or squeezing your breast improperly. This milking should not be painful even if you have a sore, cracked nipple. If it hurts, you're doing something wrong.

If your baby does not take all your milk, your supply will stay adequate when hand-emptying is done regularly and completely after each feeding. Don't spend more than five minutes on each breast—another three if they still seem full.

BREAST PUMPS. Sometimes in the first few days a breast pump—either hand, water-suction, or electric—will be helpful in bringing the nipples out, drawing some of the milk down, or relieving some of the pressure. It is a nuisance to use and cumbersome. Unless you are very engorged or distended, you will do better with hand expression. If you are using a pump, make certain you try to imitate the sucking motions of your baby with alternate suction and relaxation of the pump. Don't just suck the breast down into the pump funnel. You won't get any milk in this fashion.

NIPPLE SHIELDS. Nipple shields are used only to start a feeding and bring out the nipple if the baby is having difficulty getting hold of it. They should not be used for an entire feeding. They don't permit the nipples to be stimulated directly by the baby.

ENGORGEMENT. About your second or third day after delivery, your breasts become full, firm, and tender. They are very sensitive to touch and movement. This engorgement is the normal response to beginning milk production. It marks your shifting of glandular gears as you move into milk production.

Mild engorgement will be relieved when your baby nurses. If it is more severe, you are relieved by nursing but your breasts fill so rapidly that you are uncomfortable again very soon. You may have to hand-empty your breasts between feedings. Make certain your breasts are emptied as completely as possible at each feeding. If not, they can become hot, swollen, and throb with pain when you move about. In the most noticeable engorgement, the breasts seem stretched to bursting. They are so tight and hard your baby can't nurse from them. He can't get his jaw far enough back on the nipple. Hand-empty—or use the breast pump—to reduce some of the swelling. Encourage your baby to take the nipple by stimulating it to stand out. Get some milk on it to attract him.

Your baby may get into trouble if engorgement makes your breasts give milk so fast that he has trouble keeping up with his swallowing. He chokes and gasps, which stops his nursing. Hand-empty your breast to relieve the pressure before you let him start again. This problem fades as he gets bigger and your breasts settle down in their production.

Adequate support for your breasts is especially important now. Tight bindings to support the breasts may be needed for a few days. Warm, moist applications may relieve the aching, throbbing discomfort. You may need analgesics or sedatives to help you with the discomfort until you get it under control. Your doctor may prescribe estrogenic hormone shots to relieve the engorgement.

CAKING. Caking of the breasts means that some segment of the breast tissue has not been properly emptied out, so that the milk has backed up and is staying there. Breast massage to express the milk should take care of this. Check your breast support, and be sure you are in a proper position when nursing. Don't stop nursing. Do nurse and hand-empty more completely.

If the pain is very severe, you can apply heat, using warm, moist compresses, a hot-water bottle, or a heating pad. Try to get extra rest. Sometimes your doctor will prescribe a special medication. This won't hurt your baby.

Caking is different from mastitis, an infection of the breast tissue. You should check with your doctor if you are not certain. If your breast shows a tender spot which is sore, red, and hot, check with your doctor to make sure you are not developing an infected area. If you are, it is essential to take the baby off that breast. Continue to nurse with the normal breast, and hand-empty the infected one.

SORE NIPPLES. Your nipples can get sore from nursing. This is a common complaint for which there are various causes. Long nursing on a breast not yet producing milk may cause some trouble. Some mild discomfort is often present when nursing first starts, with sharp twinges in the nipple. This should lessen. Overfull breasts can cause soreness, as can letting your baby suck at breast too long or letting him use your nipple as a pacifier. Poor nipple care is also a common cause.

As a baby gets older, he can be rough on you. He chews, mouths hard, or clamps down hard on the nipple. Make sure that you are getting enough of the nipple and areola deeply into his mouth and that you are not jerking out the nipple too often.

A sore or cracked nipple can cause a good deal of pain. If it is really bothering you, keep the baby off that breast until the nipple is healed, but hand-empty it at the regular nursing times. You can feed the milk to him from bottle, cup, or spoon if the other breast isn't sufficient for him.

You may need to take an aspirin, a glass of sherry or beer, or even a pain pill.

Expose the sore nipple to the air as much as you can. Use loose clothing to avoid pressure on the nipple. You can use a nipple cover inside the brassiere if there is plenty of air circulation.

Pain, soreness, or redness in the nipple should be reported to your doctor. He may advise using a lanolin or an antibiotic cream. After this you will have to be scrupulous about your nipple care.

Use a lamp with a 30-watt or 50-watt bulb, or a heat lamp, two feet from the breast for ten to fifteen minutes on each side to ease a sore nipple. This makes a comfortably warm dry heat. If you use an ultraviolet lamp, be very cautious. Protect your eyes. Start at thirty seconds and increase the time by thirty seconds a day. Give no more than three minutes' exposure on each nipple. Stay 4 to 6 feet away from the lamp. Don't get too enthusiastic about this type of treatment, or you will end up with sunburned nipples—and no breast-feeding at all.

LEAKING. This can be a sign of successful nursing. It doesn't mean you have too much milk. Normally it will happen just before you start nursing, once your let-down reflex is operating. You may also leak from one breast as you nurse from the other. Use padding in your brassiere to catch the moisture. Leaking can be halted by direct pressure against the nipple for a few minutes. If you are dressed, press against the nipple by folding your arms across your breast.

TYPES OF BABIES

In breast-feeding you must consider your baby's maturity, weight, vigor, appetite, and feeding characteristics. Let me describe some of the different types of babies and their responses to the feeding situation. You can have behavior problems at this age just as you can in later years. Certain patterns seem to be part of the makeup the child is born with. Each baby has his own distinct personality, and it shows in his eating behavior at the breast or on the bottle.

MR. EXECUTIVE. This is the fellow who settles right down to business. He may hurt your nipple as he starts. He doesn't wait for the nipple reflex to take over. He nurses vigorously for ten minutes or so. Then he promptly goes to sleep. He is the active, satisfied baby who establishes sucking reflex and rhythm quickly. As he gets older he shows eagerness for his feeding with rhythmic motions of his hands and feet and with a definite rhythm of sucking. After his feeding is completed, his relaxation is characteristic of the completely satisfied individual. He may show the sensuous enjoyment of feeding that seems to increase a baby's desire to suckle his mother frequently and fully. This stimulates your milk secretion.

MR. ARTIST. This fellow gets so excited about the whole business that he just doesn't seem to know what to do. He makes a pass at the nipple, grabs it, but drops it right away. Since he doesn't get what he wants with all his jumping about, he screams. You will have to ease this guy along, or he will get so worked up about the whole thing he won't nurse. He frustrates easily because you have so much difficulty controlling him. When he finally gets the nipple working in his mouth he performs very well.

MR. TOURIST. This is the leisure lover. He lazily nurses and looks around. After a few minutes he rests a spell, then nurses again. He reminds you of the middle-aged tourist who is in no hurry to move along. He just wants to enjoy the view. If he isn't interfered with, this kind of baby nurses well, but he drags the process out. You can't hurry him.

MR. TASTER. The tasting baby has to go through a period of mouthing the nipple, rolling it around, smacking his lips, tasting a little milk, and finally nursing. If you push this guy he gets furious and screams at you. Left to himself with just a little encouragement, he does a good job after a time. You may get a little frustrated, but he does make you laugh. He so obviously acts as if he were settling down to a gourmet feast.

MR. HEDONIST. He loves the sensation of the warm breast, the touch of the skin, the smell of mother, the feel of the nipple. Feeding is secondary to him. You have to keep reminding him that he is there for business, not pleasure.

MR. CONSERVATIVE. He is a delayer. In the more extreme form he can worry you. In spite of being normal size he doesn't seem to know what it is all about. He is disinclined to move or become involved. You have to help him a good deal. Self-demand is not for this fellow. He needs a fairly regular schedule of feeding at first until your coaxing and patient guidance get him underway. You just have to let him come around a little later than you expect. If you prod or force him, he gets balky. Once he starts, he does very nicely at his own sedate pace. With his insufficient sucking, you must stimulate your milk production by hand-emptying regularly until he takes over.

MR. PROTESTER. This baby may not be a true demonstrator against the Establishment, but something makes him dislike the nursing situation. Maybe he is reacting against the "affluent society"—an overfull breast, a too-rapid delivery of milk. A rigid feeding schedule, which makes him too hungry, and overdressing, which makes him too warm, also produce anger. The most extreme form of protester can cause you a good deal of distress about your nursing. As soon as you present the breast to him he screams at you and refuses the nipple. He may suck a few times and then begin screaming. He fights and rages around at the whole process, which makes you feel very inadequate and clumsy. If he does take the nipple, he works at it like a dog with a bone. He worries it, chews hard, and bites, which makes you pull away in pain. This just makes him angry, and he continues his attack. A flat nipple makes him irritated. If you are nervous and anxious anyway, he gets worse. With this kind of baby the whole feeding is likely to be a battle, leaving you exhausted after a thoroughly unpleasant experience. If you try to discipline him, he just gets worse. Rough handling infuriates him more.

Your goal will be for the two of you to come to some common ground of understanding. This is necessary in every mother-child relationship, but it is a more difficult job for you with a baby of this persuasion. Keep in mind that there is nothing wrong with you, your breast, or your baby. After some weeks you have a settled-down association that can still have its stormy periods. This kind of baby often ends up on a formula because he tries your patience so hard—and you have a sneaking suspicion that he isn't getting enough to eat. He may fool around so much that he messes up your milk supply. This protesting kind of baby grows up into a determined, active child who may have difficulties about feeding in his early years.

MR. COLD FISH. You have an odd situation here. This rather rare bird seems to lack responsiveness in the feeding situation. He is just not warmed by the usual things. I've wondered what the attitude of those about him have to do with his lack of warmth of feeling but have never been certain. This baby almost always ends up bottle-fed. It is difficult for a mother to give in the usual fashion to this kind of baby.

Most of the situations described above adjust themselves after the first few weeks when you find out what your baby's pattern is. But you continue to deal with an individual child with his own approach to life situations. You will gain nothing by impatience with a new baby. Don't push him. He knows where the nipple is. If you try to force a baby to the breast, hold his head, work his jaw, push against his cheek to bring his head around, hold his cheeks to force his mouth open, slap him, pinch his skin, snap his feet, or shake him, you can expect upset but no nursing.

Don't stop trying to breast-feed just because you get a lazy, sleepy response. Your baby has to have a chance to learn how. Get him hungry for feedings so that he will make a good effort. A turndown of your breast is not a signal for panic. It is a signal for hand-emptying adequately and offering the breast at the next feeding as usual.

NURSING IN THE HOSPITAL

Your baby will start nursing sometime from twelve to twenty-four hours of age. Just when is determined by his behavior after he comes out of his quiet period of newborn shock. Nursing can be tried a few minutes after delivery, but there seems little point to it when the mother's breasts are not producing and the baby is often too tired.

You will start your first feedings lying down. Lie on the side that you are to nurse from, with your head and back supported so that you are comfortable and not straining. Prop pillows at your back to avoid any strain. Face the baby, who is lying turned to you. Put your arm up over his head or cradle his head in the crook of your arm—whichever feels better to you. Move your breast close to his face. Bring him toward you with your other arm until his mouth is near your nipple. Keep his legs and body close to you. If you want, you can elevate the back of the bed so that you are sitting quite straight. (See fig. 30.)

Now compress the areola about the nipple, squeezing it gently to get some fluid on the tip. (See fig. 31.) Take ad-

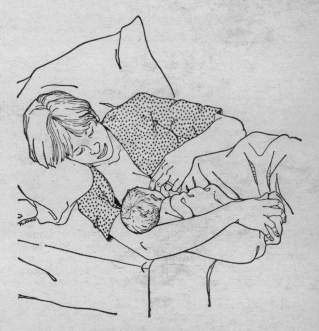

Fig. 30. Nursing in the lying-down position.

TO START MILK FLOW

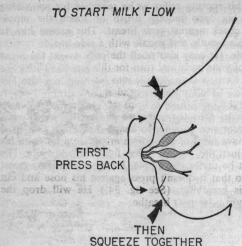

FIRST
PRESS BACK

THEN
SQUEEZE TOGETHER

Fig. 31. Starting the milk flow.

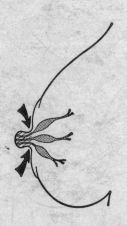

Fig. 32. Baby's jaws grasp
nipple only (incorrect).

vantage of his rooting reflex as he searches for something to go into his open mouth. Brush or touch the nipple against his cheek nearest your breast. This causes him to turn, open his mouth, and nuzzle with a side-to-side motion for the nipple. He may also smell the milk or get the sense of warmth of your body and turn for this reason. This gives you a chance to insert the nipple into his mouth. Guide the nipple to him—don't push his head into the breast! Compress the areola and nipple from above and below with your fingers so that they fit into his mouth easily. His mouth is wider side to side, so shape the areola this way. He should have most of the brown areola area between his gums, not just the nipple. (See figs. 32 and 33.) His tongue must be under the nipple. Hold your finger against the breast so that it doesn't press against his nose and cut down on his breathing. (See fig. 34.) He will drop the nipple and quit if he can't breathe.

As noted previously, these first feedings are really just for practice. Your breast milk is yet to come. So don't push at him too hard or too long. Nurse both breasts each time. Try five minutes on each breast to start. This is enough until your milk comes in. Start on alternate breasts at subsequent feedings. This gives sufficient nipple stimulation to

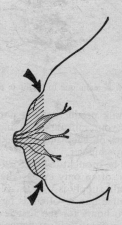

Fi . *33*. Baby's jaws compress sinuses (correct).

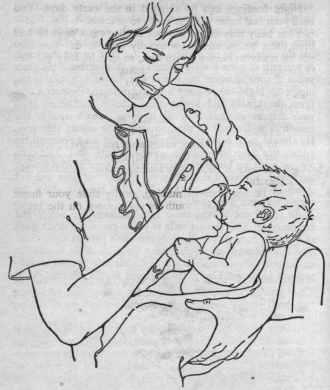

Fig. 34. A technique to facilitate nursing.

encourage your milk production but not enough to abuse the nipple. After your milk appears, increase the nursing time to ten minutes on each side, depending on your comfort and your baby's hunger.

Your baby will be brought to you for feeding every three to four hours, bu. often only every other feeding is taken well until your milk supply is well established. Rooming-in permits you to nurse him as often as he acts hungry. This may be every two hours for the first few days. Just don't nurse too long at a time. You are better off to feed oftener and not longer than ten minutes on each side after your milk is in.

Night feedings can be skipped in the early days. You need your rest more than he needs to practice.

Your baby may start right out at the breast as if he had been there before and knew exactly what to do. You may not be ready to keep up with him, so that he may get irritated with you. But give your breasts time. His vigorous nursing will take care of that. You may have the more usual baby who isn't very interested at first. You have to make things as easy for him as you can. Help him to practice getting the nipple and sucking properly. He gets his sucking reflex going by forty-eight hours, but he has to be helped to get at the breast easily and properly. This stimulates your milk production and helps prevent engorgement of your breasts. If these early feedings accomplish this, they are successful.

When he has finished nursing, gently slide your finger into the corner of his mouth or press down on the breast at one corner of his mouth to break the suction. Don't pull him off the breast. This can eventually cause soreness of the nipple.

Only glucose water will be offered after your first breast-feeding. This plus the colostrum will be enough to satisfy him unless he is the live-wire type, awake and demanding. Then you may have a hard time for a few days satisfying him until your milk comes in. Formula is not given during this time if you plan to nurse.

A little nipple pain as your baby starts to nurse is normal for the first few days, but it soon stops. If your nipples hurt all through the nursing, be sure that your baby is nursing correctly. He must have the dark area in his mouth. If he sucks only on the nipple this hurts and damages the nipple.

Unless you have breast-fed before and produce rapidly, it isn't likely you will have a good breast supply during your hospital stay. Milk comes in at two to three days but more adequate milk production does not arrive until 7 to 10 days or later. The mature milk production cycle takes a little longer than this to get established.

GOING HOME

The excitement, the emotional tension, and the physical fatigue of going home may push you pretty hard. This causes a decrease in your still-borderline supply of milk.

You must have adequate help, adequate rest, adequate emotional relaxation. Your milk supply will then come along, increase, and be adequate for your baby.

You may have to nurse more frequently at home to catch up, since your baby will act hungrier. He is at the stage where he nurses irregularly and quite frequently anyway. Feed him as often as he is hungry, but don't nurse any longer than ten minutes on each breast each time. Nurse oftener—not longer—to catch up and stimulate your breasts. Always nurse both breasts at each feeding. Empty the second breast by hand if he hasn't done so, to further stimulate your breasts. Your milk supply increases gradually and adequately so that he levels off rapidly to longer intervals between feedings. In a few weeks he even settles down to a fairly regular feeding sequence.

WHERE TO NURSE

Check your home to find a place where you can nurse comfortably. Privacy is the most important element. Nursing should not be a sideshow, although this does not mean that you can't talk with someone while nursing. You may want to read, or to turn on the radio, record player, or TV. Get clean-up materials and breast care items together and near at hand before you start. Relax for a few minutes before you approach your young charge. Don't carry the push of your everyday life to him.

POSITION

Experiment a little here to find which position is the most comfortable for you. You may prefer to nurse lying down, well padded with pillows, as you probably did in the hospital. This does limit your movements. One arm and hand are less free. More often you will like sitting up. Choose a low, straight-backed armchair to give your back support with more freedom and less strain. The old-fashioned rocking chair may turn out to be your favorite. Use pillows to get even more support for your back. A foam-rubber cushion in the early weeks may ease the strain on your tender posterior. A footstool can give your feet and legs some extra support. You can raise your leg on the nursing side for extra support. Don't forget the stool is there when you finish! Whatever position you want is fine, so long as you are comfortable—sitting with no strain on your arms, shoulders, and back—and holding your baby close.

Your baby must be comfortable, too. Check to see that he is dry, not too warm or too chilly. He should be in a semi-upright position, cradled in your arms without cramping or excessive restriction. One of your arms supports his head, and he leans back so his head is in the bend of your elbow. Your breast falls more naturally into his mouth as you cradle his back and head in your arms.

A lying-down position is easier for night nursings. However, if you are likely to doze off, you will be wise to sit up in bed to nurse if you are alone. If father is there to bring the baby to you and see that you don't go to sleep too deeply, you may catnap. Don't leave the baby in bed with you after the feeding is over, or you may fall asleep and roll over on him.

Nursing Sequence

I have already discussed how to begin your first nursings. Now that you have milk, you may find that the breast is so hard that he can't get a grip on the nipple. You can hand-milk some fluid out to soften it first.

As already noted, the nipple and areola must go deep into his mouth for sucking to be effective. If he sucks only on the nipple he will damage it, and he won't get any milk, either.

But there is more to his feeding at breast than getting a whole mouthful of nipple and areola in the proper place between his palate and tongue. What does he do when he takes in milk? He just doesn't suck on your breast—he milks it. Anything that touches his lips or the top of his mouth causes his sucking reflex to go into action. First he brings his gums or jaws down together on the areola to block the ducts and squeeze the milk sinuses in that area. Then he squeezes milk out into his mouth by pressing up under the nipple with his tongue against his palate to draw out the nipple toward the back of his throat. This empties the milk into the back of his throat. The vacuum or suction he creates in his mouth carries the milk on down.

In addition to your baby's sucking and milking, your

breasts also contribute their share to the process by secreting and expelling milk.

MILK-EJECTION. The first part of the breast performance is a muscular contraction of the alveoli, the milk-containing spaces of the breast, when your baby sucks on the nipple. This forces milk out into the ducts where your baby can milk it out. This is the early reaction of the breast when milk first comes in.

LET-DOWN REFLEX. The second part of breast activity is the let-down or draught reflex, which is a little slower in coming. Your baby's sucking on your nipple (plus the emotional stimulation associated with nursing), triggers the pituitary gland to pour out the hormone oxytocin. When this hormone reaches the milk-producing cells of the breast, milk is secreted rapidly into the alveoli where it is available for milking out. When this happens, the breast briefly becomes tight and uncomfortable. Put to breast, your baby takes a few sucks, then waits for a few seconds while the milk is secreted and pushed into the ducts, then starts his vigorous sucking. This doesn't happen in these first few days. Sometime between three and eight days, perhaps later, you can depend on these reflexes to work for you so that your baby gets his milk faster and with less effort. You see signs of this reflex response when you find milk dripping from the opposite breast during nursing, milk dripping from your breast before the baby starts to nurse, uterine cramps during nursing, and disappearance of nipple discomfort during feeding. Emotional upset or physical discomfort can interfere with this reflex.

Your doctor may give you a nasal spray that contains a substance similar to oxytocin hormone. This is to aid in setting up your let-down reflex a little faster. If you will just work a little longer and not try to hurry the process, your nursing baby will do the same thing for you.

How Often?

Once the practice sessions are over, follow a demand schedule with your baby for the first weeks—which means no schedule at all. Six to ten feedings a day are usual in the first weeks. The intervals between feedings increase to three and a half to four hours after the first few weeks when your milk supply is established, although small babies may take less at a feeding and need to eat oftener.

Night feedings are a must for the first few weeks. You need to empty your breasts at that time so they are ready for the next feeding—not overfull. A well-fed baby may start to pass up the night feeding at four to six weeks, sometimes sooner. If he is not getting enough to eat during the day, a night feeding may go on for a longer period.

If your baby is sound asleep during the day when you think he should nurse, should you wake him or let him sleep? After your milk has come in, you will find it helpful to try to feed him at regular intervals. If he is hungry before four hours are up, you should feed him. But you may save yourself some time for night sleeping if you don't let him go longer than four hours during the day without eating. Try gently to wake him. If you handle him roughly or jerkily he may wake up, but he won't be in any mood to nurse. Joggle him a little, talk to him, make a little noise. Put him to your breast and see if his rooting reflex will help you out. If he isn't hungry he won't search for the nipple or suck. If he doesn't respond, put him back to bed. He will nurse at his next hungry time.

How Long?

Not all babies nurse equally rapidly or equally vigorously. Older babies are more efficient. Some breasts are harder to nurse. As mentioned before, increase the length of time on each breast from five to ten minutes after your milk comes in. (A light-skinned blond or redheaded mother should limit nursing time especially carefully, since her nipples are not designed for heavy duty.) Nurse from the first breast for ten minutes, ease the baby off the nipple, burp him briefly, put him on the other breast. If he nurses too long on the first breast he tires, sucks badly on the second breast, and goes to sleep without enough food. On the second breast he may nurse a second ten minutes, making a total sucking time of twenty minutes. At each breast he will get 75 percent of the milk in the first two to four minutes and 90 percent in six to eight minutes. The total amount from the two breasts is usually adequate for a full feeding. Just be sure you let him nurse comfortably and continuously during his feeding time. A few more minutes of breast for lulling off to sleep may be added to the twenty minutes' total. If he wants more milk than this time allows him, he needs to be fed oftener—or some other modification in his diet must be made. If he is just sucking but not nursing, he is using your nipple as a pacifier. Don't let him chew or mouth the nipple, take him off.

He swallows just as much air as a bottle-fed baby during nursing time. If he nurses on a dry or empty breast, he will fill up with a lot more air. If you have more than enough milk, and you nurse too long, he will overfill. Then he has to spit back or regurgitate to get rid of the extra milk. Don't urge him to this extent.

How Much?

When you start to nurse, your breast may produce only half an ounce at a feeding. By the end of the first week, you may produce only as much as half an ounce to one and three-quarters ounces from each breast. This can increase to an ounce for each pound of his birth weight at a feeding by the end of two weeks in good producing breasts.

Don't start to compare notes with someone else on feeding amounts. If your baby is satisfied for three to three and a half hours and adding to his weight after his initial weight loss, he is getting enough milk. As he gets older your milk supply will increase. You have to let him decide if he needs three ounces or ten ounces at a feeding.

Don't weigh your baby daily, or before and after each feeding, to see how much he's taken. If you start this little game he may end up on a bottle because you have dried up your own milk supply by worrying. Your doctor will weigh him as often as is necessary.

How Many?

Use both breasts at each feeding time. Alternate the breast you start with so that you empty each breast completely at least every other feeding. This means that if you started with the right breast for the last feeding then you start with the left breast at the next feeding. This use of both breasts for ten minutes of nursing is important in the early weeks so that you adequately stimulate them to produce. Keep in mind that in the early weeks after delivery, your milk supply is quite irregular. Production is easily upset by lack of adequate nipple stimulation as well as by fatigue, anxiety, emotional strain. After a few weeks your milk supply becomes much more stable.

If you are producing well from both breasts, your baby may be so satisfied on one that he refuses or doesn't take much from the second breast. Hand-empty the second if it feels at all full and uncomfortable. If it isn't adequately emptied, caking or backing up of unused milk may cause you some discomfort.

BURPING

All babies swallow air when they eat, whether they are breast-fed or bottle-fed. You can burp your baby to raise the air bubble in several positions. You can hold him against your shoulder or face downward across your lap or sitting up in your lap. (See figs. 35–37.) The sitting-up position involves the least amount of shifting the baby around and therefore interrupts his feeding the least. Place him in your lap across your hand so that he is sitting upright and leaning forward somewhat. Using a gentle to-and-fro motion, rub his back or pat him gently. Don't bang on his back or sway him back and forth to get the gas bubble up. His change of position to the upright brings the air bubble to a place where he can raise it. Handling him too much and too roughly will just get more bubbles into him and can also cause him to spit up or regurgitate the entire feeding.

Burp your baby at the end of his feeding time. If you estimate that he has swallowed a good deal of air, try burping him after he has finished feeding at the first breast, or, if he is on formula, halfway through the bottle. Don't interrupt his feeding if he is going along well. This will just make him mad.

The size of his burp can vary with the amount of swallowed air. Your small baby is not a little lady or a little gentleman in this respect. The burp can be a loud, whole-hearted expression of release and comfort.

If he doesn't burp, don't worry. This isn't a cause for frustration, rage, or despair. He is not refusing in order to be mean. If you are midway through a feeding, go on with

Figs. 35-37. **BURPING**

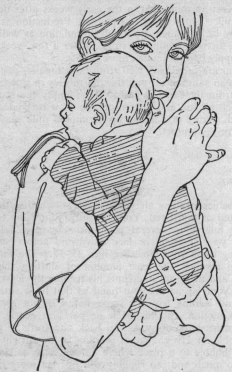

Fig. 35. Over the shoulder

it. If you are at the end of a feeding, put him down on his abdomen in his crib. Then he can handle his own burp. Don't put him on his back. He cannot burp much air in this position, and he may aspirate what he spits up.

SPITTING UP

Spitting up tells you very little by itself. Your baby's weight gain is your answer.

Most babies sometimes bring up some milk after a feeding. This may happen often or rarely.

You must expect a little spitting up when he burps. The

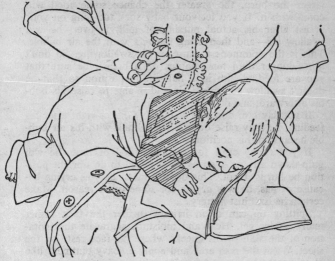

Fig. 36. Face downward across the lap

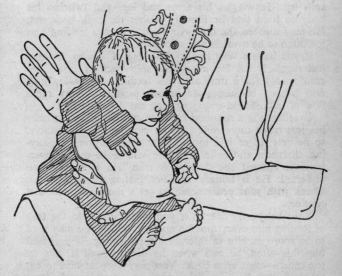

Fig. 37. Sitting up

larger the burp, the greater the chance some food will come with it. If you let your baby suck too long on your breast after his actual nursing of milk is over, he will swallow air—and then bring up milk with the air bubble. This is the commonest cause of air swallowing. So don't nurse longer than ten minutes on a breast; be sure that you are feeding him in a half-sitting position so that he doesn't swallow too much air and is able to raise his bubble afterward; and do burp him properly.

If you lay him down to change his diaper right after his feeding, he may raise quite a bit of milk with his air bubble because of his position.

If your baby cries for a long period of time, he will gulp down air. As soon as he is raised to an upright position he burps it out. This doesn't mean he was crying because of gas, he was crying for some other reason. Make certain he isn't just hungry.

Spitting up can often irritate further the face rashes many babies get. Heat and moisture aggravate the irritation of the skin of his cheeks where his face rests on the sheet. Wash the rash area and apply a heavy ointment like Vaseline, A-D ointment, or zinc oxide.

The very active, alert, wiry baby is often a baby who spits up. He wiggles his arms and legs and twitches his body so hard that he literally pushes the milk back out. He may also be the one who fools you into feeding him too often so he overfills and spits back.

If you have a very hungry little pig of a baby, he may just regularly eat too much. He spits back or fusses uncomfortably for a time after his feeding. Overeating may also happen because your breasts produce a very rapid flow of milk. Hand-emptying may cut down on this.

Overfilling is a common cause of spitting up. Your baby has just taken more milk than he can handle comfortably, so he gets rid of it a mouthful at a time. Vomiting, crying, diarrhea, and colic are often said to be due to overfeeding. Almost the reverse is true. He is more often underfed. He is hungry and not getting enough to eat. Check with your pediatrician to get a more adequate diet routine.

Your baby may overfill if you have fallen into the trap of feeding him every time he makes a noise. You may need to be more careful in interpreting his crying. If you feed him this often, he eats when he doesn't need it, fills up too much—then spits back. You may keep at him to eat so much that he cries because he is uncomfortable from the excess amount. If your baby has good bowel movements, wets his diaper regularly, gains rapidly, he is doing well. If he also spits up a lot, you may be overfilling him. So ease off. Let him take only one breast if he wishes. (Be sure to express the other.) Let him get hungry before you jump to feed him.

If your baby brings up feeding after feeding in a tremendous explosive outburst, it is essential for your doctor to check him.

CRYING AFTER FEEDING

If your baby is wide-awake and crying after a feeding, whether from breast or bottle, and you are certain he is full, it may mean that you are handling him too much. After a feeding, when he has a full stomach, is not the best time to do a lot of changing, fussing about, back patting, or rousing him out of his pleasant after-feeding drowsiness. If you must change his diaper, do it quickly.

Some babies have a period of fussing after a feeding before they settle down. Put him down. Allow him to take care of his own needs at this time.

SUPPLEMENTAL FEEDINGS

The supplemental feeding is a bottle-feeding that takes the place of a breast-feeding. You may have to use this in the early weeks to alternate with breast-feeding until your breasts produce enough milk. Later the so-called freedom bottle gives you a chance to be away from your baby for six to eight hours at a time. In the early weeks, don't use the freedom bottle unless essential. When your feeding routine gets established after six or eight weeks, you may be able to arrange your schedule so that you can use it quite comfortably. You may want to use it if you are tired and need an extra few hours of sleep at night, and Daddy is willing to pinch-hit, or if you want to be away from home. Once breast-feeding is definitely established, it isn't a bad idea for your baby to get acquainted with formula, as well as other foods. You are teaching him another technique of eating.

COMPLEMENTARY FEEDINGS

What about giving a bottle after breast-feeding if you don't think your baby is getting enough to eat? I don't recommend it except as a temporary measure. The trouble with giving both breast and bottle is that it makes more work and is almost certain to result in your baby going off the breast. A baby is not unintelligent. If he doesn't get enough at the breast and has to work hard to get that —and then he has an easy time taking what he needs quickly from a bottle with a fast-flowing rubber nipple— what do you think he will do? Right! He quits the breast. So don't use complementary feedings for long. Try instead to increase your milk supply. Also try offering the baby water after the breast-feeding.

BOWEL MOVEMENTS IN THE BREAST-FED BABY

You have been raised in a bowel-conscious society. But your baby may not follow the golden rule of the Bowel-Watchers' Society—a bowel movement every day. Let's look at this business of intestinal activity on the part of your baby.

The change to the orange-yellow, smooth stool of the breast-fed baby may take several weeks to happen until his breast supply is more adequate. During the change from meconium to this type of stool he may have bowel movements with a lot of mucus containing small curds often with some bright green color. He passes his stools with a noisy outburst of gas, mucus, and stool. He may have 10 to 12 movements a day during these adjustment weeks. Or he may have far fewer movements than this. He may have a bowel movement every 3 to 5 days for a week, then go to 5 or 6 movements a day, yet show no changes in his general behavior.

Since your breast milk is quite completely digested there isn't much bulk for the bowel to work with. Some of these liquid stools seem to pass through rapidly with no sign of distress on the baby's part.

When you feed your baby, his intestine experiences a reflex that puts it into action. This causes his lower bowel to move its contents along to produce a bowel movement. For this reason he may have a bowel movement every time you feed him, or oftener. He may also absorb the milk so completely that he doesn't produce a stool for several days at a time.

The loose, frequent stools of the breast-fed baby are not diarrhea. If each stool is quite green in color, he is not getting enough to eat. You can only call his bowel movements abnormal if your baby loses weight, shows signs of fluid loss, acts unwell and fussy, and has a sudden increase in a very watery type of stool.

Your baby is not showing signs of constipation when he grunts and strains with or before his stools. He may pass a bowel movement with relatively little fuss or he may strain and pass gas a half hour or more before any bowel movement occurs, and then pass a soft stool. Your breast-fed baby is not constipated just because he does not have a daily bowel movement.

If you think a baby is constipated, do not use laxatives, purgatives, enemas, suppositories, paregorics, or anything else to produce a bowel movement.

Enemas or suppositories are only used on specific direction from your doctor. Constipation needs correction at the food-intake level, not at the bowel level.

IF YOUR BABY JUST ISN'T GETTING ENOUGH . . .

As I have stressed previously, don't jump to the bottle without giving yourself and your baby a real chance at breast-feeding. But if your baby just isn't doing well on breast, you will have to consider other feeding arrangements.

What are the signs that tell you that your breast-fed baby is underfed? The average baby who is underfed at breast demands frequent feedings, perhaps every one to one and a half hours, even after the newborn period is passed. He may cry from one feeding to the next and search constantly for something to get into his mouth. He chews on his hands with his wide-open yelling mouth. If you try to nurse him, he may refuse the breast or take it only for a few sucks, then draw away and start crying all over again. He may suck for a normal length of time and drop off to sleep but within half an hour he is crying hungrily all over again. This kind of crying doesn't stop when you pick him up.

Your underfed baby passes more gas than usual and acts colicky. This may be the result of sucking on an empty breast or air swallowing as well as a bowel that has nothing to digest. If his air swallowing is too great, he may vomit. The hunger-pain-colic combination is frequent in an inadequately satisfied baby. He sleeps poorly. He is so concerned with his inner hunger that he can't settle down.

As an arbitrary rule of thumb based on experience, I would suggest your decision to give up breast-feeding be made on the following recommendations: If your baby has not gained over his birth weight by 3 to 4 weeks, or if he shows signs of underfeeding and gains less than 4 ounces a week, stop breast-feeding. You won't increase your breast milk enough to take care of his needs.

There is another alternative to switching to bottle-feeding, and it is one I have used for years. If the breast supply is not quite adequate, a cereal mixture is started. This method has the advantage of staying away from bottle and continuing to use breast as a milk source. (I describe this more fully later in the *First Month* section, under "The Hungry Baby.")

BOTTLE-FEEDING

A properly put together cow's milk formula, although not the same, is digested as easily as breast milk. Like breast milk, it contains about 20 calories per ounce. As discussed earlier, it is just as adequate nutritionally.

TYPES OF MILK

There are many different types of cow's milk some of which are either too expensive or unsuitable for your young baby. I will list, therefore, only those types recommended for use during his first year; only the prepared infant formula group (or evaporated milk) will be described.

PASTEURIZED WHOLE MILK. Pasteurized whole milk has been treated by heating to 145 degrees F. for thirty minutes, or 160°F for 15 seconds which kills the bacteria. The heating also changes the casein, so that the curd is smaller and less tough for easier digestion. You will always boil it again in your formula making. You cannot keep it sterile for a very long period of time, even with refrigeration and proper handling. I would use some other form of cow's milk until later in the baby's first year.

HOMOGENIZED WHOLE MILK. This is pasteurized whole milk in which the fat droplets of cream are broken up into finely divided particles by forcing them through small openings. The fat or cream doesn't separate out and rise to the top. This milk is more easily digested than pasteurized whole milk and causes a less tough, smaller curd —and it may be the only way you get whole milk in your area. Check to see if it contains Vitamin D. You won't use this form of milk until later in your baby's first year.

EVAPORATED MILK. This is cow's milk that has been treated so as to lose more than half of its water content. It is homogenized, fortified with Vitamin D, and sterilized in the canning process. Evaporated milk has a number of advantages. It is available almost everywhere. The unopened cans will remain sterile and in good condition for months without refrigeration. They do need to be turned at monthly intervals. It is cheaper than fresh milk and your baby can digest it more easily. You can feed evaporated milk in higher concentrations than you can whole cow's milk.

After you open a can you must refrigerate it and follow sterile precautions. If it is not contaminated you may use it for several days. Wash the top of the can with soap and water and rinse it. Then punch two holes in opposite sides of the top with a clean opener. After you use what you need, flip the can to bring milk up to the opening to form a film that can be used as a sealer. Cover the can with plastic, waxed paper, or a clean cover, and refrigerate. Make the formula with equal parts of evaporated milk and water unless instructed to do otherwise. Such a formula has about 20 calories per ounce.

DRIED WHOLE MILK. This comes from fluid milk with a 3.5 percent fat content. Only the water has been removed. It can be kept for months in a closed can. It does not keep well after the can is opened, since it picks up water and turns rancid. Keep the opened can tightly covered, dry, and cold, and don't contaminate the contents by dipping an unclean spoon into it. Look on the can for directions in making a milk solution with it that contains 20 calories to the ounce. Usually three and one-half tablespoons plus seven ounces of water equal 20 calories to the ounce. Dried whole milk goes into solution poorly. You have to stir or mix it vigorously. You will not use this type of milk often.

DRIED SKIM MILK. This has up to 1.5 percent fat, and it is prepared like dried whole milk. There are instant nonfat dry milks available that go into solution easily. Most milk of this kind comes in boxes or packets and keeps well as long as no moisture gets into it. Pouring from the box avoids the contamination of dipping in with a spoon. This is the least expensive form of cow's milk, and you will use it later in your feedings. It is not a first milk for your baby.

PREPARED INFANT FORMULAS. Special milks modified for infant feedings are sold under many different trade names, such as Enfamil, Modilac, Similac, Carnalac, SMA. Fresh milk is altered in various ways by evaporating, drying, adding sugar, vitamins, some kind of minerals, by making fat or protein content higher or lower, by substituting other fats for milk fat, by adding iron or balancing calcium or phosphorus. These prepared infant formulas come in powder, concentrated, and ready-to-use liquid forms. They can be mixed into a formula rather easily. They do cost more than evaporated milk, but they are the best choice for your baby's formula in the early months because they cause fewer digestive problems and they save your time.

MILK SUBSTITUTES. These are sometimes necessary if a baby cannot tolerate milk. Soybean milk is one such substitute. There are also formulas using meat as a base. Don't ever use a milk substitute for your baby until your doctor has given you careful instructions for its use.

FORMULA PREPARATION

You will be given directions about preparing formula when you leave the hospital. Your doctor will probably recommend that you start out with one of the prepared infant formulas discussed above, or with a formula made with evaporated milk. He may choose any one of the prepared infant formulas. They are all quite similar. Your baby can do as well on one as on another. If he is colicky, gassy, crying excessively, or showing any other intestinal problems, don't try switching formulas. Find out first if he is hungry. Ninety percent of the time in his early weeks these symptoms are caused by hunger. An occasional baby may be sensitive to cow's milk, but shifting cow's milk formulas around certainly doesn't answer his problems.

You may be given the details for preparing special formulas by the aseptic method or the terminal method when you leave the hospital. If your pediatrician chooses one of the various prescriptions requiring special formula preparation, you can ask for a more detailed description from him.

I am suggesting that it is more economical in the long run, as well as better for your baby and less time-consuming for you, to follow these suggestions for the use of the prepared infant formula or evaporated milk mixture. I will describe only a simplified method of prepared infant formula (or evaporated milk) for use, since laborious formula-making can be avoided entirely by the use of modern conveniences. There are some basic ground rules for you to follow in the abbreviated easy-to-do system I am suggesting.

You won't be able to use this method if you have no equipment, dirty surroundings, poor refrigeration, or an inadequate set-up. Under such circumstances you must obtain information on formula preparation from your pediatrician or institutional clinic for terminal or aseptic methods of formula preparation.

STERILIZATION. In any formula use sterile conditions are very real considerations. Cleanliness is basic to the preparation and giving of any food item to a baby. If food, either milk or solids, is to be stored, even if refrigerated, it must be kept in clean, sterile containers to insure safety. To anticipate a little, baby canned foods left in the cans are sterile unless contaminated by a dirty spoon. Packaged dry

foods are sterile unless soiled by a dirty or wet spoon. Any
utensils or pieces of equipment used in the preparation or
storing of food must be of the type that can be thoroughly
cleansed, or sterilized if necessary. The very useful food
blender, used later, is in this category. Any clean dry
utensil used for brief transportation of food and not for
storage is acceptable.

An automatic dishwasher in the modern home or apartment can be a satisfactory unit for preparation of equipment or feeding items if the hot water supply is adequate,
proper detergent is used, and thorough draining and drying before use is accomplished. Only properly cleaned bottles should be used in the dishwasher, since it cannot be
expected to remove old, adherent food or milk particles
from the inside of the bottle. The utensils must be placed
for full exposure to the sudsing and rinsing spray with open
ends down for proper drainage and drying afterwards.

In the practice of this suggested method the only items
of equipment that require sterilization by boiling are the
nipples, cover discs, and nipple collars. The sterilization of
these items stops only when the nipple use is stopped. Clean
bottles are always required whether you later use evaporated milk, skim powdered milk, or whole milk. In the
later menus clean dry utensils are indicated.

BOTTLES. There are small-mouth and wide-mouth bottles
with snap-on nipples that seem less than satisfactory in
comparison to the medium-size-mouth screw-on type of
nipple holder bottle. Any type of heat-resistant glass bottle
that can be easily scrubbed and thoroughly cleaned is acceptable. A similar plastic bottle, unbreakable and heat re-
sistant, is available. The small-mouth bottle cannot be dishwasher cleaned. A plastic bag formula holder with a rigid
screw-on plastic nipple unit is also available. If you live
near a town of any size, you can buy ready-to-use formula
in disposable bottles with disposable nipples. It is almost
a must when you are traveling. You will have to balance
the value of your time against the extra pennies it will cost
in considering it for everyday use.

The four-ounce size bottle is a handy one, particularly
if you are going to follow the feeding schedules described
later. You can always use or offer a second four-ounce
bottle if the first is used up. In the early weeks the four
ounce size may be ample. As a baby's hunger increases
other diet changes are made. As you use more and more

formula in the solid food, you will be offering less than four ounces to drink afterwards.

If you wish to make up eight ounces of formula at a time the large eight-ounce bottle size will work out better for you. Hopefully you will later use most of these eight ounces in his solid foods and not for drinking alone.

After the bottle has been used, discard the remaining formula (see page 150 for leftover formula) and thoroughly rinse the bottle out with cold water, leaving it standing filled with cold water until the next daily clean-up time.

NIPPLES. Nipples are chosen to suit the type of bottle used. With the medium-mouth screw-on nipple type there is a nipple unit made up of a nipple, a plastic screw-on collar to hold the nipple in place, and a plastic closure disc that covers the bottle opening when the stored nipple is inverted. At feeding time the disc is removed from the screw-on collar and used to push the nipple into the feeding position in the collar before it is discarded and the collar screwed back into position.

The nipple shape is not too important as long as it flows freely with little effort on the baby's part. Usually you will need more nipples than bottles. Most nipples have one or more holes. Some have cross-cut openings.

Nipples (with screw-on collar and disc) should be treated with scrupulous care. Used nipples should always be thoroughly cleaned inside and out and adequately sterilized for use again. This is particularly important in the feeding routine suggested here.

In sterilizing, if they are not treated with the bottles, the nipples (with screw-on collar and disc) are boiled in a pan of water not less than three minutes and not more than five minutes. It will save you time to boil a day's supply at a time, storing them in a sterile covered glass jar with perforated lid ready for use. When you are handling the unit don't contaminate it. It is best to use clean dry tongs to assemble the unit.

After a nipple is used it should be thoroughly rinsed, cleaned, turned inside out and cleaned, and water flushed through the holes, then put in the used-nipple jar with the used collar and disc to wait until the next clean-up time.

Set a special time of the day for equipment and/or formula preparation. Avoid interruptions so that you won't make mistakes. You'll find it a great help to have a special place to work. Keep all the equipment you will need together in one place. You should be able to sterilize or thoroughly clean every piece of equipment you will use. If you can't, don't use it.

EQUIPMENT. Listed below are the articles needed for preparing formula.

Sterilizer: Standard eight-bottle sterilizer with wire bottle rack or any deep kettle or pail with a tight-fitting lid. If there is no bottle rack, a wire mesh or folded cloth should be placed at bottom of kettle to hold the bottles off the bottom. The receptacle must be deep enough so that the bottles do not touch the lid. A pressure (steam) sterilizer is satisfactory. Electric types are available.

Bottles (6–12): four- or eight-ounce size

Nipples (6–12): with screw-on collars and closure discs

Bottle brush (1): long-handled with stiff bristles, and shaped to reach the edges of the bottom of the bottle

Nipple brush (1): small, but tapered to reach inside the nipple

Nail brush (1): for cleaning your hands and nails

Can opener (1): punch type

Nipple jar (2): glass, preferably pyrex, with perforated lids, one for storing used nipples, collars, and discs, the other for sterilized nipples, collars, and discs

Funnel (1): with built-in strainer, if you are using the aseptic method described below

Tongs (1): long-handled

Teakettle or covered saucepan with a good pouring spout

Covered saucepan: to boil nipples in

Clock with alarm, or timer

Preparing Equipment. This will be easier if you have rinsed bottles, nipples, nipple collars, and closure discs thoroughly with cold water right after using them. Leave the bottles standing filled with cold water. Turn the nipples inside out as well, clean them, and flush water through the holes. Leave the nipples in the used-nipple jar with the used collars and discs.

Before you start the day's clean-up, wash your lower arms, hands, and nails with soap and hot water. Use your nail brush. Cover any infected cuts or sores. Work in a clean apron or housedress.

Wash all utensils to be used as well as the work area (table top or sink). Scrub thoroughly, both inside and out, bottles, nipples, screw-on collars, closure discs, or other utensils, using hot, soapy water, or detergent solution. One to two tablespoons of vinegar in the wash water will loosen the lime scum on the insides of the bottles. Be sure to clean the insides of the bottles and nipples with a bottle and nipple brush.

Rinse each piece of equipment well in hot water to remove the soap or detergent. Squeeze water through the nipple holes. They must be open.

Let the bottles drain upside down on a clean surface. Don't wipe them.

Aseptic Method. Prepare the bottles and nipples by the aseptic method. With this method the bottles and other equipment are sterilized before the addition of any formula.

1. Put bottles upside-down in the bottle rack and lower the rack into the sterilizer. If you have no bottle rack, put the bottles upside-down on wire mesh or folded cloth in bottom of receptacle to be used as sterilizer.
2. Put nipples in the pyrex jar, screw on the perforated lid, and put upside-down in the center area. If you prefer, you can boil the nipples separately for not less than three minutes and not more than five minutes in a small pan, then store in a sterile jar.
3. Add two to three inches of water, or amount indicated for that type of sterilizer, to cover equipment (not bottles).
4. Put lid on sterilizer. If there is no tight lid, put bottles on their sides and cover everything with water.
5. Bring water to a boil and boil actively for 10 minutes by clock or timer. Longer boiling weakens the nipples.
6. Turn off the heat and let cool. You can pour off the excess water for quicker cooling. Leave everything in the sterilizer.
7. Remove the sterilizer lid after the initial cooling. Turn it upside down on the table or counter.
8. Use tongs to remove all of the items onto the inverted sterilizer lid or clean towel or diaper. Place the bottles upside-down to drain and dry thoroughly. Leave nipples in the closed nipple jar, turning the jar upside down to drain.
9. After draining and drying turn bottles upright. Don't touch the tops, insides, or rims of the bottles. With tongs place the nipple, disc, and collar in place and screw on loosely. Store until used.

Dishwasher Method. If you have a properly functioning

automatic dishwasher the aseptic method is modified as follows:

1. After properly preparing the equipment items, put bottles upside down in rack for glassware. Do not use this method with small-mouth bottles. Do not include in the load dishes or other items that have not been prepared in the manner described above. Include the other preparation utensils in the load.
2. Nipples are treated separately as described in "Aseptic Method." The screw-on nipple collars and closure discs can be placed in the silverware rack for washing.
3. Add adequate detergent to the machine and start the cycle. Do not interrupt the cycle but allow it to run its full course.
4. Allow the bottles to cool, drain, and dry before removing them from the dishwasher.
5. As they are removed, put screw-on collars and closure discs in place with tongs. Sterilized nipples may be added at this time or at the time of feeding. Attach the collars and store ready for use.

If you are using ready-to-use prefared infant formula proceed with the following steps:

1. Prepare and sterilize bottles, collars, discs, and nipples as described under "Preparing Equipment" and "Aseptic Method" and store ready for use.
2. At feeding time shake the formula can thoroughly to mix.
3. Scrub the top of the can with hot, soapy water, then rinse off with hot water. Punch the top with the sterilized can-opener, making two holes at opposite sides.
4. Remove the disc, collar, and nipple from the bottle.
5. Pour from the can to fill one bottle with the prescribed amount of formula.
6. Cover the can and put it back in the refrigerator at once.
7. Replace the nipple in the feeding position, screw down the collar, and feed.

If you are using the concentrated prepared infant formula or evaporated milk:

1. Prepare and sterilize the bottles, collars, discs, and nipples as described under "Preparing Equipment" and "Aseptic Method" and store ready for use.
2. At feeding time shake the can of formula thoroughly to mix.
3. Follow the can-opening instructions previously described.

4. Remove the nipple, collar, and disc from the bottle.

5. If the water is from any other source than the city or suburban water supply, it must be boiled for five minutes before it is added to the bottle. *This is most important!*

6. Add an equal amount of a concentrated prepared infant formula or evaporated milk from the opened can. Cover the can and return it to the refrigerator at once.

7. Replace the nipple in the feeding position and seat the screw-on collar, ready for feeding. Be careful not to contaminate the bottle, cap, or nipple when removing it or putting it back on.

8. Shake the mixture thoroughly and feed without delay.

If you wish to make up a day's formula at one time:

1. Sterilize a quart container with good screw-on cover as well as prepare and sterilize the bottles, discs, collars, nipples, and other equipment as described under "Preparing Equipment" and "Aseptic Method."

2. Add thirteen ounces of sterile (boiled ten minutes) water to the quart container.

3. Add an equal amount of the prepared infant formula or evaporated milk. Remember milk into water, not water into milk.

4. Replace the cover and shake to mix. Store in refrigerator.

5. At feeding time pour formula into bottle and place the nipple as described previously. Take care not to contaminate the supply jar, bottles, caps, or nipples. Return supply jar to refrigerator.

If you are using powdered prepared infant formula you will have to include a measuring pitcher (heat-resistant, graduated in ounces), a measuring tablespoon (metal or heat-resistant plastic), and a long-handled spoon or stirring rod (for mixing formula) to the other equipment to be sterilized as described under "Preparing Equipment" and "Aseptic Method."

1. At preparation time pour the required amount of hot boiled water from the teakettle into the measuring pitcher.

2. Open a can of powdered formula. These usually come with snap-on covers which fit back on the can to seal it well. Avoid contaminating the powder with a moist spoon or with material dropped into the open can.

3. Add the prescribed amount of powdered formula with the measure.

4. Stir thoroughly to dissolve the powder. You may have

to use a sterilized wire whisk or egg beater to accomplish this.

5. This made-up mixture is then placed in the sterile quart jar, covered, and refrigerated until ready for use. The same procedure is followed here as is done when using a 24-hour formula mix described above.

LEFTOVER FORMULA

You can avoid wasting formula if you leave the bottle nippled at the end of the feeding. Keep it untouched in the refrigerator until the next feeding. Then remove the nipple and use the leftover formula in the baby's cereal mix, or add it to the next bottle to be used. If you do not leave the nipple in place or do not refrigerate the used bottle at once, you will have to discard the leftover formula. In any case, don't save the leftover formula beyond the next feeding.

NIPPLES

Nipples are made of rubber. Keep this in mind in your cleansing, sterilizing, and storage of them. You will find that excessive heat, sunlight, butterfat, or greases are damaging to rubber goods. Too-aged or too free-flowing ones will have to be discarded. As soon as you use a nipple, turn it inside out and clean it thoroughly before tossing it into the used-nipple jar. Nipple holes should be of the right size for your baby's easy sucking. Milk should drop in an almost continuous stream when you turn the bottle upside down. If your baby works too hard to get the milk, he tires too soon, gulps too much air, or doesn't get enough food. The age of the nipple has something to do with the degree of force that he will have to use.

ENLARGING HOLES. Start with a new nipple which usually has one or two holes. Pinch the nipple close to its tip between your thumb and forefinger. Use the point of a sharp scissors to make a small slit. Squeeze the nipple slightly. You should be able to see light through the cut you have made. Turn the nipple and hold it to make a second cut like the first to form a cross-cut. Nipples with a cross-cut opening are available.

You can enlarge nipple holes by burning with a needle. Insert a large-size darning needle into one of the holes so that an inch protrudes from the nipple tip. Hold a lighted match to the end until the needle glows red-hot. This burns a larger hole into the nipple. Dispose of the match and put the nipple and hot needle into cold water. Remove the needle from the hole and check hole for proper size. This can be done with all the nipple holes. Sterilize the nipple before you use it again.

CHECKING HOLES. To make sure feeding holes are clear, fill nipple with water, hold between the first and second fingers with thumb over the opening at the base of the nipple. Press with thumb, and water should squirt through all feeding holes.

CLOGGED NIPPLES. A pinch of salt cuts butterfat and unplugs clogged holes. After a feeding, remove the nipple from the bottle. Rinse thoroughly, then shake salt down inside the wet nipple to form a paste. Squeeze and roll the nipple between your fingers, forcing the salt paste through the holes. Rinse again thoroughly, and it is ready to sterilize for use.

WARMING AND TESTING THE BOTTLE

If you wish to warm the bottle at feeding time, place it in a pan of hot—not boiling—water. As you heat the water, shake the bottle several times so that it warms evenly. Don't boil the formula. You may have an electric bottle warmer available. Don't have the nipple collar on too tight. When the bottle is warm enough, remove the cap or cover and arrange the nipple for feeding.

Test the warmth of the formula. Let a few drops fall on the inside of your wrist or forearm. They should feel warm —not hot. You can also hold the lower part of the bottle against the inside of your wrist to test the temperature. Shake the bottle thoroughly before you do this.

You may not wish to warm the formula. Some babies prefer cold formula from the first—others want it warm.

You can gradually shift your baby either way you wish. There is no appreciable difference between babies fed cold formula and those fed warm formula. Sleep patterns, crying, and activity are the same. Food and fluid intake, weight gain, and degree of food regurgitation are the same. There has been no evidence that the traditional procedure of warming the bottle is in any way an advantage for the baby.

GIVING THE BOTTLE

After the first feedings with glucose water in the hospital, your baby is fed on bottle much as he is on the breast-feeding pattern. He is fed with a dilute formula to start. This is increased in amount and strength as he wants more. By the time he goes home he probably will be taking one and a half ounces to three ounces at a feeding, about every three to four hours.

Many of the suggestions about breast-feeding at home apply to bottle-feeding too.

WHERE TO FEED. Pick a quiet place for feeding. This is not the time for your baby to entertain a big audience. Get everything you need at hand before you sit down.

HOW OFTEN? As with breast-feeding, you let your baby set the frequency of his feedings at first. Feed him when he is hungry.

HOW MUCH? Always give your baby as much formula as he wants. Don't try to get him to take too much too soon —if you do, he will spit it back at you. Always have more in the bottle than he usually takes. You don't know when his hunger will increase. Don't be surprised when the amounts vary from feeding to feeding. And don't worry how much he takes each time.

HOW LONG? Your baby may be a rapid, vigorous feeder and finish off his feeding in a very short time, like five to ten minutes. If your baby is the dawdling sort, don't drag out his feeding time too long. Too-frequent or too-long feeding times will tire him so that he doesn't get enough at each feeding—and is too tired to do well at the next. A thirty-minute feeding is certainly the total time you should allow your baby. (Look back to the material on "Breast-Feeding" to see the various types of babies and their eating behavior.)

You must try to keep him awake—or at least half-awake during the feeding. You may try tugging slightly on the bottle, turning it around in his mouth, or rubbing behind his ear. Vary your pressure as necessary to rouse him enough to suck. Be as rapid as you can. Your baby may rest between spells of nursing.

HOLDING THE BOTTLE. Keep his bottle at right angles to his face. Don't let it drop down. Let him get food—not air! He develops his lower jaw by pushing it out to nurse. If you avoid upward pressure on his palate he is able to nurse more effectively.

Don't take the bottle out of his mouth repeatedly to regulate the milk flow. This is annoying to him. It destroys his feeding rhythm. He will usually regulate this pretty well himself. If necessary, you can regulate his milk flow in some other way. Gently rotate the bottle in his mouth—perhaps with a gentle tug. This will often start him sucking again after he pauses.

HOLDING YOUR BABY. Always hold your baby for feeding. Don't prop the bottle and leave him. This is not only inhuman but dangerous. When the flow of milk does not correspond perfectly to his sucking-swallowing rhythm, he must get rid of the nipple to avoid choking. If the bottle holder has no give, or the weight of the bottle is on the nipple, he will be flooded as he struggles to get free. In his struggling he may regurgitate milk. He can actually drown in milk. Don't prop him up in an infant seat. You need to give him the security and warmth of your arms, your voice. Try to make him feel secure and comfortable. Either one of the two positions given below is good.

1. The breast-feeding position is the one that imitates a baby being fed at breast. Hold your baby in your lap with his head resting in the curve of your arm. He is in a semireclining position, with head higher than his body. Hold the bottle so that the nipple and the neck of the bottle are kept full of milk. (See fig. 38.) Sit

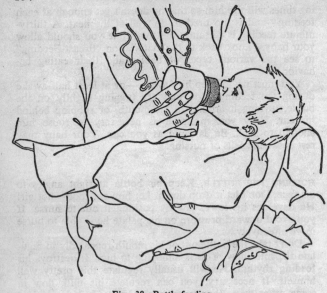

Fig. 38. Bottle-feeding.

him upright on your lap for a few minutes once during the feeding and once again after the feeding. Pat him gently on the back, or gently move him back and forth to help him to get up any air swallowed during his feeding.

2. Hold your baby on your lap in a more upright position. Cross your left ankle on your right knee (or vice versa), or put your feet up on a stool in front of you to support his back. Hold his head cradled in your hand, with your thumb behind one ear and your fingers behind the other. Rest your elbow on the chair arm or a table to take the strain off your shoulder. Feed him with the bottle in good position. Hold him upright to bubble him.

Don't modify this second position as is sometimes done. If you prop your feet up on a chair, your upper legs can form a seat much like an infant seat. Your baby's feet are toward your stomach and he faces you. He is too far away from you. You are holding him, but there isn't much closeness or cuddling.

AIR SWALLOWING. Look back to the material on breast-feeding for suggestions on how to burp your baby. If your baby is showing a good deal of air swallowing, even to the point of vomiting, you need to check what can be causing this much difficulty. Probably the commonest cause in the bottle-fed baby is too small a nipple opening, so that he has to work too hard to get the milk out. Improper bottle holding can also give a good deal of air rather than food in swallowing.

SELF-DEMAND FEEDING

There are several approaches to feeding schedules. There is the strict schedule, the self-demand schedule, and the self-regulation schedule. You can use any of these methods you find most convenient for you and your baby. There is no evidence whatever that the manner in which you feed your baby, whether it is strict or permissive, has any long-range psychological effect on him—as long as you don't go to extremes in either direction. You will find, though, that you will have a lot quieter time with the average baby in these early weeks if you feed him when he is hungry.

STRICT SCHEDULE

Before the 1900's, when breast-feeding was the rule, it was taken for granted that a baby was fed when he was hungry. With the start of substitute or artificial feeding, chemical mixtures were devised to supply known basic needs. It was necessary for the baby to be fed exact amounts of a carefully calculated formula at exact times. Over-feeding was considered dangerous and was avoided at all costs. As nonhuman milk became available with better health controls this type of precise formula-making was found unnecessary. With clean cow's milk sources formula-making was simplified until today it involves little effort in preparation.

At that time it was also felt that if a baby was fed in an orderly fashion he would develop orderly habits. Even mothers who breast-fed were given exact instructions as to time, amount, and length of feedings.

Although a strict feeding schedule is no longer required for health reasons, it still has the advantage of regularity. Large numbers of babies adapt to an exact schedule easily. Regular schedules are also good for small, immature, or premature babies, the ones who never demand to be fed.

The trouble arises when the baby varies from the prescribed pattern. The prolonged crying of a hungry baby can upset his family and can tire the baby so that he eats poorly and swallows a good deal of air, giving him gas or making him vomit. Any baby probably feels overwhelmed by the utter devastation that comes with feeling neglected. He goes out of control so that he doesn't see, doesn't hear, doesn't feel—he just screams, because he has gone hungry too long.

So your baby needs some leeway, since he may get hungry between feedings and need more food at shorter intervals. This may mean that he needs an adjustment in his diet, but it also means he can be fed if he is hungry.

STRICT SELF-DEMAND

Strict self-demand is the method whereby you feed your baby whenever he wants to be fed. This method may sound just the thing to make your baby happy and contented. The advantages actually are tremendous for some infants. Their needs are met quickly, so that they don't come to associate long crying with feeding time.

But there are difficulties with strict self-demand. Crying is a baby's only way of talking at first. He tells you he is hungry by crying. But he also tells you that he is wet, cold, trying to burp, getting ready for a bowel movement, sick, tired, or fussy. You have to live with your baby for a time before you know what he is saying. As a result, crying is not a reliable sign of hunger if you're trying to follow a self-demand schedule. If your baby stops crying when you pick him up, he is not hungry. If he keeps on crying, he is either hungry or uncomfortable—or both. If he doesn't stop crying when you offer him food, he isn't hungry. He may be doing afternoon fussing or evening social sound-off.

Another difficulty is that any baby fed every time he cries will end up being fed too much and too often. He ends up uncomfortable—then he really has something to cry about.

Self-demand feeding can cover up hunger in a baby who is getting insufficient food. With a weak formula and a hungry baby, you can end up feeding him every one to two hours. But what he really needs is an adequate diet—not more frequent feedings.

The mother who stops whatever she is doing to feed her baby every time he cries is giving him too much responsibility for decision-making. The infant whose actions control the household routines will be a burden on any family and will quickly come to be resented. He finally becomes a domestic tyrant if he is not helped to learn something about coping with frustration. What began as an attempt to give him security can make him so uncertain in his dealing with frustration that he is not socially adequate.

Another point to consider is that there are easy babies and non-easy babies. The non-easy babies have a harder time fitting into a pattern of family living in all areas of activity, not just feeding. This kind of baby is unpredictable, and most disturbing to his parents. With a complete self-demand schedule, a baby like this gets more and more out of control. He demands so much of his parents' time and attention that they do little else. Both mother and father feel guilty and inadequate and eventually wind up blaming themselves or each other. They try to follow the baby's lead. They hesitate to impose a schedule on him. Yet a reasonable schedule is the very thing he needs most.

It is just as important that feeding systems be adapted to the mother's personality as to the baby's. If self-demand is held out as the only good way, a mother feels guilty if she just isn't ready to handle this type of scheduling. Some mothers may misunderstand the self-demand goals. If so, they are better off with a strict schedule. An unhappy, confused mother is not the one to follow strict self-demand. She is being given responsibility that she doesn't want and can't take. Another type of mother may find it very irksome to try to adjust to her baby's irregular feedings. For her also a regular feeding pattern for her baby is desirable.

SELF-REGULATION

Under the self-regulating plan, you don't have to rush to feed your baby whenever he cries. You do feed him whenever he is really hungry. Gradually a mutually satisfactory arrangement is reached between mother and baby.

With an adequate food supply, he begins to establish a more predictable pattern. This you can modify to fit in with your own needs.

During the first weeks you feed your baby as often as he is hungry. You don't watch the clock. If he is hungry before feeding is due, you feed him. If he has gone four hours without eating, wake him and feed him. Let him sleep as long as he will at night. This gives you some chance to plan your time. If for some reason you have to wake him to feed him, do so.

It doesn't take long for a well-integrated infant to get his own pattern set up. Ninety percent of the babies on self-regulation will be on a fairly regular schedule of their own choosing by one month. They gradually develop their schedules as they gain the capacity to shift to three meals daily over the following months. (Look ahead to the material on "Eating," in the month-to-month descriptions of development and baby care, for more about feeding times.)

If your baby doesn't set up his own pattern after a month or so, you should begin to impose some regularity. This may be done by allowing three and a half to four hours to pass between feedings and by not picking the child up during the defined rest periods. With this regime, mothers must expect crying at first and be willing to tolerate it. The amount of protest will vary, depending on whether the baby is intense and persistent or mild and nonpersistent. A more practical routine finally becomes established, although there may be considerable irregularity in the amount of food the child takes from one feeding to another.

Some irregular babies adapt quickly to a regular routine once they're set on it. Others continue to be more or less erratic about hunger and sleep. Even if they continue to fuss and cry an hour before feeding, there's no cause for worry. As mentioned before, these irregular babies usually fuss just as much on self-demand as they do on a schedule.

THE HUNGRY BABY

How can you tell and what do you do if your baby is not getting enough to eat? After the first weeks your breast-fed baby is not getting enough to eat if he shows signs of underfeeding (see "Underfeeding at Breast," pp. 139, 140) and wants to nurse oftener than every three hours after the first two weeks. Similarly your formula-fed baby is not getting enough to eat if he shows the same signs, regularly takes over four ounces at a feeding, and wants to eat oftener than every 3½ to 4 hours.

The answer to his need is to start a ready-prepared, precooked, fortified, high-protein infant cereal with his feeding. Rice is an easy-to-use cereal but barley and oat may be used, too. Mixed infant cereal preparations can be introduced later.

ADDING CEREAL TO BOTTLE

If your baby is on the bottle you will probably find it easier in the first few weeks to add cereal to the formula in the bottle. In a small, weak baby this may be necessary at first. Sometimes a thickened mix from a pitcher or cup works better for your small baby who sucks poorly. If you are breast-feeding, or are an old hand at baby feeding, you will start spoon-feeding at once.

Add one teaspoon dry cereal to each ounce of formula (four teaspoons for four ounces) and shake the bottle well. Remember that this will be a thicker mixture so check the nipple opening. Make it large enough so that your baby does not have to work to get the formula. As you thicken the formula by adding more cereal, you may have to use scissors to make a large cross-cut or cut off the tip of one nipple for easy use. Don't do this to all the nipples since this method of feeding cereal is only temporary.

INCREASING CEREAL

Increase the amount of cereal mix as rapidly as your baby needs it. You will have to feel this out as you go along. No two babies behave the same. You can conclude that he is getting enough if he seems satisfied when he finishes the meal. If you are giving your breast-fed baby enough cereal mix, he will nurse ten minutes on one breast, take very little of the other afterward, then fall asleep for four hours. Hand-empty the other breast, or both, if he hasn't taken much. Use the breast milk in his next cereal feeding. If your baby is on formula, feed enough of the cereal mix first so that he doesn't wish to take more than one to two ounces of formula from the bottle afterwards. If he does take more than this amount of formula after the cereal, he needs more cereal mix first. In this fashion you can adjust the amount of food (cereal, etc.) he needs to meet his requirements. Infants differ widely in how much it takes to make them comfortable. It is fairly safe to assume that your infant is getting enough to eat if he takes his solid mix, then 1 to 2 ounces of milk (or 10 minutes of breast), and will then go 4 to 5 hours until the next feeding without fussing, wakefulness, irritability, colic pain, or constipation. Avoid pushing milk at him after his cereal feeding. You can overfill him, and make him lose the entire feeding. Let him decide how much he wants of the formula. If he takes more than 2 ounces, at the next feeding increase the amount of cereal mix that you give first. If he nurses longer than 10 minutes at breast and is hungry too soon, increase the cereal mix. Whenever he loses the entire feeding and acts hungry, refeed him the entire amount. Use a little more caution with the second feeding. If you give him four tablespoons or more of the cereal and he acts hungry, he is still hungry. Make a further change in his diet by adding fresh mashed banana, one teaspoon to one tablespoon of cereal. (Look under *First Month,* "Eating," for further discussion of foods.)

SPOON-FEEDING

By the time you are adding two tablespoons of cereal or more to 4 ounces of formula, you will find that it is easier to start spoon-feeding. You may even have used spoon-feeding to start with. Once you have switched to spoon-feeding, you can leave the cereal out of the formula in bottle, or you can keep the formula thickened as well. Give this bottle mix after you have spoon-fed what you can, if you are formula feeding.

Spoon-feed the cereal mix before you offer breast or bottle. Your breast-fed baby may wish a few minutes on breast before you give him solids, but don't make this a full nursing period. Occasionally a formula-fed baby will want a few sips from the bottle or cup before he settles down to his food. But don't let him have it all. He won't satisfy his hunger well enough with what solids he will take after a full nursing. With formula, it is better to offer the bottle only after a cereal feeding.

Make the cereal mix by adding formula (or breast milk) to the cereal in the feeding bowl. Start with a cup or custard-cup-size container, but it won't be long before you will need a larger bowl. A bowl which can hold 8 ounces of mixture or more is fine. Plastic is better than glass or china if it can withstand heating in a dishwasher. Make a smooth, moist paste which you can handle easily with a teaspoon. Don't make it so runny that it won't stay on the spoon. Use an ordinary teaspoon for the feeding. Don't use a demitasse or infant's spoon. They are too small to control easily and you can't deliver much of a spoonful at a time.

There is a technique to spoon-feeding that you can quickly master. The baby eats purely by reflex movement at this time. Anything that hits the back half of his tongue automatically goes down. What is on the outer end of his tongue is thrust out. Take advantage of this mechanism in feeding the cereal mix by spoon to move the food from the front of his mouth to the back of his tongue. Fill the spoon with some of the cereal, then slide it over the lower lip and tongue so that it lands in the middle of his tongue. Then, with an upward wiping motion, bring the spoon out against his upper lip as you remove it from his mouth, leaving his mouth loaded. Respoon what is left or add it to the next spoonful. Your goal is to move the food rapidly to his mouth so that he has a continuous supply of cereal on his tongue. Don't sit there with a spoonful of drippy food and try to dribble it into his mouth. You are not asking him to use his sucking action, as he does on breast or bottle. He won't get enough in by sucking. You are using his tongue reflex for swallowing. Move the food rapidly and he will have no cause to complain. The secret of success in your baby's feeding is a rapid filling before he tires.

Don't expect success right away unless you have a ravenously hungry baby. Your skill with a spoon will improve as you lose your new-mother jitters. Expect half of each spoonful to come back. You will be very messy at first, but much neater as your skill increases.

SCHEDULE

If he is adequately fed the average baby will eat at four-hour intervals, possibly 6 A.M., 10 A.M., 2 P.M., 6 P.M.,

10 P.M., and 2 A.M. Don't let him go longer than this at first or you will be awake more frequently at night. If your baby seems satisfied at the end of the feeding, sleeps three or four hours before he wants to be fed again, seems in good health, and is putting on weight, then he is getting enough to eat. If he wakes oftener than this, you will feed him and remind yourself that he probably needs more to eat. (Check back to "Self-demand Feeding" under *Breast-Feeding and Bottle-Feeding*.)

Between-meal feedings are not needed at this time. Don't get in the bad habit of giving your baby a little something every hour or so. This way, he never gets really hungry or really full. You only exhaust him and yourself, too!

Don't make him wait for his food. If he wakes early go ahead and feed him. There is method to this kind of advice. You are aiming for a schedule even if you have nothing like one in these early weeks. You will be ready when your baby is ready for more regular routines next month. Now you know that if he is hungry more often than every three or four hours you need to increase his food. If he begins to stretch out the intervals, you start some type of scheduling. You offer him juice or water to help him hold off until his next feeding time. After his regularity is well-established there is no harm in waking him for a feeding. If he regularly sleeps through certain feeding hours, you know that his schedule needs adjusting.

A larger baby will probably set himself up on a four-hour routine in the first few weeks. If he is eating well, his night feedings will be ready to drop out of his feeding pattern after the first few weeks. You give him a late evening feeding like 11:30 P.M. instead of 10 P.M., then put him down to sleep. Don't waken him at 2 A.M. but let him go until the next morning.

The only schedule that is right for your baby is the one which you and he approve. You have to follow his lead now to find what his individual requirements are for food, sleep, and play. Once he has shown you his tendencies, follow them with as much regularity as possible.

VITAMIN

Whether your baby is breast- or formula-fed, from the very first he needs a multiple-vitamin preparation that contains vitamins C, D, and A. Vitamin D is not present in adequate amounts in either breast or cow's milk unless it is added. Vitamin C will not be available in his diet until you start citrus juices later. Even then it may not be adequate. As a precaution a multiple-vitamin drop with vitamins A, D, C, and B-complex should be a regular part of his diet.

A prescription for a multiple-vitamin drop is given to you at the time of your discharge from the hospital. If not, get any standard multiple-vitamin drop in a water-miscible base. The preparation should be continued daily during the child's growing period through adolescence. The dosage is not varied during winter or summer whether breast- or bottle-fed. If fluoride is not in your water supply, use a multiple-vitamin preparation which has added fluoride or give fluoride drops separately in a dosage recommended by your pediatrician or clinic. These drops may be put in his mouth along the side of his cheek (not squirted down his throat), or mixed in his food at the time of his feeding. Give extra amounts of Vitamin C (ascorbic acid) at the time of any infection.

6.

The
New Parents

In the previous section I discussed feeding and the feeding routines you will use for your new baby during the early weeks at home. There are many other aspects of baby care you will be dealing with now that you are home. Perhaps by the end of your hospital stay you were eager to get home and take care of your baby. Tending to him seemed simple: clothes, food, bath—all routine. You expected him to sleep a lot of the time so that you could get caught up on your household chores. But now that you have him home, a lot of questions about baby care begin to come up. You are not as certain as you thought you were, or as strong.

SETTING REALISTIC EXPECTATIONS

Being the mother of a new baby, especially a first one, can easily throw the most efficient woman off-base. There suddenly is so much to be done, so many adjustments to make. You are in for a terrible letdown if you cling to an unreal, romantic picture of what it should be like to be a mother. Every minute of every day with your baby is not going to be a happy time! You will have periods of fatigue, irritability, anger, none of which is mentioned in the movie-script version of motherhood you may be trying to follow. I have said this before—don't try to be a perfect mother.

If you set up impossible standards for yourself and your baby, you can't avoid failing.

Don't try to deny the hostile feelings you will sometimes have for your baby. You won't fool him anyway—the tightness of your voice and your movements give you away. You will be spending so much energy on control that there's none left over for loving attention. It is better to express your irritation or anger and get it over with. If you can realize this, you will save yourself a great deal of distress. Your ability to love grows with understanding and tolerance, not only toward others but toward yourself. So accept your own feelings, even though some of them won't be very nice.

Don't expect too much of your baby, either. You can't demand that he fit a preconceived image of what a baby should be like. Accept him as he is. His development has a definite pattern. (Look ahead to the section on *The First Year*.) Try to help him follow that pattern at his own speed and in his own way. Don't demand that he grow, learn, or act like anyone else but himself.

Your baby will learn a great deal about family life by watching his parents together. His attitude toward his home will be determined, to a large extent, by the way his father and mother feel about each other and about him. This isn't to say that everything has to be sweetness and light between you all the time. Every husband and wife have quarrels. You have mixed feelings about each other as well as about your child. An occasional spat isn't damaging to your baby if there's a steady undercurrent of affection in the family.

THE "BLUES"

The blues can come with your first baby, your third, with each one, or not at all. Not all new mothers get the blues, but enough do so that it is advisable to prepare you for the possibility. To know that other mothers have had the new-baby blues and come through all right is reassuring. This let-down feeling often comes on your second or third day in the hospital. It used to be called milk fever, as it can coincide with the beginning of your milk production. More frequently it occurs when you come home and face full-time motherhood. You feel depressed, not hungry, tense, wide-awake, restless. You often find yourself crying for no reason. You may be quite unreasonable in your demands and quite unrealistic in your interpretation of events and people's reactions. You may feel ugly and unwanted, misunderstood and picked on. If you are in the hospital, you find the nurses lack understanding. You brood over your husband's "indifference."

The cause of your blues may be no more complicated than the feeling of anticlimax that often comes after a long-awaited event. Hormonal changes that take place in the mother's body after the baby is born can set the stage for the blues. Sometimes just simple physical exhaustion is the cause, especially in a mother who has had successive pregnancies, or is in poor health, or who faces inadequate help or exhausting emotional demands at home. A mother may have a good deal of physical discomfort after delivery from painful stitches, sore breasts, bowel and bladder difficulties. These keep her from resting well in the hospital and may still be bothering her when she goes home, especially if she goes home on the third or fourth day after delivery. The weakened mother suddenly has to face the grim reality of increased household chores and the care of her new baby. Her nighttime sleep is interrupted by baby feedings. If she uses the baby's daytime napping periods to race around ironing and polishing floors rather than resting, exhaustion is sure to set in.

The first-time mother is often shocked at the total commitment motherhood demands. She begins to feel isolated and tied down. She resents her loss of freedom. In addition, she is faced with the fact that her new baby upsets the most well-ordered household routines. If she tries to run her household just as she did before he came, she is almost certain to be frustrated. Exhaustion and frustration lead to depression. You may not be able to avoid the blues entirely, but certain commonsense procedures may help you to minimize them.

Try to get your house in basic order before your baby's arrival. If you are going to have a temporary housekeeper, make your arrangements before you go to the hospital. Plan ahead also to find a good baby-sitter, so that you and your husband will be able to go out together occasionally without worrying.

Try to keep your days as simple as possible. If you don't have outside help, do the essential household tasks and let the other things go. It may help to plot a rough schedule of the main things you need to do. Keep it flexible, and include plenty of time for rest and sleep.

If you're feeling blue, pour out your troubles to someone who will make no moral judgments, someone who will understand that no matter how little real basis there is for your depression you nevertheless feel it strongly, but who also knows that with a little help you will manage nicely before very long. Try not to wallow in the blues, but don't be ashamed to express your feelings. You don't have to act like a cheerful cherub when you feel like Pitiful Pearl.

MOTHER CARE

Good mother care is essential whether you have the blues or not. One of the most important features of good mother-care is to remember that you are also a wife and an individual.

Your obstetrician will tell you how soon you can resume marital relations after delivery. Six weeks is often the specified waiting period.

Keep yourself looking attractive for your husband. Try to arrange your daily schedule so that you will have some free time together, even if it's only a few minutes for a cup of coffee or some diaper folding or a shared involuntary laugh as your baby burps with that bewildered look on his face. Arrange for an occasional evening out together with friends your own age. After the first weeks, resume some of your community and church activities. You will have to plan, but you can fit in family life, married companionship, and your own development as an individual. You will need your husband's cooperation.

REST AND SLEEP

Adequate amounts of rest and sleep are musts. Catch a few winks when you can during the day. Rest when your baby rests. If you have other children, try to keep them occupied elsewhere or napping at the same time. You need to regain and retain your strength. Give yourself one day a week without any planned tasks.

DIET

Follow the diet outlined in the *Pregnancy* section, with emphasis on the protein foods. If you are nursing, look back at the recommendations listed under *Breast-Feeding and Bottle-Feeding.*

HYGIENE

Full tub baths will not be part of your routine for the first six weeks after delivery, but daily showers are a must. You will perspire more freely in these early weeks as your body readjusts to the nonpregnant state. Make a special effort to keep yourself free of the odors of stale milk and perspiration.

WORK LOAD

Return to your usual work load gradually. What you can do, do. But avoid fatigue. Stand erect as you work and walk. Stoop over, lift, and bend as little as possible until you are back in shape. Rest your back when it gets tired. Give yourself three months for full recovery. If your back gets tired, here is a good position for rest. Lie flat on the floor with your knees flexed at right angles to your body, your heels supported only by a coffee table or low chair. This helps all the joints of the pelvis and curve of the back to settle into their usual position after the loosening of these joints in pregnancy.

CONSTIPATION

Constipation is very common in the new mother. It is best to regulate your bowels with foods and exercise, as described in the *Pregnancy* section.

EXERCISE

Walking is still your best relaxer and body toner. The following five exercises should be done regularly. In three months you should have regained your pre-pregnancy fig-ure—if you have watched your diet, too.
Stand against a door, with your back, heels, calves, hips,

Figs. 39-43. POSTNATAL EXERCISES

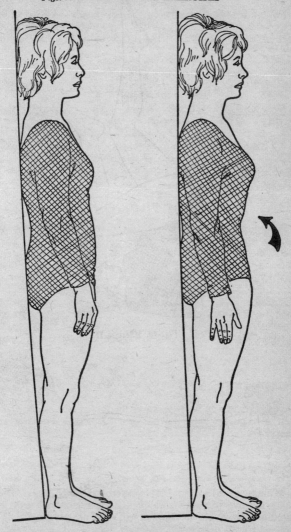

Fig. 39. Exercise I (A) (B)

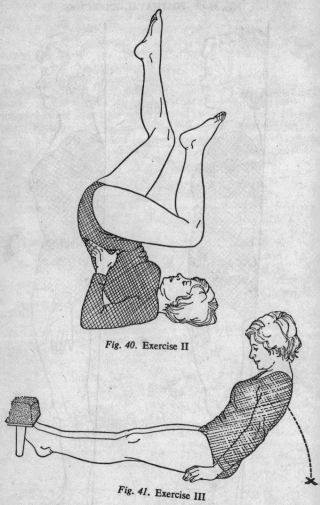

Fig. 40. Exercise II

Fig. 41. Exercise III

shoulders, and head touching it. Tilt your pelvis upward and pull in your abdomen until you cannot get your hand between the door and the small of your back. (See fig. 39.) Demonstrate this to yourself as you stand sidewards looking in a mirror.

The rest of the exercises are done on the floor, without any padding. You can use a pillow under your head.

Bicycle for two minutes, raising your hips off the floor. (See fig. 40.)

Lie on your back, legs straight with toes hooked under some heavy object, arms at your sides. Pull yourself up to a sitting position without using your hands to give you a start. (See fig. 41.)

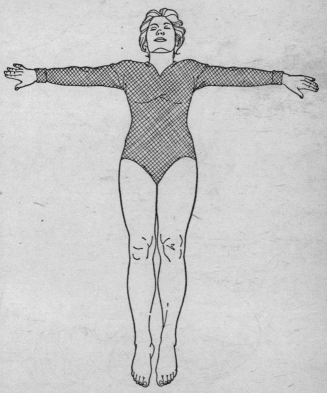

Fig. 42. Exercise IV (A)

shoulders, and raise your right foot, with knee straight, as
still (with toes pointing away from you). Swing it to the left
slowly. Touch the floor beyond your left hand (see Fig. 42,
position X). The toes can twist outward in the process of bringing in a curve.

Start at the centre-line again. Swing your right foot slowly
any good in the ...

By now, if you have been ... do this exercise ...

Exercise V

Lie on your back, legs and arms loose. Press the lower
part of your chest ... raise your feet off ... your knees
a sitting position without ...

hips. Holding ...

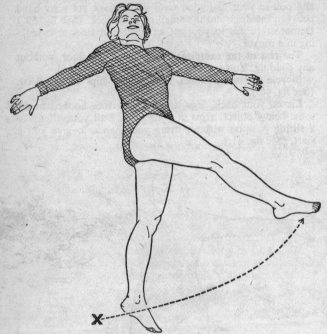

Fig. 42. Exercise IV (B)

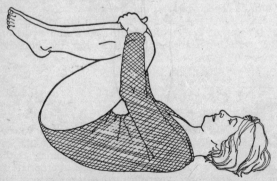

Fig. 43. Exercise V (A)

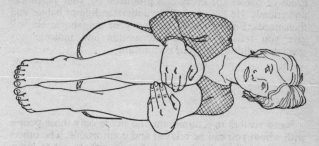

Fig. 43. Exercise **V** (B)

Lie on your back with your legs straight, feet together, arms extended to the side, shoulder-height. Bring the right leg over, touching the left hand. Keep both hands and both shoulders on the floor. Bring the right leg back into position and repeat, this time bringing the left leg over, touching the right hand. (See fig. 42.)

Double your knees up under your chin and hold them there with your locked arms. Roll over and touch one knee to the floor; then roll to the opposite side, touching that knee to the floor. (See fig. 43.)

HELP

The length of time you will need extra help depends on your speed of recovery and the general state of your health. A week is a pretty short time; ten to fourteen days is better. Perhaps you can get by after the first week with a part-time helper who can come in and take over the household chores.

ADVICE

Whatever else you may lack as a new mother you will suffer from no shortage of volunteer experts on the care and upbringing of your new baby. Well-meaning as they usually are, their suggestions may not be appropriate for your baby. Remember, your doctor has taken care of hundreds of babies for every one produced by your neighbors and friends. He has a scientific understanding of babies and their needs. Follow his advice, not your neighbor's. He will give you reliable general information and indicate any special conditions for your own infant.

VISITORS

Keep visitors to a minimum and invite only those people with whom you can be relaxed and comfortable. The others can wait until you've had a chance to rest, to get to know your baby and your job. The whole idea is for you to try to get back to an easy and regular life without too much emotional upset.

When people come to visit, by all means let them see the baby. But that is all. Make it understood that visitors may "see" but "not touch." You may be laughed at for treating your child like a zoo inmate, but it pays off. As discussed earlier, your young baby is highly susceptible to infections. By cutting down the number of people who handle him, you cut down the chances of his exposure to a variety of illnesses.

No one with a fresh cold, not even a grandparent, should hold the baby or go into his room. Not even your own mother should pick up a newborn without first washing her hands. Don't let anyone—including yourself—kiss your baby on the lips. No one should lean over your baby's crib and cough or talk.

FATHER'S ROLE

As a new father, you may find yourself facing problems of adjustment just as your wife is. You may be disturbed by loss of freedom, by your increased responsibilities—financial and otherwise. In addition, you may feel isolated, left out of this rearranged household of yours. You might try to get back into the swing of things by involving yourself in some of the aspects of your baby's care. Certainly you will feel awkward and out of place if you have never done any of this before. But as time goes on you will find that your positive involvement with your child is a great big plus in your enjoyment of life. If you are a father who shares actively in the care of his baby, who plays with him, bathes him, carries him around, the bond between you becomes very strong.

Don't let yourself be shoved aside. Don't take second place to the practical nurse, the relatives, or any other helpers. This baby is a very important product of you and your wife. You both have top priority. Perhaps this can be a valuable learning time for the two of you.

A father's closeness and friendliness to his children has a vital effect on their characters and lives. It is well to start early so that you can learn together. You should not assume a mother's role, just as a mother should not have to be a father to the children. But you stand in contrast to his mother from the very start of the baby's life. Together, you provide a balanced view of the world. Children need both a "mothering" person and a "fathering" person.

7.

Your Other
Children
and the Baby

Perhaps your newborn baby is not your only child. What about the older child or children in your family? The two-child family group often has the most difficulties. The first child has had center stage to himself. Now he has to share. Subsequent children usually have less of a problem in adjusting.

The ages of your other children will play a large part in determining both their response to the new baby and your approach to the problem. One overall observation: If you worry too much about preventing jealousy in your older child, you actually defeat yourselves. You show so much guilt and uneasiness about the new baby that you make your older child feel anxious, too. An appeasing, apologetic attitude on his parents' part actually cues him to be jealous and apprehensive.

Your child from one to two years has a memory like a sieve. If you tell him months ahead of your new baby's arrival that "Mommy will go to the hospital and have a baby," he will only forget it. Since he will be concerned about a separation from his mother, do start preparing him one to two weeks ahead of your due date. Say it simply and use the same words each time. "Mommy will be going to the hospital. She is going to have a tiny baby. Then she and the new baby will come home."

Plan to have someone your child knows come into your home to care for him. If father can stay at home and have some familiar person come in to do the housework, this is of course best. The child will be in his familiar bed and surroundings, even if his mother is gone. If a new housekeeper can come a few days ahead or drop in for several visits before your actual departure, this will make the whole process smoother.

If he is to be taken away from his home for the period of your absence, your child should be with people he knows and likes. It is best if he has already spent some time in the other home before being separated from his own. Whoever is taking care of him should know him, his schedule, his favorite toys, words, the signs he uses, and so forth.

Anxiety about separation from his mother is a basic fear at this age, although he may not show it openly. Some extra cuddling and attention will help. Father should be available as much as possible. If both his important people are taken away at the same time your child can really feel abandoned, and it will effect his attitude toward his mother and the new baby.

When you do come home, try to arrange to have father bring the new baby in unobtrusively while you are greeting your first child and reestablishing your relationship with him. Don't be surprised if he is reluctant to forgive and forget. After all, you did leave him—even though he had a good time in your absence!

Try to avoid disrupting your older child's life any more than necessary. If he is to be moved to a bed or a different room to make a place for the baby, make the shift well before the baby arrives. Don't try to push him into more grown-up ways so that he can take care of himself when you have your hands full with the new one. Pressure will just make him balk.

The two-to-five-year-old is the most likely to feel angry and resentful. He needs to feel part of what is going on and to get answers to his questions. This is a normal time for him to ask about the origins of babies. If he asks the common question, "Where do babies come from?" he definitely doesn't need a stork story or one about a doctor's black bag. He needs to be told "from inside their mothers." Give him the facts adequate for his age, no more and no less.

You can explain to him that you don't know if the baby will be a boy or a girl. Pictures of newborn babies will help him to realize that "his baby" will be small and helpless, so that he won't expect a full-grown playmate.

As with the younger child, prepare your two-to-five-year-old for your impending departure for the hospital, and make the same type of arrangements for your absence. Separation from the mother is less anxiety-producing for this age group. If he is already well established at a nursery school, home changes may be less upsetting for him. But don't throw this experience plus a new baby at him at the same time, or he will just feel he isn't wanted at home.

While you are in the hospital you can maintain daily telephone contact with him. Father can also relay details to him about you, the hospital, and the baby.

When you and your baby come home, follow the procedure already suggested for the younger child. Try not to have the new baby around while you greet your child, and talk about how fine it is to have the family together again and the things that he did while you were away. After this he may ask to see the baby, or there may be a natural lull when the new baby can be mentioned. Whatever his reaction, accept it as the normal thing. You don't have to force the baby on him. If he isn't much interested, leave well enough alone. If he wants to touch and examine the baby, you can help him. Show him how you hold the baby. Indicate where the family can kiss him to show their affection.

In the early weeks, try to keep your older child's routines much the same as usual as far as bath time, eating, bedtime, and play time. Insofar as you can do so without too much strain, try to care for the baby when your firstborn is occupied elsewhere. When he is present, let him help if he wants to. He can bring a diaper or a clean sheet, or hold some article of clothing while you are dressing the baby. But there is an element of danger in this. He may overestimate his ability with the baby once he has helped. He may decide to take him for a walk, give him a bath, or feed him. So be watchful. Set limits for him. He may safely hold the baby when he is sitting down, preferably on the floor.

Don't use the same songs, the same pet names, or any of your older child's toys for the new baby. If he offers them himself, fine.

Many of the tight moments with your older child will center about the feeding of the new baby. This is especially true about breast-feeding. Be as natural as you can. The child can be told that the breast produces milk for the baby just as it did for him when he was little and that this is the way a baby eats to begin with. Tell him this whether he asks questions or not. When he hangs about as you are getting ready to nurse the baby is a good time. He may want to push in closely. Set limits on his interfering with nursing, but don't prohibit him from being present. Read to him or talk with him. Remember special times when he was the central attraction. He will like sharing the memory. He can be better occupied elsewhere if he seems upset by the whole procedure.

Don't be shocked if he wishes to nurse at the breast too. Explain that breast-feeding is for tiny babies only. It is not for big boys who take their milk from a cup. Emphasize his maturity, but don't lose your patience if he doesn't always respond. If you are bottle-feeding, he may ask for a bottle. He usually cures himself after a taste or two. You will have to set limits; if you are too lenient you will force him back into bottle-feeding.

Understanding your older child's resentment of the baby is no guarantee that you can avoid it entirely. You will find it can be a problem in spite of your enlightened point of view. Your child may demonstrate his anger by taking direct action against the baby. You do need to keep him from hurting the baby, but you can indicate that you know how he feels and that you love him just the same. Or he may try to substitute himself for the new baby on the theory that since you wanted a baby so badly he had better be one too in order to be acceptable. He may go back to crawling, messing his pants, asking for a bottle, using baby talk. Or he may show you how angry he is by suddenly becoming very destructive. Perhaps he will be so hurt and angry that he tries to punish his family by withdrawing into silence. Actually you will find it easier to deal with the child who expresses his emotions than with the one who bottles them up.

Give him attention and praise whenever you can. Let him be the star if possible. When he is helpful, thank him, but be sure he doesn't get the feeling that he is just there as an errand boy. Let him see your pride in him and what he is. His father should do so, too. He needs to know that both his parents enjoy talking to him and being with him.

Interfere as little as possible with the relationship between your older child and the baby. If you think he is squeezing the baby too hard but the baby doesn't seem to mind, let it go.

Give your firstborn a chance to let off steam. Perhaps he can have a wooden block and mallet to pound and a hammer with nails to drive. Dolls can help both boys and girls to act out their feelings.

Sooner or later your preschooler will have to reach some

kind of acceptance of the baby. If this can be done without any more supervision from you than absolutely essential, it will probably go more quickly and smoothly.

The school-age child probably adjusts more easily to a new baby, though he, too, may have problems. He is developing more outside interests and companions. His mother and father are becoming less and less the center of his world. He may resent or be irritated by the new addition to the family. A new baby is a lot of work for everyone. Try to avoid putting off things for the school-age youngster because of the baby. Too many answers like "Just a minute," or "Not now, I am busy with the baby," can produce trouble where none might have existed. Some school-age children will be eager to help with the baby. Others wish to have no responsibility as far as the new one is concerned.

Teen-agers are an interesting group to observe in relation to a new baby. Some of them will have been particularly affronted by mother and father demonstrating their youthful vigor in producing another offspring. These are the ones who have the "Oh, mother, how could you?" attitude. Other teen-agers will be very enthusiastic. These are the ones who make the best substitute mothers and baby-sitters.

You mustn't go so far in protecting your older child, of course, that you neglect the legitimate needs of your baby. In some homes everyone is so busy protecting everyone else's psyche that the baby takes a back seat. This means that he spends the first weeks of his life, when he is most susceptible to infections, being lugged around by kids with runny noses, picked up and kissed by visitors, and even licked by the family dog. You don't need to feel guilty toward your older child when you insist on reasonable restrictions and adequate protection for the baby. Your attitude should be a very natural one. You love the baby and you want him to be safe and happy.

Fortunately, in the early weeks your baby sleeps most of the time, and it is during these early weeks that your older child needs the most attention. If during this period you can give him enough reassurance, he will gradually get used to the baby and begin to build a more constructive relationship.

8.

Grandparents

Grandparents can be a blessing to both grandchildren and parents. Affectionate grandparents increase your child's feelings of security. If he is important to others as well as his parents, he has added assurance of his value. The new mother can get a great deal of help and support from the grandmother about baby care. If their relationship is a mature and secure one, the new mother can ask for advice without any thought of being belittled or dominated. If what she hears doesn't seem applicable, she tactfully turns it down, without argument. For her part, grandmother is pleased to be asked for her opinion and advice. While she doesn't push her views about baby care, and is considerate about the frequency of her suggestions, she isn't afraid to offer an unsolicited comment if she thinks it necessary, nor is she upset if not all her suggestions are accepted.

In most families the relationships between the generations are not as ideal as the one described above. There can be mild to severe disagreements about the new baby, particularly about a first child. While more of such conflicts seem to center around the new mother and her mother or mother-in-law, the new father and grandfather can also play a part. There are, after all, six adults involved here, which allows ample opportunity for all sorts of clashes.

One source of possible conflict is the difference in the relationship between child and parent and child and grandparent. The grandparent is in the highly enviable position of having all of the fun and none of the responsibilities of parenthood, none of the burdens of day-to-day care and discipline. The grandparent has no other duty than to enjoy the grandchild. This is the reason grandparents and grandchildren can have such special, mutually rewarding relationships. But sometimes it can also create problems, such as spoiling.

One such problem involves the grandparents' role as gift-

181

bearers. Their aim is to give pleasure to the child, but the appetite-destroying sweets and the overwhelming number of complex and frustration-producing toys they often bring become your problem. If you can arrange for the nonedible, simple toy gift, given at reasonable intervals, you will have achieved a major victory.

You may have been lured into another of the possible problem situations: using grandparents as baby-sitters. It seems so simple! Here are two perfectly good grandparents just panting to take care of your baby. You may think they want to give you a chance for some pleasure, and they do. But your after-party homecoming will be a mixed pleasure indeed if you're confronted by a wide-awake, tired, unhappy young fellow exhausted by the demands made on him by his grandparents.

Your problems can really be compounded when both sets of grandparents are available and indulge in a tug-of-war as to who will come first with the baby. This frantic competition can be corralled or slowed down if parents stand fast together. Each will have to set limits on his own parents.

Conflict can spring from the relationship between parent and grandparent. This is a very subtle, all-encompassing sort of thing. It can be very obvious, or complex and hidden. The mother-daughter-child triangle can be one of the most ticklish of human relationships. Unresolved problems of dependency and competition between mother and daughter can produce all sorts of tensions and conflicts when a new baby comes on the scene.

The most obvious example of dependency is the new mother who clings to her own mother. She runs back home to consult her on the most trivial problems or conflicts in her own home. For her, a grown-up married womanhood is never achieved. A stable, emotionally mature home situation is never reached for her child.

The new mother may have achieved some independence after her marriage, but with the tensions created by a new baby she wants to run back to her little-girl role. At first she seeks help from her mother. Only later does she reject it, with hurt feelings all around.

A less obvious kind of dependency occurs when the new mother depends on her mother for help with the children apparently only for practical reasons. Her hidden anger at her own dependency will come out as constant disagreement. The baby is the battlefield.

In some situations, the more dependent the daughter has

been, the harder her struggle to discard the relationship. This leads to her over-reacting to minor frictions. There is a touchiness about the way she reacts to everything that suggests that she is still dominated by her mother.

Unconscious feelings of rivalry with her mother, dating back to the daughter's adolescence, intensify the problem. She may carry the battle to grandmother without waiting for any sign of disapproval on her mother's part. She is the aggressor in making the conflict. She views all grandmother's opinions on child care, whether sound or not, as old-fashioned, opinionated, or meddlesome. She is very adamant about the infallibility of her own views. She may carry permissiveness with her child to an extreme—delaying toilet training, allowing a poor eating routine. At heart she may not believe in such extremes, but with them she accomplishes several things. She upsets the grandmother and gets even with her for past disapproval. She proves how old-fashioned and out-of-date her mother is and what a modern, therefore superior, mother she herself is. Her behavior implies how inadequate the grandmother was in her role as a parent.

Such difficulties are increased when in-law problems are added. Rivalry between a wife and her mother-in-law is not uncommon. When a wife has been engaged in a contest with her mother-in-law for the affection and loyalty of her husband, the stage is set for trouble when a baby arrives. A mother-in-law may constantly disapprove of her son's wife—her appearance, her outside activities, her housekeeping, her attitudes, and now her methods of baby care. The new mother recognizes the nature of the contest. She is highly sensitive to any suggestions on the part of her mother-in-law; to accept them would merely strengthen the grandmother's belief in her inadequacy. Even when there are no genuine differences of opinion about the grandchild's care, it is often used as another battleground in the running war.

The dominating grandmother can pose a real problem for any young couple. It takes great understanding, patience, and strength of character to deal with such a person, whether it is one's own mother or a mother-in-law. One of the main problems here is the inability of the young, vulnerable mother to stand up to an interfering grandmother. Her lack of confidence, her sensitivity to criticism, and her fear of making the grandmother angry make her a perfect victim. The grandmother also knows how to make her feel guilty by taking any difference of opinion as a personal affront.

The best solution in any of these conflict areas is the one that eliminates the frictions. This calls for emotional maturity from the adults involved. None of the conflicts described can be resolved unless there is some degree of emotional maturity to call upon.

It can be difficult for an uncertain young mother to free herself from a dominating grandmother, but it can be done. If you have doubts as to your own methods of baby care, discuss them with your husband and pediatrician. When you have developed confidence in your own opinions you will be better able to speak up for yourself. A matter-of-fact, confident approach is usually the most effective way to convince a grandmother that you have the courage of your convictions. Listen to what she has to say, but don't get into long arguments.

Remember that it requires extraordinary flexibility on the part of any grandmother to be able to accept the changes made in child-care practices over the last twenty to forty years. When she was a young mother, it was believed that to feed a baby off-schedule caused indigestion, diarrhea, or spoiling. Regularity of the bowels was a cornerstone of health. Early toilet training was necessary. Now grandmother is suddenly expected to accept the idea that flexibility in feeding schedules is not only permissible but desirable and that toilet training should not be imposed against the child's will. It is hard to make these ideas sound drastic to a new mother today. To understand grandmother's alarm you would have to imagine some fantastic new advice about child care, such as feeding a newborn baby fried pork or bathing him in ice-cold water.

Both of you, the new mother and new grandmother, must recognize that people have differences of opinion. It is also a fact that two women who in actual practice would handle a child about the same can still argue endlessly about theory.

So to young parents: Remember not to live with grandparents—either in your home or theirs. Don't expect them to give regular help as nurses, housekeepers, or sitters. They are usually happier to have it that way. Remember, too, that for the most part grandparents try to give you the best that they have. All interference is not malicious, even if it is ill-timed or ill-advised. Try to decide what is helpful and what is not. And bear in mind that sympathy, courtesy, and respect are musts in a good relationship between parents and grandparents.

9.

Crying
and
Rhythmic Patterns

CRYING

As new parents you expect your baby to cry. Nevertheless, you may be surprised to find out how loud and long
he can do it—and how disturbing it can be. Babies do cry
a tremendous amount, even healthy, "good" babies. A
baby's cry is hard to ignore. It is loud and wholehearted.
It competes with other sounds and drowns them out. The
crying baby is completely occupied with what he is doing.
He uses his whole body at first. His chin quivers, his lips
tremble, maybe his arms and legs shake. His fists are tight
and waving about. He takes big, sobbing breaths and lets
out loud, piercing shrieks.

If your new infant's crying bothers you a great deal, you
will have a hard time being a good parent. Crying is like
traffic noise, rain, or the endless chatter of people you don't
like—unless you learn to take it in stride, it can make
you become irritable enough to act unwisely. The less your
baby's crying annoys you, the better off he is.

CAUSES OF CRYING

In the early months the baby cries in much the same way
for different reasons, which makes it harder to determine

the cause. You can say that there is always a reason behind your baby's crying, but this doesn't mean you will always find it or that you spend all your time looking for it. It does mean that you will look for the obvious cause of the trouble.

Sour tastes, gagging, sneezing, or pain sensations can produce tears, but your baby may not cry at the same time. Tears do not have the same emotional meanings in children as they do in adults. When a baby cries with tears, it just means that his body is able to produce tears. Crying during the early weeks of life, with or without tears, has no great association with emotion.

Do consider crying as a signal—a way of talking. At first it is the baby's only way to let you know something about how he feels. He is able to let you know about what displeases him long before he can indicate his pleasure in anything. But healthy, contented babies don't cry for extremely long periods of time—certainly not for an entire day or even the greater part of a day. So you have one lead here—prolonged crying in your baby is a sign that something is wrong. You need to look for the cause. The age of your baby makes some difference in what you will look for. In these early months his crying primarily reflects body or physical needs or hurts. In the second six months, crying more often indicates emotional needs.

Soon after birth, your baby's crying begins to serve as a response or a reaction to his body needs. As his demands are met and his needs are satisfied, you condition him. His crying becomes a learning process. He learns from your response. His cries become more and more purposeful.

What are some of the more specific causes of crying? Let's examine them.

PERSONALITY? One baby may cry as though he is deeply wounded—and all he has is a wet diaper. Another smiles happily at you with overloaded diapers. One fellow waits patiently while you get his food ready. Another can't wait a second after his stomach says it is empty. This doesn't mean that you can regularly blame your baby's disposition for his crying. But each baby has a built-in set of traits. After a while you will get to know what kind of baby you have. Also keep in mind that babies have good days and bad days—just as you do.

Often the baby who cries a great deal for no reason is

just an active, vigorous type of baby letting off steam. The quieter baby spends more time lying awake and sucking on his finger.

There is also the crybaby type of infant. I don't like to call him this, but I don't have any better name for it. After about six to eight weeks, a new kind of crying begins in a particular kind of baby. This is crying for other than his immediate needs. It is a reflection of the baby's personality. It is an habitual crying which is uniform, weak, lacks variation, and has many pauses. It calls for no immediate action but perhaps shows a need for reassessing handling procedures.

PHYSICALLY INSECURE? Your newborn may find being out in the world an upsetting affair at first. In the early weeks he may have a feeling of physical insecurity. His sense of safety in your uterus ended with his birth. This sudden change affects prematurely born or small infants in particular. Old-fashioned swaddling may help such a baby. (Look ahead to *The First Month*, "Baby-Care Routines.")

STARTLED? A young baby's startle-reflex cry can be set off by very mild stimulation. (Check back to *The Newborn*, "Reflexes.")

HUNGRY? The commonest and most important cause of crying in the young baby is hunger. During the first two months his crying is automatic when he is hungry. After this time he begins to replace crying with fussing. He has longer intervals of quiet as well. He shows interest in other ways of acting. Other things besides hunger determine his behavior. His crying by this time doesn't last as long. It occurs less frequently. Hunger crying has almost disappeared by four months. Morning may be the only period you will see it.

A well-established hunger cry is seldom a spasmodic, jerky cry. Typically it begins loud, gradually dies down, then stops altogether. After a brief pause it not only starts all over again but usually grows even louder than before. Often it goes hand in hand with loud screaming. The baby's agitation and movements increase as he goes on. Of all the infant cries, the hunger cry is the most nasal. As it grows louder it becomes shrill. During the first weeks it is usually accompanied by sucking movements with quivering of the mouth, chin, or cheeks.

INDIGESTION? Indigestion is one of those vague terms that can mean almost anything. It is used to describe hunger pains, colic, and fussy periods, among other things. What has been called indigestion can be caused by an immature gastrointestinal system, an immature nervous system, an intolerance for carbohydrates or fat, a food allergy, or flatulence, which is just gas. Most of the conditions described as indigestion seem to fall in the group of colic conditions or of hunger.

THIRSTY? This isn't too common a reason at first. It could be a very common cause after his early months. It is always worth a try. Offer your small baby a little sweetened water. Offer your older baby fruit juice.

TOO HOT? TOO COLD? The former is more likely than the latter. He may feel a little warm and start to fuss. He gets hotter by the minute from his crying exercise. Then he really has a reason to sound off. Don't overdress him and make him perspire. When you put him to bed he may feel just right to your touch, but a full stomach and a snug bed may overheat him. His temperature changes are very rapid. Feel his body, not his hands or feet, to check his temperature.

IS HE HAVING A BOWEL MOVEMENT? Your baby usually cries before, during, or after a bowel movement. Many a young baby will start fussing half an hour before he has any gas to pass or any stool to get rid of. He does this less as the weeks go by. Especially during his first six weeks he may cry when his diapers are wet or soiled. (This may cause crying in his sleep, too, which can be confused with bowel-movement fussing.) After this initial time many babies accept a soiled diaper with nonchalance. A diaper rash or other irritation can also cause crying.

Your baby may cry when he urinates or is about to do so. He may not like the feeling of his full bladder. He can be mildly bothered by passing his urine. If the tip of his penis is irritated at the opening, he may have some pain. Use Vaseline liberally until the irritation heals.

UNCOMFORTABLE? He may be feeling mild discomfort about something—his position or something else. Is his bed uncomfortable? Some babies will fuss when the sheets are cold, wet, or wrinkled. Is there too much noise or light? Is he fussing to get into a favorite position? Is he physically restrained so that he can't move his arms and legs? Check his position, his clothing and bedclothes.

ANNOYED? As mentioned before, a new mother trying to do everything just right at feeding time may fuss over details until she has her sleepy baby thoroughly irritated. Poking a bottle nipple or the breast in his mouth just to get a little more in, wiping too vigorously or too slowly at the little dribble from his mouth, changing a diaper put on only a few minutes before, adjusting his clothing—all these things serve only to rouse your baby from his sleepy contentment.

FATIGUED? Overtiredness is a common cause of anger crying. If you have waited too long to get your baby to bed, or exposed him to too much stimulation—too many voices, too much handling—he may begin to cry and take a long time to settle down.

LONELY AND BORED? The newborn may sense the strangeness of his new surroundings, but he doesn't know enough to miss anything in particular. When the baby is older, he knows very well what he misses. If he is closed away alone when he isn't sleepy, he protests his separation from people and household activities. His attention span is so short that he needs a variety of interests. The older baby left alone with his toys may very soon sound off about your neglect.

The basic feature that distinguishes his cry of loneliness is his reaction to handling. Crying from hunger or discomfort doesn't stop for any length of time when you pick him up. The bored, lonely baby stops crying as soon as you handle him. His cry of boredom can be recognized by noticing what produces it. It often has a sharp, staccato pattern. It may carry an overtone of a whine.

In the older baby, night crying during the first year indicates not fear of the dark, but a wish for companionship. Familiar surroundings, or things such as his own hands and feet, give him something to focus on. To him darkness is emptiness, so a very soft light may help. He will be a year or more before darkness will frighten him.

From three months on, boredom is a more and more important cause for crying. And the baby's body and mind develop, his needs develop also. If his needs are satisfied, you will find him crying less as he grows older. The older he is, the more he wants to see and hear what is going on. He cries when the family leaves the room. Try to put him where he has an opportunity to see and experience.

While it is important to respect his growing abilities and give him what he needs, keep it clearly in mind that this does not mean that you are required to give him constant attention. If he is regularly overstimulated in his early weeks, he will be much more susceptible to boredom later. Just as every baby requires care and protection, he also requires some setting of limits. With a less easily adaptable baby you may have to be quite definite in setting these limits. His development benefits from a little time to himself, a few islands of quiet which permit him to look and listen and feel on his own.

REFLECTING FEELINGS? Your baby is sensitive to the moods and feelings of the people around him. Fatigue and tension are contagious. He may cry because you are tired, tense, and cross. If you think there may be a chance of this with your baby, you had better take a good look at your home situation.

SICK? Crying can be an early sign that your baby is coming down with a cold or some other infection, especially if he is usually happy and contented.

SETTLING DOWN? Some babies have to fuss to settle down to sleep. They spend ten to fifteen minutes fussing, then are gone into the Land of Nod.

CYCLIC (RECURRENT) FUSSING

There are certain kinds of crying during the first three months that can be grouped together under the term cyclic or recurrent fussing. The differences between them are a matter of degree, so that I have described them as normal fussing, P.M. fussing, and paroxysmal (colic) fussing.

NORMAL FUSSING. Most babies have regular crying periods that seem to be part of their daily living. This can be true of any baby, whether he is happy or unhappy, passive or hyperactive. It comes whether his mother is anxious or calm, soft-voiced or a screamer. This regular, recurrent, or cyclic crying is not associated with any real physical problem or trouble. It may serve a useful purpose in his development.

There are differences in babies. The quieter baby spends more of his awake time looking about and sucking or waving his hands. The more vigorous one spends his awake periods in more active behavior like crying and exercising his head, arms, and legs. Some babies need a more vigorous activity pattern, others are more sensitive to accumulated tension.

There is a relationship between the total amount of crying and finger-sucking in the young baby. A typical light-fussing baby sucks his finger for a longer period each day than the heavy-fusser. Heavy-fussers cry three to four hours daily but suck only for one hour a day. Light-fussers cry one hour a day but spend two to four hours sucking. The really intense fusser cannot substitute sucking for crying. He is not able to discharge his energy and tension in any way but by crying and vigorous physical activity in his early weeks. A finger-sucking, less fussy baby is able to obtain satisfaction with this activity rather than crying or movement. This may be related to his ability in his hand-to-mouth action.

In his early weeks his fussing is irregular and scattered during the twenty-four hours as his living settles down into some pattern. By three weeks his fussing is less scattered but has about three peaks of more concentrated fussing activity. By six weeks he has brought his scattered crying periods together into a morning and evening period, usually with the evening time the more intense. This is usually the time of the greatest complaining. Although he continues two periods of fussing at ten weeks they are of less intensity. He concentrates his major activity in the evening time. By twelve weeks his fussing is subsiding to a total of an hour or so a day, or has even disappeared. At each of these intervals the baby is developing more outlets for his energy which sucking or crying had satisfied in earlier periods. He can reach out to his surroundings in more ways to make contact and relieve tensions.

P.M. FUSSING. When the usual type of baby fussy period is replaced by a more noticeable and bothersome type of crying, it may be labeled P.M. fussing. The name indicates the time of day your baby picks to sound off most vigorously. He concentrates his efforts at one period of the day.

Unfortunately his most intense fussing occurs more often in the late afternoon (4 to 6 P.M.) or early evening periods (7 to 10 P.M.) when most households are at the low point of the day. Father and Mother and the older children are tired.

The description of the usual P.M. fussing period is as follows: At about the same time each day, often after an adequate feeding, your baby wakens from a sound, contented sleep. He begins to whimper in a fussy, discontented fashion. He sounds unhappy. It sounds like an uncomfortable hunger cry, but you know that he has been well-fed. If you pick him up he will burp, because fussing or crying has made him swallow air, but this is not the cause of his fussing. It is not caused by any severe distress, even when it is loudest. Nothing you do helps for long, although you will temporarily halt it with most anything you do. He is not hungry. He will refuse food or take only a small amount. He is not wet or dirty. He won't suck his fingers. A pacifier doesn't help. If you hold or rock him, walk the floor with him, sing to him, he slows down briefly. If you put him down, he starts all over again. This more concentrated type of fussing episode appears after four weeks. The duration of his P.M. fussy period gets a little longer as he grows older, to reach a peak at eight to ten weeks. Then it shortens and finally ceases about twelve to fourteen weeks.

PAROXYSMAL (COLIC) FUSSING. The more severe and dramatic form of fussing is the paroxysmal fussing syndrome called colic. "Colic" is a catch-all word, a wastebasket in which you can throw any kind of crying. It means different things to different people. Some consider it colic when a baby awakens at night, fusses, and eats poorly. To others, a baby is colicky only if he cries uninterruptedly for a number of hours, seven days a week. The name comes from the long-standing idea that crying is due to intestinal cramping, but there is no actual evidence the baby is suffering this kind of pain. He does have long periods of hard crying, air swallowing, screaming, drawing up his legs, with red face, hard and tense abdomen, gas passing but no evidence of any organic disease or physical abnormality. He continues to cry after he's picked up. In spite of all this, he gains weight and progresses normally in other respects.

Colic can occur in either boy or girl babies or in one or all babies of the family. The heavy-fusser baby is probably a colicky baby if his reaction is the violent kind. He is colicky because of the intensity of his response. His crying increases in duration and intensity until his sixth week. From about two weeks of age he cries about four hours a day before it lessens. Maneuvers to relieve him don't help. He acts as if he is under great pressure. After the third month, even severe colic crying lessens, and ceases by the fourth month. This is why it is called three-months' colic, although it can end before three months or last longer.

After the first six months, crying decreases considerably, but the reasons for it increase.

REFUSING SLEEP? Bedtime crying in the older baby may come from a number of causes or a mixture of them. The wonderful world of wakefulness has a good hold on him by this time. He gets tremendous satisfaction from new skills. He has contact with people. When he laughs and babbles, they share in his fun. Even when he is tired and sleepy, he may be too wound up to let go. In dealing with going-to-bed crying, it helps to keep in mind that the older baby isn't as independent as he seems. The same kind of loving and living that appealed to him earlier will help him now. If he has trouble letting you go out of his sight, he may need some substitute comfort like his teddy bear or favorite blanket or toy.

DREAMING? Your baby may start dreaming in his second six months of life. You will find it difficult to be certain about this. Eliminate other causes and then relax. You can't stop him from dreaming, but you can ease off on his daytime activities. See that he gets more rest. Tiredness may be a cause.

TEETHING? Teething is blamed for so many things during infancy that I am reluctant to let you blame anything on this natural event. Your baby can be uncomfortable as his teeth are coming up in his gums. You can rub the gums vigorously with your finger to give some relief. A hard rubber bone or toy for him to chew on will help. Aspirin quiets this kind of discomfort. But remember—aspirin is to be swallowed, not rubbed on the gums. Check with your doctor as to the amount.

STRANGERS? When your baby is seven or eight months, or possibly younger, he may surprise or embarrass you by suddenly crying and clinging to you at the sight of an unfamiliar face—or even one that is familiar. A new place or voice can set him off, too. His crying is "developmental," or a step in growing up. He is beginning to know the differences between people and things. He clings tightly to you to make certain his safe home base is there. He cries when anyone other than his mother comes toward him. Even his grandma may suddenly seem strange to him, although a few weeks before he cooed happily under her management. A new sitter may need to get acquainted with a baby of this age before she takes over.

UNHAPPY? After six months emotional crying is seen. This can be the result of anger, jealousy, a bid for attention, crying when another child cries, or similar feelings. The amount of this kind of crying is always increased by fatigue, boredom, and hunger.

FRUSTRATED? The second half of his first year produces many changes in his crying. He will cry with greater feeling than he did earlier. He cries when any pleasant experience stops. He cries when there is any change from the usual. He has his likes and dislikes in food, clothing, and places.

Because he is so intensely single-minded about his interest of the moment, any frustration or blocking of his actions is hard for him to bear. He has no patience with any thwarting of his developing abilities. He wants to do the next thing he can do. Now it isn't just loneliness he cries about, but a chance to do. He puts tremendous effort into maneuvering himself to a strategic position and grabbing hold of something—and instantly someone takes it away from him or it slips away from his grasp! No wonder he cries. If he is learning to crawl or roll, he will cry if he is restrained or confined.

As you can see, frustration can be a frequent cause of crying. There's the leg-stuck-through-the-bars type of frustration, easy enough to take care of. A not-so-simple type for you to cope with is the crying your baby does when he has almost, but not quite, mastered a new skill. You may not be able to guess what he's fussing about. A few days later you will see his frown and tears suddenly give way to smiling pleasure. He has finally managed to roll over—or maybe sit up—all by himself!

His cry of anger is often hard to spot at the time of its appearance. It is generally tearless unless he carries it on for some time. Some of your baby's anger is unavoidable. Living and learning involve certain restrictions and disappointments for all of us.

HURT? The older baby is more active and more likely to have accidents. Crying may be due to a banged head, a fall, or some similar cause. It is a good idea to check and see what has happened. He probably needs your calm reassurance and a comfortable degree of sympathy. A cry of pain is shrill, loud, and lasting, or it is made up of short, single cries. This crying is interrupted by whimpering or groaning. The more severe the pain the longer it lasts and the higher the pitch.

WHAT TO DO ABOUT CRYING

It is comforting news, if you are having trouble interpreting your baby's cry language, that the first two or three months are the hardest. It is nice to know that even if you can only guess at the reason behind his fussing, trying to soothe him will by and large cut down and not increase his crying. Don't be afraid of spoiling him by answering his legitimate needs. It is more likely that your baby will get spoiled not when his cry is answered but when it is misunderstood or ignored.

When your baby cries, look first for hunger, then for pain or discomfort, then for fussing.

The manner of his cry is a further clue. Sharpness, loudness, high pitch, and long duration reflect a greater urgency than do his soft, low-pitched cries of short duration. Since any baby in these early weeks cries not only with his voice but with his face and whole body, the violence of his movements is a further clue to the seriousness of his crying. Keep in mind, as already noted, that some children make a greater fuss about a small matter than others do with great provocation.

When your baby is neither hungry nor in pain, you will have to judge the reason for the crying by noticing under what circumstances it appears. This is particularly true if it comes repeatedly under the same conditions.

To begin with, you don't seize your little one up in your arms every time he lets out a chirp. This may be the settling-down type of crying already mentioned. Wait at least ten minutes. If by then his crying has become a lusty demand for action, look the situation over. Try to determine if his crying falls under any of the causes discussed in this section.

Sometimes just your matter-of-fact "shush" may help him to control himself. Patting him and telling him how nice he is may soothe him. Avoid too much socializing if this is at the time of his normal fussing.

If his crying is of the normal fussing or paroxysmal type, then what can you do? Just as feeding is no answer if he is not hungry, neither is putting a pacifier in his mouth. It has been suggested as an answer to any type of crying your baby may do, but you have to take responsibility for more than this. If you feel he is asking for cuddling and human closeness, then sit and hold him and let him use the nipple. But it is dishonest to leave him to the cold mercies of a pacifier without holding him, in an effort to shut him up. Your non-sucking fusser refuses consolation from a pacifier anyway. Your sucking, nonfussing baby already has his own built-in pacifier, his thumb.

Check on your handling routine. As discussed previously, any approach you make to your baby should be quiet and relaxed. And don't annoy him by overhandling him.

Some families try motion routines—rocking, walking the floor, tossing, jiggling. Some babies respond to the sound of the radio, the TV, the vacuum cleaner, or other noises. The difficulty with motion routines in particular is that it is so much easier to start them than to stop them. Your baby doesn't want to give them up. Rocking, patting, car riding, or any other form of motion may certainly be used *briefly* to soothe the tired or unhappy baby, but I would suggest you don't start something you can't finish. Car riding is one form of motion treatment, but do you want to ride around for three hours every night for the first three months?

Switching feedings around, setting different bath hours, or making other schedule changes can be tried. My impression is that such changes don't make much difference.

A finger has been pointed at mothers as a cause—if not the main cause—of paroxysmal fussing. I think that there is no evidence for this. I would like to turn the finger in the other direction. There is no one type of mother who has a colicky baby. Calm or jittery, tense or relaxed, young or experienced, any mother can find herself faced with a baby who indulges regularly in paroxysmal fussing. It is not directly related to his mother's emotional makeup. Parental tension may aggravate colic symptoms, but it does not cause them.

Medications of many different types have been used. Lime water, barley water, peppermint water, or gruel are old standbys. Whiskey, paregoric, brandy, and opiates unfortunately have been used. Antispasmodic doses of belladonna, phenobarbital, and atropine have been used with varying success. If these are effective, then probably there has been some intestinal spasm. Enemas are used, but I would suggest this only rarely, if ever. It can start a pattern of dependency that can grow to unfortunate proportions. Generally, I would say no medications except under special circumstances, usually when there are other signs of intestinal difficulty. Sedatives should be reserved for special sleep problems. Don't give any medications without consulting with your pediatrician.

Perhaps you will just have to put your baby down and let him fuss. Keep in mind that his prolonged crying isn't your fault—it is common—it won't hurt him—it will stop.

It is difficult for most parents not to feel upset with a persistently crying baby. You may find yourself irritated enough to reject him to the point of refusing to help him as much as you can. Try to keep a calm, friendly attitude toward him and to avoid too much preoccupation and concern. You need time away from him to refuel your emotional engines. A baby-sitter who is prepared can tolerate your fussy baby for short intervals.

When your older infant cries a lot, look for troubles in the area of feelings as well as physical discomfort. See what you can do to relieve his loneliness, his frustration, his inability to do something.

RHYTHMIC PATTERNS

These are rhythmic motions of one sort or another, such as thumb-sucking, ear-pulling, blanket-stroking, or others, which the baby or young child uses as a release for built-up energy or tension. When you see them you can usually assume your baby is tired, bored, or tense. They are used most of all for inducing sleep. As he gets older and is better able to release his energy into physical activity and satisfactions from the outside world, they become less important to him.

These rhythmic activities are harmless, natural patterns of behavior for the baby and young child, but they can disturb parents who have been taught to view them as bad habits. Parents may also see them as indications that the child is insecure, maladjusted, or unhappy.

Many adults have some favorite rhythmical method to release tension or relieve anxiety. Smoking, gum-chewing, foot-swinging, and finger-tapping are examples. If you call these bad habits, then perhaps the child's rhythmic activities are bad. But why single out the child?

The fact is that these rhythmic activities are useful to your child at certain points of his life. If they are treated as normal patterns of growth, and not as sins, they will tend to disappear as your child develops and matures.

The course of a child's rhythmic activities will undoubtedly be influenced by the attitude his parents—and their relatives and friends—take toward them. If you consider them as normal devices your child uses to help him manage his tensions, you will act in one way. You will accept them calmly, courteously, and with consideration for his needs. Your relaxed, accepting attitude allows your child to develop out of them in his own good time.

If you consider such rhythm motions as bad and degrading habits, you will act entirely differently. You will approach your child with the idea that he has a bad habit that you must break him of. This then presents him with a nagging, punishing, tense parent who is out to change him. No matter how well intentioned you are, it is a destructive thing to do. It tells your child that he isn't acceptable as he is, which only increases his need for his rhythmic release.

THUMB-SUCKING

Thumb-sucking is such a common practice in babies under a year that it seems to be an almost universal method of satisfaction. The amount of it varies a good deal from one baby to another, but you will see a good deal of it in many babies after the first few months. It may start earlier. This type of sucking reaches its peak at about seven to twelve months. It appears partly as a stress-and-tension response and partly as a developmental process. It disappears as other things occupy the baby more. The amount and type of sucking your baby does depend on his temperament.

Thumb-sucking has been blamed for malformation of the jaws and teeth. In most cases such malformation is the result of heredity or poor nutrition. However, very persistent sucking after the first year can give one-sided irregularity of the jaw as the baby's thumb and finger push against it. More often it pushes the upper teeth out and the lower jaw in. They later fall back into line as growth occurs and sucking diminishes.

Changes in the jaw shape can be brought about by prolonged sucking beyond the time of the first set of teeth. It should be stressed again that prolonged sucking is more likely to occur when a child is urged to give it up before he is ready to do so.

If there is no interference, the usual pattern is that thumb-sucking is used off and on as tensions in the baby's life dictate. As he grows into more mature ways of acting, thumb-sucking drops out as a useful tool. You may see it at intervals up to four or five years, but it does not occur constantly or even very often, and produces no serious dental problem.

Many people dislike seeing a child sucking his thumb or finger. Just why is not entirely clear; it seems to be a cultural attitude. It used to be that a good baby was a baby who sucked his thumb. However, thumb-sucking came into ill repute some twenty or thirty years ago. It was falsely blamed as the cause for any one of a variety of disorders, from a curved back to adult digestive disorders.

Some of the prejudice about thumb-sucking may have to do with our cultural attitudes about manliness. Little girls can get away with thumb-sucking much longer than little boys, because it is considered to be babyish and little boys are supposed to be little men.

Certainly thumb-sucking is a baby habit. But if a baby habit persists beyond the age of babyhood, then you look for the reason for the habit, not at the act itself.

This brings mention of the so-called sucking instinct that you will hear about. This has been given great status in child care. Much like colic, it has been used to describe a variety of activities. My own feeling is that you will do best not to push this idea too hard. If you do, you may misinterpret what your baby is trying to tell you. As discussed under *Crying,* a small baby may or may not get pleasure out of sucking.

Sucking in the early weeks is generally associated with hunger. Thumb-sucking should really be considered as a normal type of reflex in the early weeks. The baby's rooting and sucking reflexes are the ones that he is using when his thumb or finger is sucked. As your baby develops, his mouth is used as an exploratory organ. After the first few weeks, everything has to be put in his mouth to be tested and identified. He does a lot of sucking, chewing, and mouthing on anything he touches. He moves out of this stage when he can use his eyes and hands for such exploring and identifying. Perhaps one might call this type of sucking an instinct, but I prefer to consider it as part of the baby's natural development in learning his world.

So approach this idea of a sucking instinct with caution. There is no set rule as to how much sucking any baby should or shouldn't do. There is no reason to believe that a baby won't get as much sucking as he needs with his own finger.

The pacifier, a rubber holeless nipple fastened to a disc, is supposed to be an answer to the sucking instinct. My feeling is that there are more objections to the use of the pacifier than there are good reasons for its use, particularly in view of its all-too-common misuse. I have tried to indicate that the rooting and sucking reflexes of your new baby are automatic responses centered about his need for food. He will suck on anything that hits his mouth. In my opinion, the commonest reason for your new baby to chew and suck vigorously is hunger. I believe this to be a much more common cause than is a sucking need. You are being unfair to your baby when you give him a pacifier instead of food. Just as you are unwise to pick him up every time he makes a peep, so you should not stick a pacifier into his mouth with every whimper.

As I have said earlier, if your primary aim is to comfort your baby, you can use the pacifier while you hold, talk to, and cuddle him—once you are certain he is not hungry. Most babies are done with this sort of thing by the time they are starting cup feeding. Mouthing is then becoming exploratory, and the pacifier is an interference. If the pacifier is discarded at that point, then the normal course of development is not obstructed. The real objection to the pacifier lies in the fact that parents continue to use it after the baby no longer needs it. Then a habit pattern is set up.

An argument advanced for the use of the pacifier is that the baby needs to suck other than at feeding time, that the pacifier gives you control over when he sucks because, unlike his thumb, you can remove the pacifier from his mouth. But, as I have stressed, thumb-sucking in the early weeks is a normal reflex used to indicate hunger or physical discomfort. After the first weeks, it is used as part of the normal developmental process of exploration. As another part of normal development many babies will use thumb-sucking as a rhythmic pattern, with or without other rhythmic activity. A thumb or finger is certainly more available for instant use to the baby. It is not a plug for his mouth when he sounds off. It is under his control as a built-in pacifier.

OTHER RHYTHMIC PATTERNS

Many rhythmic activities are often associated with other rhythmic patterns, most frequently with thumb-sucking. Examples are ear-pulling, navel-pulling, and lip-biting. So are hair-twirling, twisting, or pulling (although these activities in the older child are often associated with anger or frustration). Stroking or holding a soft object also falls into this group of comfort devices often associated with thumb-sucking. The favorite object can be anything, from a favorite blanket to a cloth doll. It is the baby's friend in times of stress, fatigue, or sleepiness. The satin edge of the blanket, the furry feel of his toy dog, the roughness of a Raggedy-Ann doll—these are samples of friends.

So many of these motions are a combination of activities. You may see a child lying in bed dreamily sucking his finger and twisting a lock of hair—or stroking his nose with one finger while another is thrust into his nostril as he sleepily sucks on the other fingers—or sucking one thumb while the other hand is stroking some other area or a blanket.

Tongue-sucking, tooth-grinding, head-banging and -rolling, body- and bed-rocking, and genital play are rhythmic patterns too, but are usually not associated with the thumb-sucking group of comfort devices. They seem complete and satisfying acts in themselves. They are all quite common in the first years, often accompanied by sound effects. They have no more long-lasting significance than the other rhythmic patterns already described.

Tongue-sucking is a rhythmic activity many parents are not aware of, since unlike thumb-sucking it isn't readily apparent. This tongue-sucking or tongue-thrusting often causes more orthodontic problems than finger-sucking. I know of no good way to prevent this even after the child gets older. When he is old enough to cooperate, speech exercises may help in retraining his tongue use. Tongue-sucking may be quite noticeable if the child rolls his tongue around in his mouth and makes a loud, sucking noise.

Tooth-grinding may happen during sleep, but the day-time type is very often associated with parents' reactions. The greater the parents' concern, the greater the child's grinding. Perhaps it can be called an attention-seeking device more often than a rhythmic pattern. You don't need to do anything about it except ignore it.

Head-rolling is the mildest of this group of rhythmic body patterns. The child may merely roll his head back and forth as he readies himself for sleep. This is very often done while he is lying on his back, and may be associated with some humming or singing to himself. His singing or noise-making may attract more attention than his head-rolling, which might go entirely unnoticed by itself.

Body-rocking is the same kind of pattern. The child does this on all fours rather than on his back. Body-rocking turns out to be bed-rocking as well, since it is a vigorous activity and usually quite noisy. The child gets up on his hands and knees and rocks back and forth. He may grunt at the same time. This activity appears at about eight months and may stop after a few months or last longer. It is an effective way to demolish a crib over a period of time. The crib literally goes to pieces with the heavy beating that it takes. The baby may rock hard enough to move the crib back and forth about the room. Don't try to stop the rocking itself, but you can muffle the sounds by using casters, or you can keep the crib in one place by putting a pad or rubber furniture cups under it.

Head-banging is an even noisier and more noticeable type of rhythmic action in this same group. It usually comes during the last half of the first year and is another activity found mostly at sleep time. It may be an attention-getting device too, since this is what it usually gets from parents. The baby bangs his head against anything hard that is handy, like his mattress or the side of the crib. The activity can go on anywhere from half an hour to four hours. The rhythm of the banging can be slow—about one bang every three to four seconds, or fast—about two bangs per second. It is usually combined with some other rhythmical activity like head-rolling, which usually comes first. Most youngsters are done with this type of rocking or motion activity by about three or four years. Some do keep it going in the school years. No permanent damage comes from it, and any attempt to stop it is futile or worse. Make it as noiseless as you can—and as safe, too. Bumper pads, heavy padding on hard surfaces, casters and rubber cups, pads on the outside of the crib, or bolts holding the crib to the wall will noiseproof the activity.

Genital exploration is rare before six months. The baby has to get some arm and hand control before he begins to explore the parts of his body. In grasping various objects, he grasps his genital area as just another act of curiosity. With this type of investigation there is no evidence of excitement or of any particular satisfaction.

Nail-biting, nervous twitches or mannerisms, fidgeting, playing with the fingers or hands, are tensional releases not seen in children under one year.

What to Do About Rhythmic Patterns

I indicated earlier that you should consider these activities as normal patterns during the early years of life. If you do so, they will follow a normal developmental course and disappear by three or four years, or at least become so inconspicuous that they bother no one. My recommendations for their treatment turn out to be a series of negatives for parents:

Don't use restraints or restrictive devices.

Don't use mittens or cuffs or apply bad-tasting stuff on his thumb.

Don't use mechanical aids.

Don't use dental appliances.

Don't nag or fuss.

Don't shame or ridicule.

Don't threaten, punish, or force.

All of these say don't make a big issue about something natural. However, you can do something positive. Attempt to ease his fatigue, boredom, and tension. It is better to get him to bed when he is tired than to try to correct what you consider a bad habit. If your baby does a great deal of any rhythmic activity, especially thumb-sucking, you need to look for causes. Hunger is the usual one in the very young baby. The older baby may need more attention in some area, or perhaps he is getting too excited and tired. He needs exercise and interesting activity, and he also needs a relaxed bedtime at a reasonable hour.

If thumb-sucking or any of these other rhythmic patterns has not largely disappeared by three or four years of age, then you have to look at the situation again. A child of four who uses thumb-sucking or any other rhythmic pattern often during the day as well as for long periods at night is trying to say something. Such prolonged rhythmic activity is an indication of worry or troubled living.

10.

Well-Baby Care

Every child should have the benefit of well-baby care. As its name indicates, this kind of medical care is for the healthy child. The emphasis of the pediatrician is on the prevention of illness. He looks for early signs of trouble in all areas—physical, mental, and emotional. By checking your baby on a regular, continuing basis, your pediatrician will get to know him well and be better able to estimate his progress.

You do not need to ask about fees and discuss budget terms with your pediatrician. Perhaps he has a year's care plan which furnishes complete well-child care for your baby during his first year.

Look for a well-baby clinic in your area if you feel you are unable to afford private care.

During his first year you will probably take your baby for checkups monthly for the first six months and every six weeks for the second six months. Special laboratory procedures will be carried out at intervals to estimate your baby's condition. Immunizing vaccines are given at appropriate times. Effective immunizations are available for smallpox (variola), whooping cough (pertussis), diphtheria, tetanus (lockjaw), poliomyelitis, measles (rubeola), mumps, and German measles (rubella).

Your pediatrician will want details about your baby's progress since the last examination, and will discuss with you any problems that have come up.

At the end of the examination you will be given advice about diet and general care, suggestions for any changes.

and prescriptions for any medications that may be necessary. You will also receive an explanation of new procedures to carry out.

When your pediatrician recommends something, try to understand clearly what he is saying and follow through on his recommendations. If it is difficult or inconvenient to do so, explain this frankly to him so that he can find a compromise or substitute. Feel free to ask questions if you are unclear or doubtful about some suggested procedure.

When you are ready to leave, stop at the receptionist's desk to make your next appointment. Between visits you can use the telephone for consultations with your pediatrician about problems that don't require an office visit but that do require professional advice.

Call your pediatrician promptly when you have questions, but try to do it during the day. He may have a telephone hour. Don't wait until the middle of the night to call after your baby has been ill all day. Don't wait until your pediatrician has left his office. He may need the office chart. He may want to see your baby in his office.

Call yourself. Don't try to have a third person give the information. Always identify your baby accurately, so the doctor knows whom he is talking about. Be prepared to tell him the baby's temperature and other significant details. Get his instructions accurately and write them down.

Call immediately any time you have an emergency. You will be told where to take your baby for further care.

As mentioned earlier, as you think of questions between visits, jot them down. This way you won't leave the doctor's office still groping for that important question. Any question, no matter how foolish you think it is, can be of concern if it remains unanswered. This book may help to answer some of your questions, so that you can make some decisions on your own without calling the pediatrician.

11.

The

First Year

From the moment your baby is conceived he undergoes a constant process of change. I have described the changes during his uterine life in the earlier part of the *Pregnancy* section, and those immediately after birth in the section on *The Newborn Baby*. In the following sections dealing with the first twelve months of life, I will describe each month's progress in the various areas of your baby's growth, as well as outline your continuing role in baby care.

You will notice that in each month's descriptions the areas of development often overlap. Changes in one area are linked to changes in another. That is because your baby's developmental plan can't be neatly divided into categories labeled "physical," "intellectual," "emotional." These are so closely allied they can't be easily separated. Your baby grows as a unit.

You will find that the most obvious measurement of his development in this first year is his physical progress. If this is satisfactory, then appropriate sensory and mental growth must also be all right. His motor accomplishments are very much influenced by his sensations and emotions. All his physical acts depend on his mental control as well as on his muscles and bones.

Although the baby will follow a certain *sequence* of developments—e.g., he will sit before he can walk—the *rate* of development varies from one child to the next and from one developmental area to another within the same child. When the baby will sit and when he will walk cannot be determined simply by age. While most infants will roughly conform to the norms for various ages, many will show unusual patterns.

A baby's rate of growth is often uneven and irregular. There are lulls and spurts. As he is actively learning one skill, he may stand still in another until the first is mastered. As an example, there can be a slowdown in his speech development when he is learning to walk.

The baby's developmental progress depends on the maturation of his central nervous system. This can't be speeded up by your training or by his practice. If he is ready, then training and practice can improve his performance. This readiness concept is demonstrated in the month-by-month descriptions. When your baby is ready to perform, you should encourage him. If he is not ready to perform, you should leave him alone. He can be considerably slowed down if he is ready for a particular skill and does not get to practice it. However, his central nervous system continues to mature, so that when the interference ends he makes up for lost time.

Thus the individual matures according to a biological pattern, but there must be adequate environmental stimulation so that he is able to organize various skills into action units so that he can use them.

The baby's growth process is from head to foot. You find him using his sucking reflex well before he can do much with his extremities. He gains head control, then neck and trunk muscle control, and finally gets strong enough to hold his head up and sit. You see him do a great deal with his hands before he is able to walk. He pulls himself forward with his hands and creeps before he actually gets up on hands and knees and crawls. (See pp. 371-372 for further discussion of creeping and crawling.) This extension of control follows the manner in which the nerve cells mature. Growth goes downward from the brain and out to either side around to his front from the spinal cord. Thus the face muscles develop first, since they are nearest to the brain. Then growth continues on down the body. One part of this type of growth is a bridging effect. As your baby goes from one phase to another, there is a carry-over of the old pattern into the new pattern before the new pattern becomes well set up.

In his newborn period the baby operates almost entirely by reflexes. His actions are for the most part involuntary. These primitive reflexes have to be lost before corresponding voluntary movements can come about. For example, his walking reflex will have to disappear before he is able to walk. These primitive reflexes come from the midbrain and spinal cord. His voluntary control comes from higher brain centers. These higher centers are where reasoning and other intellectual activity come from. There will be a gradual take-over of control by the brain proper during the months and years ahead. Actually, this take-over is never completely achieved, not even in the adult. This should be kept in mind so that you don't expect perfect behavior from young children. It just isn't possible. You should be aware when these changes from lower to higher levels of control come. In the sections following I have tried to describe them at each month's level.

Another pattern to notice is that your baby moves from a general body response to a more specific one. For instance, he first expresses pleasure with a massive general response when he sees something he wants. His eyes widen, his respiration increases, he pants with excitement, his legs kick, his arms wave around wildly. The older infant just smiles and reaches for the desired object, or makes a noise to attract your attention. He has lost the need for allover wiggling and jumping. He makes a specific response to get what he wants. The aimless arm and leg movements of the early months of the first year are replaced by specific movements of locomotion and manipulation in the later months. These are not completed until sometime after the first year.

In his intellectual and emotional growth, your baby shows the same kind of growth by succession. His development has pattern and shape to it, just as his physical growth does.

Consider your baby as being in the middle of a rapid growth period during this first year. He is constantly learning. He will show an extraordinary ability to learn by experience. He may fumble a good deal, but in his first few months he will start to show his abilities. He will demonstrate his very complicated forebrain when he begins to learn coordination between his eyes and his marvelously adept, grasping hands. Then he will begin to demonstrate in a crude way the first evidences of his inborn power. A first sign of thinking will be substituting a thought process for action. He will relate what he hears to the sounds that his own voice can produce. From this comes his delicate speech skill, so intricate that someday he may be able to speak several languages. He will start to show that his brain can absorb a variety of things. He will take in sense perceptions. He will construct a large variety of abstractions. Put together as ideas, he can arrange these in patterns. He will draw conclusions from these arrangements and move, often clumsily, toward answering a variety of questions. He will also pose new ones.

He will be exposed to social experiences from birth on. You, his parents, pass on to him your own values, ideas, habits, and interests. He will be exposed to our American culture because he lives in it. He learns to adjust to the life around him. So his environment comes to exert influence on his growth.

The temperament of the child has considerable bearing on his development. His particular pattern of response to new situations plays an important part in the process of mastering and shaping his personality. His initial reaction to social situations may affect the response of the other people involved and influence the whole character of his interpersonal interactions. Each child approaches a situation in his own characteristic way. This is not due to variations in social or cultural factors and is not due to parental child care factors. It represents differences in the built-in characteristics of behavior of that particular child. This factor that I am calling temperament is your child's ruling pattern of functioning. It represents the basic style that characterizes a person's behavior.

Generalizations about good and bad child care, good and bad children, good and bad parents, all blur the fact that each child is an individual. It is essential to acknowledge human differences, although there are different approaches to explain them. Why does one person develop differently from another? Why is one strong, another weak? Why does one grow up stormily, while another moves along placidly in his development? Over the years there have been two differing viewpoints about individuality. One approach is that all human differences come from inborn qualities that are assumed to be inherited. The other approach is the environmental one, which says that individual differences come from the influence of environment and experience.

These two approaches are the nature versus nurture viewpoints. Neither by itself really answers all the questions that arise. What it really comes down to is that a child's makeup results in part from heredity and in part from his surroundings. His basic character may be inherited from his parents, but his environment has a profound effect on the character he gets from them.

His basic mental equipment cannot be changed very much. Any changes in the way of improved functioning reflect the type of surroundings in which he lives. His early experiences with the people about him in his home are important not only for his emotional development but even more for his intellectual progress. You may have heard that a mother should be in attendance twenty-four hours a day with her baby—this is supposed to assure his normal emotional development. It does not appear to be her presence or absence which is the important factor—it is the stimulation of her person, the handling, the body contact, her voice, which makes the difference. The child who has no one to talk to, no toys—in short, the baby to whom nothing interesting happens—is the child who gets into difficulty. It is the quality, not the quantity, of the stimulation to which the baby is exposed that is valuable.

This means that the mother substitute, as well as the mother, is important. It also means that a mother doesn't have to be in constant attendance so long as she leaves her baby with the right kind of person. Father, too, can feel valuable in these early months if he knows how much he can contribute to his baby's development.

Physical factors play a part in your baby's development. His type of body configuration may very well be inherited, but it does predispose to competence or lack of skill in many areas of development. The muscular child can do well at physical sports, while the skinny one may never get himself coordinated enough to play well. Just so it is with physical handicaps, unusual growth patterns, illness, poor nutrition, lack of practice—they lead to variations in getting the skills that lead to normal maturity.

Don't forget that your child's temperamental characteristics may strongly influence your parental feelings and behavior. If he turns out to be an easily adaptable, quiet child, any parents will be pleased with him, whether they are old and tired or young and vigorous. If he turns out to be a loud, forceful, active, irregular, poorly adaptable fellow, you will need to be lively and energetic parents to keep up with him—and you may wish you didn't have to. It isn't that some babies are good and others are bad. It is that some are easy to look after and some you never seem to be able to satisfactorily take care of. The mother of the difficult baby too often thinks she is doing something wrong and ends up overhandling, overfeeding, or the opposite, overleaving alone. So keep in mind that there are two parents and a baby. Each acts on and is acted on by the other.

As you read the month-to-month sections that follow, you may find that your baby does not always fit into my descriptions of the development of the average baby. You must remember that the average baby is just a make-believe person who does everything at a time when most of the children his age do them. There have to be many children who do a thing sooner and many who do it later to obtain an average. So don't try to force your baby into the patterns I describe. Each baby has his own pattern, which can be quite clear if you read his growth map accurately.

12.

The
First Month

Let's take a look at this new baby of yours in this first month at home. Small, self-centered, demanding, inconsistent—this is your baby! Your job? To help him get accustomed to living with others in a home.

WEIGHT

*Ranges:** Boys   7.4–12.2 lbs.   Average 9.2 lbs.
          Girls   7.1–11.2 lbs.   Average 9.0 lbs.

After your baby regains his birth weight by about ten to fourteen days, he may gain one to two pounds or more by the end of his first month. His weight gain changes his appearance radically. At birth he may have a scrawny look. By the end of his first month he will be considerably filled out. He begins to look plump. His weight gain isn't consistent, so don't weigh him daily and expect to see a weight increase each time.

HEIGHT

*Ranges:** Boys   19.6–22.7 in.   Average 21.2 in.
          Girls   19.7–22.3 in.   Average 21.0 in.

*Figures given each month for weight and height represent weight-and-height ranges at the beginning of that month.

MOTOR DEVELOPMENT

I will point out the changes that occur month by month as your baby develops his control over the large muscles, the ones that he learns to use step by step so that he can finally stand and walk erect. You can test each of these steps as you go along by placing him in situations that present him with the best possible position to use his nerves and muscles to perform.

By the end of his first month your baby is not only bigger and stronger than he was at birth, he is also better put together. His physical development has moved ahead so that he is less limp and floppy. There is more tone to his muscles. His muscles tighten when he is picked up. His breathing is deeper and more regular. He doesn't choke as easily. He holds onto his food better, with less spitting back. There is less jaw-trembling, shaking of the arms and legs, and sneezing. His temperature is steadier, less affected by external change. His sweat glands are working. Although you will still see some signs of unsteady control, such as fitful waking, choking, and sneezing, his basic body functions are under better control. He is coming to better terms with his surroundings.

REFLEXES

You will see some actions you feel he controls, but most of what he does can be described as automatic. He is still pretty much a creature of reflex. He cries, he sucks, he empties his bladder, he has bowel movements, without his conscious control. (Look back to The Newborn Baby for a fuller description of his reflexes.) His basic brain structure and his nervous system, though developed at birth, are not yet mature enough to control his body movements. He hasn't gained enough experience to know what sensations mean or indicate. But he is starting to learn. He seems to watch your face and listen to your voice.

His sucking reflex is still very much in evidence. By this time you recognize and use this valuable reflex at feedings. You touch his cheek or his lips and you get a rooting and sucking response.

Most of his other reflexes found at birth are also still present. You may wish to test some of them at this time.

The grasp reflex described on page 94 is still present but will gradually be replaced by a grasp response that appears in stages in these following months. His grasp reflex is duplicated in his foot as his toes curl to try to grasp your touching finger.

LYING, SITTING, STANDING, AND GETTING ABOUT

When he is on his abdomen, he still stays curled up, his bottom high in the air, his knees drawn up. (See plate 17B.) Some babies, however, will already have begun to stretch out little by little so that they lie flatter.

He can turn his head from side to side. He will try to raise his head to get his nose off the bed. He may even hold it straight up for a second or so, but he doesn't really have any control of his head. He may try to push up on his arms to rest more weight on his forearms. His arms and legs move about quite actively, but without accomplishing very much.

He won't do much on his back except thrash around and push out with his legs. He may not like to stay in this position long—unless you train him to back sleeping—because he can't lift his head up. His front neck muscles are just too weak.

Let him grasp your fingers to demonstrate his pulling up. His grasp reflex lets you gradually raise him to a sitting position, but he doesn't make any active effort. When he grasps your fingers and comes up, his head falls backward. (See plate 18.) Then his back curves and his head sags forward. (See plate 19B.) His legs are bent up on his abdomen. He makes no effort to lift his bottom up from the table. He lifts his head up, only to have it drop again. This doesn't bother him, but it may bother you. He leans over your hand as you hold him upright. Naturally when you are moving him about you will support his head and shoulders, as I describe under "Lifting and Holding," page 230.

When you support your baby in the standing position he pushes to stand, but then he seems to be trying to bend back into his fetal position. (See plate 20B.) His head droops, his neck, arms, and legs are flexed or bent. One baby may rest no weight on his feet, another may seem to push down against the table as if to hold himself upright. He may do reflex walking if he is on a hard surface.

He moves about now with a wriggling, squirming movement which often seems to move him about surprisingly well.

HANDS

He holds his hands in a tight fist position a good part of the time—but not as much as he did at birth. He may open them to clutch aimlessly. They aren't usable articles as yet.

EYES AND OTHER SENSE ORGANS

In line with the head-to-feet pattern of development discussed in *The First Year* section, your baby's eyes are the first areas he begins to control. By the end of this first month you will find him starting to reach out with his eyes. The aimless eye rolling of the early weeks is lessening. He will look steadily at your face. You are convinced that he sees you—but not yet! Much of the time he is just staring without seeing much. He is able to hold his eyes in a fixed position for a little longer. He blinks at a close bright light, but stares at a more distant one. He will follow a moving light or your face, but you have to bring it directly in front of him. He doesn't look side to side or up and down yet.

He listens as you talk to him. He is aware of noises. You will see him stop crying or moving for a moment when he hears a new sound. A soft whisper comforts him.

TEETH

The crowns of all his first teeth are present. You may be able to see some of the outlines of his teeth in his gums. Shortly after a month many babies begin to do a great deal of drooling. This is not teething. He won't be teething this early. (Look ahead to *The Fourth Month*, "Teeth," for a fuller discussion of teeth and teething.)

EATING

During your first weeks at home, you may have started cereal mix in bottle or with spoon if your baby needed it. (Look back to p. 158 to the section on "The Hungry Baby" for details of starting solids in spoon-feeding.) There is no exact time for starting the cereal mix. This will depend upon your baby, his hunger, his feeding intervals, his comfort, his bowel movements, his weight gain. One baby may need such additions very early in the first weeks while another is comfortable much longer. Your baby's hunger is the determining factor.

As a rough rule, I would suggest that you start solids if your baby is getting hungry too soon, going less than 3 to 3½ hours, has "colic," has hard stools, has loose frequent stools often colored green, cries a great deal, or is just not a happy, contented baby. This would apply whether he is breast-fed or a formula-fed baby.

My experience has been that starting your baby early on solid feedings results in a baby filled more adequately, for a longer period of time, and who is more comfortable. The feeding sequence not only goes well but your baby becomes accustomed early to a variety of ways to receive food by spoon, pitcher, cup, bottle, breast. He may have a preference, but he still can be offered food under a varied pattern. Later he will accept change and variations much better.

The use of solids also makes it possible to construct a diet which has a wide variety of food sources with a relatively small volume. This is especially important in the protein group where it is so valuable to furnish a complete array of amino acids from natural sources.

Protein and starch in the diet are well-tolerated by the baby after his first few days. Fat may take a little longer but not significantly so.

Your very young baby can certainly survive on milk and vitamins alone. But human beings are omnivorous. They can eat both animal and plant foods. I believe that your baby is better able to build healthy tissue if you give him a variety of good basic food elements in his diet. This means primarily protein. He is able to do this in much better fashion with a variety of good protein food, and these are what I will emphasize in the coming months. Milk alone is not a complete answer to his nutritional needs.

There will be a great deal of variation in the amount of food any individual baby wants or needs to be satisfied. Beginning this month, I will suggest a menu for you to follow in feeding your baby. In this and succeeding months, whenever a new food group is added, a revised menu plan will be given, along with explanations about new food items under "Menu Comments." There will also be some description of the development of your baby's eating patterns to give you an overall picture of eating behavior in babies. This will help you see the sequence of events and be better prepared to accept your baby's appetite variations as part of the varying pattern of change he goes through. Thus you will be in a better position to handle your child's ups and downs in eating behavior and needs without excessive concern or interference. Your calm handling of these variations will do much to avoid difficulty centered about eating.

As you look at your baby's menu, you will see that portions are indicated for each food group. These will serve as a guide, not as a rigid rule, in building your baby's menu. A smaller baby may need one-half of what a larger fellow will require six times a day.

The information in the month-to-month "Eating" material is intended to help you meet your baby's nutritional requirements during his first year. Naturally, your pediatrician is the one to consult about specific problems and needs in your particular baby.

MENU

cereal	1 portion
fruit	1 portion
meat	1 portion
milk	1–2 portions

This diet is given at each feeding of the day. The foods are put together in one mixture. Milk (breast or formula) is added to form a smooth moist paste. Feeding at breast or with bottle follows after spoon-feeding the solid mix.

CEREAL. Start or continue to use the precooked infant cereals, preferably the single-grained cereals, rice, oat, or barley. They are convenient, no more expensive, and nutritionally better balanced than regular cereal. You may rotate them. If you have to cook cereal for your baby, use one of the fortified or enriched products. Follow directions for preparing it for an infant. These are not the same as for an adult or older child.

one portion = ½ cup (8 tablespoons) infant cereal (dry)
= ½ cup cooked cereal

FRUIT. Raw fresh banana is a good first fruit to use. You may already have used it this past week. It is easy to get and to prepare. Peel it, mash thoroughly and beat it with a fork to make a creamy smooth mixture. Then add it to the cereal. Strained fruits, either in jars especially prepared for babies or stewed and home-homogenized in the blender, are the next to add. Apple, pear, or pineapple can be given. Avoid prunes or peaches until later. Use only the plain fruits, not mixtures. Don't give raw fruits except for banana. Mix the fruit directly with the cereal as you did the banana. Leave the unused portion of the fruit in the jar. Refrigerated in the jar with the top covered, it can be used for several days. Do not put it in another receptacle. Try to rotate the fruits you use. Use a can of one, then a can of another fruit. Preparing your own foods is very easy if you have the use of a blender or osterizer. Home-cooked, homogenized fruits or other foods are adequate and less expensive than commercial products.

one portion = ½ small banana
= ½ cup cooked fruit sauce
= 4 ounces (1 jar) baby food

MEAT. The meat group is added this month as a source of protein in addition to the milk group. It gives high quality proteins to round out the diet in iron and amino acids. If your baby has been very hungry, you may add meats to his cereal-fruit mix before this. Use them in rotation, beef, veal, lamb, pork, ham and chicken, or fish to start. The canned baby meats, not mixtures, are readily available. If you prepare and homogenize your own, use lean cooked meat and cut off any excess fat.

one portion = 1 (2x1½x½) ounce lean meat
= 2 ounces (½ jar) plain baby meat

MILK. Continue to use one of the prepared infant formulas. They are nutritionally balanced. Each company has its own brand like Enfamil (Mead Johnson), Similac (Ross Laboratories), Modilac (Gerber, SMA or Carnalac (Carnation Company). You may use any brand of evaporated milk diluted equal parts with water for your formula.

one portion = 4 ounces (½ cup) diluted formula
 = 4 ounces (½ cup) diluted evaporated milk
 = 4 ounces breast milk (10 minutes)

As a rough guide for the nursing mother, 10 minutes of nursing has been called a portion similar to 4 ounces of prepared formula. Most of the 4 ounces of formula will be used in the cereal mix. Breast milk may be used if it is available. Whatever is left over is offered after the cereal feeding. Always offer as much breast or formula after the solid mix as your baby wants. Don't push this encouragement too far unless you want to get it all back.

VITAMINS IN THE MONTHS AHEAD. Always give a multiple-vitamin preparation, like Poly-Vi-Sol (Mead Johnson) or Vi-Daylin (Ross), in appropriate dosage. You should have started this last month when your baby came home from the hospital.

WATER OR JUICE. Except in hot weather, a well-fed baby usually doesn't want extra fluids between feedings unless he is hungry. Offer plain or sweetened water between his feedings if he seems to act hungry. You may offer diluted fruit juice (apple) if he doesn't care for the taste of water. If he refuses, he doesn't want or need it. Don't warm fruit juice. Any Vitamin C present is destroyed by heating. Give it cold. Use tap water if the water supply is safe. Otherwise, use boiled water.

WARM FOOD OR COLD

As discussed in *Breast-Feeding and Bottle-Feeding*, it is not necessary to warm formula. The cereal mix will probably be at room temperature by the time you feed it whether you warmed the formula or not. A warming dish for the cereal mix is not necessary.

WASHING UTENSILS

Use soap and hot water to wash any utensils you use in spoon-feeding and cup-feeding. Dishwasher care is ade quate. Since you are not storing food in them, sterilization is not needed. Cleanliness is. Keep your baby's utensils separate. Don't dump his used dishes into a sink piled high with dirty dishes and remnants of food unless you are prepared to sterilize them before you use them again. (Look back to "Formula Preparation" for nipple and bottle care.)

LEFTOVERS

The storing of leftover formula has been discussed previously. (See material on "Bottle-Feeding" under *Breast-Feeding and Bottle-Feeding.*) Leftover cereal mix can also be kept for the next feeding. Keep it refrigerated and adequately covered.

In handling foods, take precautions in regard to cleanliness. Don't open a can or jar until you are ready to use it. Don't transfer it to a dish if you are not to use it right away. Leave it in the can or jar where it is sterile. Use a clean, dry spoon, or pour from the container to transfer food. Cover the container with plastic or foil and return it at once to the refrigerator. Don't leave it standing about. Don't heat the can or jar of food and use it for more than one feeding. Don't feed directly from the jar or can unless you use the entire contents. With home-prepared foods your precautions must be even more scrupulous in order to avoid contamination and spoilage. Use your nose and eyes before you use any food.

The prepared strained baby foods that come in small jars are convenient, economical, nutritionally balanced, varied, available, and uniform in quality and sterility. You can also prepare your own baby food, but it is somewhat more work unless you have a blender. Acquire a good one, since you will use it a good deal in these next months. This is probably more economical than buying baby foods. If you pay attention to your food preparation then the nutritional value will be preserved. Always pay attention to good care and cleaning of your blender.

FEEDING MIX

You may want to mix all your baby's solid foods together. This saves you time and effort. You can prepare his day's food supply at one time with the use of the blender. For instance, assume he has stopped his night feeding and is now on five feedings a day. Put five meals together in the blender, which means

cereal:	5 portions
fruit:	5 portions
meat:	5 portions

This mixture is then transferred to a sterile or clean dry quart jar. At feeding time one-fifth of the solid mixture is removed with a clean dry spoon to the feeding dish. Enough formula is added to it to ready it for feeding.

CUP-FEEDING

Try offering the water or juice in a cup or small pitcher with a spout during this first month if you wish. If you are breast-feeding this may be a real time-saver since no bottle or sterilization is required. If you have the occasional baby who seems to care very little for a nipple, you may find that he takes formula in a cup very well. (See plate 22A.)

BREAST-FEEDING

By this time your breast-feeding cycle has settled down to a normal production pattern. Your let-down reflex swings into action quickly so that your baby gets milk easily and in good supply. Already you will notice how much he has grown and changed. He still uses his primary rooting and sucking reflexes, but he shows increasing control of his actions.

Make sure to empty your breast completely after each feeding. This stimulates milk production and avoids caking. (Look again at the material on "Breast Care" in the section on *Breast-Feeding and Bottle-Feeding*.) Hand-empty your breast. If you're feeding solids, use this expressed milk for his next cereal mix. Collect and refrigerate it in a sterile container until you are ready to use it.

As discussed previously, don't consider weaning until you are certain you can't nurse. Too often your decision will not be based on an adequate reason. If you can continue, your baby may wean himself in three to four months.

If your baby is not getting enough to eat, try increasing

the amounts of solids you give first so he is full and satisfied. If he doesn't get enough in this fashion, you may have to consider discontinuing breast-feeding entirely. Don't jump this way too fast, but try to increase the solids to compensate for any lack of breast milk, temporary or otherwise.

BOTTLE-FEEDING

Use most of the formula in the cereal mix. If he is getting enough solids beforehand, your baby will take one to two ounces from the bottle. You may be able to feed him enough so that he isn't interested in milk afterwards. But don't force too much milk on him after solids.

APPETITE

In most babies appetite is not too great a problem at this stage. Your baby probably has a good one. Your problem is to keep up with his hunger. A feeding should be taken adequately in twenty minutes. Thirty minutes may be too long for many babies. The amount he takes may vary from feeding to feeding.

As noted previously, increase spoon-feeding solids to the point where he takes no more than ten minutes at the breast or two ounces of formula afterwards. He should be satisfied for at least four hours. Your baby may eat enormously. You may be worried about the amount. Or your baby may eat much less than another baby and still be quite content. The test of an adequate diet is in the reaction of your baby. He should be full, satisfied, and contented.

SCHEDULE

Now that your baby is settling into his own pattern you will find a five-feeding schedule like 7:00 A.M., 11:00 A.M., 3:00 P.M., 7:00 P.M., and 11:00 P.M. suitable for most households. Start your day earlier or later if you wish. But keep a four-hour interval during the day. Wake him if you have to. Let him go as long as he will at night. He may be skipping that night feeding entirely. If you have given enough food, toward the end of this month he will be ready to shift himself to four feedings like 7:00 A.M., 12:00 noon, 5:00–6:00 P.M., and 11:00 P.M., but schedules are flexible. If you have a swing-shift family, the whole family schedule for meal time can be shifted to this with no difficulty. You know the time period. Your baby can't read the clock yet.

I talked about permissive feeding in his early weeks. (See "Self-Demand Feeding.") You may discover you have allowed yourself to get caught in a pocket of permissiveness. This may be the result of misunderstanding what was suggested. You find that you are confused, desperate, and tired. Your baby isn't happy either. He whimpers, whines, and stays wakeful. He just can't seem to settle down. You pick him up, change him, talk to him, change his position, but he still fusses. If you offer him food, he takes a little and then seems drowsy. By the time he is back in bed he starts all over again. You and he may never experience a comfortable full feeding together, or rarely do! If you have managed to get yourself into this state, make sure you are offering him enough food. Changing his formula isn't the answer. Increasing his food, plus leaving him alone for longer intervals is the best solution. Check back to the section on *Breast-Feeding and Bottle-Feeding* as to your feeding techniques and routines. If there is a question of illness, have your pediatrician see him to rule out any trouble.

You will be unusual if you aren't anxious to eliminate the middle-of-the-night feeding by this time. Anyone can use a good night's sleep, you especially. Wake him and feed him during the day at four-hour intervals if he isn't awake sooner. Don't let him go too long. Then feed him as completely as possible in the late evening. After this let him go until he awakens in the early A.M. (4:00–6:00 A.M.). This will often happen by about his third week.

FUSSING

A word of caution as you are starting out. Many babies have fussy periods of settling down. (Look back to *Crying* for this.) Don't assume that this fussing means that he is hungry. If you have fed him adequately a short time before, leave him alone and let him settle down.

BOWEL AND BLADDER FUNCTIONS

I have talked about bowel movements in the very young baby before. (Check back to the sections on *The Newborn Baby, Breast-Feeding and Bottle-Feeding,* and *Crying.*)

Many a new mother is puzzled, sometimes frightened, by the intestinal activity of her new baby. When your baby is fed he is stimulated to empty his rectum. He may stop eating temporarily and perform this function. It may squirt out quite noisily, with the passage of quite a bit of gas. Babies are continual gas-passers, anyway.

After his first few weeks, loose green stools usually mean your baby is not getting enough food. If most of his stools are like this, adjust his diet to give him more food. Solids are best. If the stools are mainly watery material, more frequent than usual, and your baby is very fussy and seems ill, check with your pediatrician. Your baby, especially if he is formula-fed, may show a too firm, pellet-like stool. He needs more bulk in his diet. More solids in his diet will relieve this problem better than giving him irritants like prune juice or sugar in his formula. In other words, don't try to produce a laxative effect, but take steps to encourage his normal bowel action.

I have said this before, but it is important enough to bear repeating: Don't use suppositories, enemas, or laxatives. Take such measures with your baby only on very definite direction from your pediatrician. Don't give oily preparations such as mineral oil. If your baby chokes on them, he may draw the oil down into his lungs and get into severe trouble.

During these early weeks you may occasionally notice a small streak of blood in your baby's stools. This is not necessarily associated with a hard stool. It indicates an irritation at the opening of the rectum, such as a small split or crack in the lining membrane. Clean the area with soap and water and cover it with Vaseline or similar heavy ointment such as A-D ointment, Desitin, or Polysorb. Try to get a plug of Vaseline up into the opening. If there are large amounts of blood in the stool, or a dark, "tarry" stool, save the stool and have your pediatrician check on what is happening.

An occasional baby will fuss when he passes his urine, perhaps even if he is asleep. This does not mean trouble.

By now you may have been hit by a stream of urine when

you were changing your baby boy's diaper or dressing him. You will just have to dodge faster—or cover him faster. His bladder emptying is a reflex act, which may occur when you uncover him, handle him, or just stroke his abdomen when he has a full bladder.

If your baby is a girl, you may have been surprised to discover that she can produce a urine stream too.

SLEEPING

The month-old baby sleeps a great deal, although not as much as he did at first. His total sleeping time during the first three months ranges from fourteen to eighteen hours. At the end of this first month the number of his sleep periods has dropped from the seven to twelve of the early days to four or five a day. The longest of these sleep periods will be about four and a half hours. In addition, he will sleep a little more quietly and soundly, although he is by no means a quiet sleeper yet. You will still hear many snuffles, snorts, squeaks, gas-passing sounds, or other sounds of one sort or another.

His fussy periods have now started to narrow down to two periods, with his usual time of fussing at about six to eleven P.M. By six weeks such fussing will have reached its peak. (Look back to *Crying* for more about this.)

His sleep habits are not of much concern at this point. His main requirement at this stage is adequate food intake. If this is supplied, his sleeping largely takes care of itself.

The type of baby he is will influence the amount of sleep he will need. There are wide variations in sleep patterns among different individuals, just as in everything else I have talked about. If he is an on-the-go type, he will require less sleep than the passive, easygoing type. The wide differences in early sleep patterns are said to be a prediction of future behavior differences.

While you can't make your baby sleep, you can provide him with the best opportunity for it. Good sleep habits will come more easily if you do so. Be sure that your baby is not too hot, that he is not restrained, that he is in his own bed in his own room, that he is on his abdomen, that the sides of his crib are raised and locked into place. (Look back to *Preparing for the Baby* for a fuller description of good sleeping arrangements.)

In his early months he will keep the TNR fencing position when asleep, with his arm and leg extended in the same direction in which his head is turned.

He may begin to show a preference for a certain side. Change his position in his crib at intervals so that his head will not always be turned the same way.

In the early weeks your baby doesn't pay too much attention to his surroundings. He can sleep soundly amidst normal household noises. He should be expected to adapt to the household, not the household to him. However, there are limits to what he should be expected to tolerate. He should not be disturbed frequently by someone tiptoeing in to see if he is asleep, wet, or in the proper position. Keep the light muted when you go into his room. He doesn't need a bright light burning constantly.

You must start early to be consistent and firm about bedtime routine. Your baby should expect to rest or go to sleep when he is put in his crib. You may want to rock him or sing him to sleep. But as I have said before, if you set up this pattern you must be willing to live with it for a long time to come. So don't start something you can't finish. You will find that changing a habit you have set up is much harder than you may think at this point.

If you go in to check your baby after he has been asleep for a time, you may be startled to find his head wringing wet. During sleep many children perspire a great deal. This does not indicate any serious physical disturbance. It takes time for him to slow his metabolism down when he goes into a sleeping pattern. You may see the same thing when he eats.

Many normal babies show a considerable amount of mucus in the nose. This is not due to infection. The shape and size of the air passages may be partly responsible. He sounds snorty and snuffly, but appears—and is—perfectly healthy. He may sound very noisy after he goes to sleep or when he is first awake. If there is much mucus, he will swallow, sneeze, or cough it out of his way.

You may be alarmed if you pick your baby up in the morning and find an arm swollen, cold, and blue. This is probably partly due to position and partly to temperature. No treatment is required since the condition disappears in a few hours. Don't be surprised if it recurs.

EXERCISE AND PLAY

Play and exercise are pretty much one at this time. Even a month-old baby should be stimulated by periods of play and exercise. You can do a few minutes of exercise with him each day. A pad on the floor is a good place for this. Brace his feet against your hands and gently push his knees up to his abdomen a few times. Grasp his hands or let him grasp yours and pull him up gently to a sitting position. Roll him from side to side and turn him over on his tummy. Your baby will enjoy the exercise if you aren't too vigorous. A good time for his exercise period may be the late afternoon or early evening. This is often his fussy time, when he wants attention, and it coincides with the time Father arrives home. Both Father and baby may be ready for play.

Many of your baby-care routines will involve some playing. Bath time is a natural playtime for your baby. Every diaper change can become a playtime for him. You bend over him, talk or sing to him, smile, nod your head. He begins to respond by watching your face.

AWARENESS AND SOCIAL RESPONSE

I have mentioned before that the very young baby is concerned mostly with his insides, but this doesn't mean he doesn't respond to his surroundings to some degree. His first give and take with the world comes through his senses. During his first month he gets a message from the way he is touched and handled. He is soothed by being picked up, held, and talked to. This is his first social response. He enjoys cuddling and motion.

By a month his social responses are developing. He probably can't quite smile yet as a means of response. He will do some grimacing, working his mouth. By six weeks he will probably be giving you a real smile.

By a month he begins to get along as a member of your family. He will probably begin to eat and sleep at somewhat more regular intervals. You have a fair idea of what to expect from day to day—although he is not too predictable yet!

When you come home from the hospital, someone is bound to tell you, "Now, be sure to train your baby to have good regular habits." This is certainly what you want to do. But how do you do it?

Realize that your baby is born with the ability to develop habits. Habits develop as a result of doing or experiencing the same things time after time. You can't start too early to help your baby into reasonable habits through your calm and consistent way of handling him. His nervous system may be immature in these early weeks, but it is working! It is receiving sensations. Discipline in the early weeks is mainly habit-training in eating and sleeping, which has been discussed earlier.

ORAL COMMUNICATION

Toward the end of this first month your baby may make some small mewing or cooing noises in his throat, sometimes with sounds resembling vowels or consonants along with sighs and grunts. They have no definite form or meaning. Most of the time crying is still his favorite means of expression.

As I have told you before, by next month he will focus more on you and your words. Your verbal relationship will be on the way. As the months pass, your child comes to recognize language as a medium of contact among people.

But what do you say to your young infant? Your conversation doesn't have to be on a high intellectual level. You need no specialized subject. When he is to have a bath, start telling him about it. As he is put in the bath, tell him about the water. Ask him if he thinks the water is warm enough. You can comment on his bottle being warm or cold, his toy being funny or cuddly, from his earliest days. Your baby is ready to develop concepts at an early age.

IMMUNIZATIONS

Your newborn baby will be immune to measles, German measles, chickenpox, and mumps, and perhaps polio, diphtheria, and scarlet fever, only if you are immune to them. Such protection lasts only the first few months. I wouldn't trust it after three months. Your baby has no immunity against anything else. His own defense processes or immune mechanisms won't be operating for several months. This makes him even more vulnerable. He is a sitting duck for any infection to which he is exposed. So don't take this risk! He is durable but not invulnerable. Usually I start immunizations when a baby is two months old. The schedule I outline in the coming months may differ somewhat from that of your baby's pediatrician, but it will give you an approximate idea of what to expect when.

You may want to keep a record of your baby's immunizations. A record form is supplied at the back of this book. Be sure to have it signed by the physician who gives the immunizations.

BABY-CARE ROUTINES

LIFTING AND HOLDING YOUR BABY

One of the first skills you will need is that of lifting and holding your baby. In handling him, always support his head and back to give him a feeling of security. All babies have an inborn fear of falling. He needs to be held gently but securely. If you hold him loosely and uncertainly, he is uncomfortable and he is sure to cry.

To pick him up from his back, assuming you are right-handed, grasp his ankles with your right hand, separating them with one of your fingers. Lift him slightly and slide your left hand up along his back, spreading your fingers to support his head, shoulders, and back. Shift your right hand on his ankles to his buttocks, raise him up to lean against you. Cradle him in your arms if you are to sit with him.

When you carry him, use the football hold—just like a player carrying a football. His legs will be tucked under your arm, with your forearm supporting his trunk and your wrist and hand supporting his head and shoulders. Pick him up as described above to start, but then bring him up

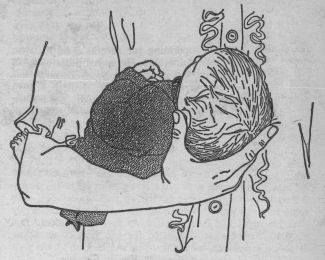

Fig. 44. The football hold.

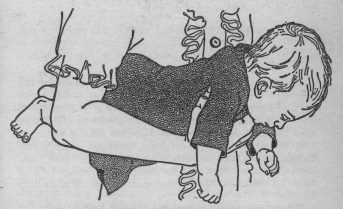

Fig. 45. The fireman's hold.

under your arm. (See fig. 44.) Another method of carrying your baby, somewhat the reverse of the football hold, is known as the fireman's hold. (See fig. 45.)

WRAPPING IN A BLANKET

The howling, restless baby whose arms and legs constantly thrash about may be quieted by being wrapped snugly, or swaddled, in a thin blanket. You can try it if you have one of these restless babies who needs some external control. You may also want to wrap your baby during feedings in the early weeks if he waves his arms about a great deal. Always keep a wrapped baby on his side or abdomen—*not on his back!* You will have to be extra diligent in watching a wrapped baby. (I said *watching*—not *bothering!*)

To wrap your baby in a blanket, lay the blanket on a table or bed with one point to the top. Lay your baby on the blanket and fold one corner over his feet. Don't hold his legs straight. He won't like it. Let him lie in his accustomed fetal position, legs drawn up and knees bent, with some room to move. Wrap both sides of the blanket firmly over his arms and body almost up to his shoulders. You may pin the blanket. The need for this type of wrapping usually disappears after the first few weeks. Don't train your baby to it. He needs to move and do on his own.

You may want to wrap your baby loosely in a light receiving blanket when you are carrying him about the house. Don't put him down wrapped up.

BATH TIME

When your baby leaves the hospital, he is ready for full soap and water baths at home. Even if the stump of his umbilical cord has not yet fallen off, this does not prevent a full bath, although it does mean that you need to use good care about the base of the cord after you get it wet.

You will probably be worried about giving your new baby a bath. You may have been given a demonstration by a cool, efficient nurse at the hospital. Watching her give a baby his bath convinced you that there was really nothing to it—you wondered why any instruction was necessary. Now you are faced with doing the job yourself you find that you are apprehensive. You may be all fingers and thumbs during the first few baths, but you will be surprised how experienced you become in a short time. A tub of warm water and a warmhearted bath-master with a cool head are all your baby really needs.

Your infant should have a daily bath. He will like it if he is securely held and comfortable. It helps to talk to him quietly throughout the bath. You will see how the bath helps him to relax. He will enjoy moving about without confining clothes.

WHEN TO BATHE HIM. The time you set depends on his age and your family's routine. You can vary it according to your needs. Choose a time when there is the least hurry and bustle in your household. Your baby doesn't have to be bathed in the morning, when the urgency of other duties tends to make you rush things. Sometime during the afternoon may be better. By then formula-making and other household duties are usually done. Don't give him a bath when he is extremely hungry, though, or right after a full feeding. The moving about may bring his meal back up. And don't feed him *immediately* after he has been given a bath. The bath procedure is tiring as well as relaxing. If he has a restless period, an unhurried bath may soothe him and ready him for sleep.

WHERE TO BATHE HIM. Your baby isn't fussy about the place for his bath. Any warm 75°–80° room should suit him fine. It may be in the kitchen, the bathroom, or his bedroom. Be sure there are no drafts. Don't keep the room warmer than 75°–80° unless there is a special reason for doing so, or you will make him hot and uncomfortable. The room temperature for older babies may be lower. Wherever you bathe him, make this your rule: *Never leave your baby alone while he is in his bath.* This goes for children up to school age.

CLEANSING AGENTS. Use a mild toilet soap or a medicated detergent like Phisohex. Ordinary detergents, castile soaps, highly perfumed soaps, medicated soaps, cleansing oils, or soap substitutes like demulcents can act as irritants and are not suitable for your baby.

OILS AND POWDERS. Oil left in the baby's body creases will cause trouble. It is better to avoid using oils after the bath, especially vegetable oils, like olive oil. These get rancid and become irritants. A water-soluble baby cream, lotion, or silicone lotion can be used if your baby has a sensitive skin. Apply it with your fingertips and smooth it into the skin. Gently remove any excess with cleansing tissues or a soft diaper.

Special baby powders are available. Any nonmedicated, nonperfumed talcum powder will be all right if you watch how you use it. Medicated or perfumed talcum powders may irritate. Ordinary cornstarch or baking soda will powder your baby effectively. Put it in an ordinary salt shaker. Special water-resistant medicated powders may be prescribed for special conditions. Don't let your baby inhale any powder. Small amounts of cornstarch or baking soda in his eyes or breathed in will not be serious. If you need a more absorbent material, try flour—browned in the oven.

BATH EQUIPMENT. Keep your baby's bath equipment in a convenient place. Have everything ready before you begin.

Bathtub. The bathtub should be baby size, oval, preferably plastic; a dishpan or similar pan of enamel, plastic, or heavy-duty metal serves the purpose well. This can be put on a table. The kitchen sink with a built-in counter can be used. Always check for a convenient height. For your older infant or child the family bathtub can be used. Don't try to use the family bathtub at first since you can't stoop or lift too well yet and you probably won't feel secure enough.

Bathinette or other bathtub-dressing table combination. This has an advantage over the built-in sink. It can be folded and put out of the way. Some well-meaning relative may have given you the latest streamlined model. You may never use all of the attachments. You may wish to strip down the apparatus until only the bath part remains. Keep the drainage tube in place, or it may get away from you and drain the water out, usually all over your carpeting. The dressing-table top is a good table top, but it does tip and must be securely fastened. Don't leave your baby unattended on this or on any other table, even when he is strapped on. There is a gadget rack in the shelf below, which is usable for storage supplies.

Bath Towels (3–4): Large cotton terry-cloth towels are quite soft and absorbent. Soft diapers can be used, too. A small towel for drying is also a help.

Washcloths (3–4): Use soft cotton terry-cloth, cheesecloth, or knitted types.

Bath Tray: This should contain the following items, all in their own jars or other form of container:

Cotton balls

Cotton wisps, swabs, or Q-Tips

Safety pins, large size. Open safety pins can be stuck into a cake of soap for easy reaching. They should not be kept within reach of your baby.

Soap or medicated detergent. Shampoo, if you want to use it.

Powder

Cleansing tissues

Ointment. White Vaseline, or A-D ointment, Desitin, or other heavy ointment.

Alcohol. Seventy percent denatured (rubbing) alcohol.

Sterile gauze squares, 2″ x 2″ x 3″ x 3″.

Rectal thermometer

Nail scissors (blunt), or clippers

Toothpicks. For nail cleaners.

Sponge

Brush and comb

Bath pad or folded blanket, and bath-towel cover

   Bath Table: This should be the right height for dressing and undressing the baby. It must be large enough to put equipment on as well as the baby himself.

   Paper bag, newspaper, or waste can with step-on cover. For used supplies.

   Diaper Pail. For soiled diapers.

   Hamper, for soiled clothes.

   Fresh diapers and clothes

PREPARING FOR THE BATH. Thoroughly wash your hands, wrists, and fingernails with soap and water. You should keep your fingernails relatively short and rounded to avoid scratching your baby. Wear a coverall apron or housedress (one without sharp buttons). Short sleeves or elbow-length sleeves are best. Remove any jewelry, such as pins or rings, that can scratch your baby's tender skin. If you have a cold, cover your nose and mouth with a surgical mask or a large handkerchief. Have the hamper nearby, or spread newspapers on the floor near the bathing area so that dirty clothes and used bath equipment may be discarded at once for later care. The diaper pail should also be handy. Check the contents of the bath tray. Remove the covers from the jars you will be using. Arrange his diaper, pins, clean clothing, and receiving blanket. Cover the bath table with the bath pad or folded blanket. Put the bath towel over this. If you are right-handed, have the tub to the left with the bath table and supplies to the right. Reverse this if you are left-handed.

Put water in the tub to the desired amount—anywhere between 2 and 3 inches deep or half full. Place a towel on the bottom so your baby won't slide along the bottom so easily when he is slippery with soap. The water should be comfortably warm to your elbow. Never put your baby in his bath without first testing the temperature. You can use a bath thermometer, but it is not a necessity. If you do, the temperature should be 95 to 100°.

Pick up your baby from his crib. If you use the football or the fireman's hold described above, you can hold him and use your free hand to strip his bed. Discarded linens can be put on the refuse newspaper on the floor. The portion of the crib linen to be aired is thrown over the crib side or end while the bath is in progress. Place your baby on the dressing-table top or on your lap to undress him. Discard soiled clothing in the hamper or on the newspapers. Leave his used diaper on (if it's not too soiled) during the bathing of his special areas—his eyes, ears, nose, and mouth. If he is soiled, wipe the bowel movement off with cleansing tissues. You will probably want to wash his special areas before you put him in the bath until you are experienced.

BATHING SPECIAL AREAS. A word of caution. Don't invade or irritate these areas with excessive diligence. You will interfere with his natural protective devices. So be careful. Don't go beyond the skin margins any more than you would do with an adult. *No cotton on sticks*. No going where you can't see.

Eyes: The covering of his eye is bathed constantly by moisture. The eyes of your healthy baby need no medications or eye drops. Irrigate his eyes with warm water only. His eyelids can be cleaned at the time his face is cleaned. A wet washcloth or cotton ball squeezed over the inner corner of his eye will irrigate it sufficiently. Gently wipe from the inside corner of his eye outward. This clears out any material. Massage of blocked tear ducts that are causing tearing is done by gently "milking" with your fingertip from the side of the bridge of his nose toward the inside corner of his eye.

Ears: His ear canal is lined with invisible hairs. These push the wax slowly along the ear canal and out. This wax is formed in his ear canal to protect and clean it. The wax and debris collect and gradually move to the outside. In small babies this material is quite liquid and light in color. As your child grows older, the wax becomes drier and darker in color. Don't probe into his ear canal. You can't see what you are doing. His outer ear and the entrance to the ear canal can be adequately cleaned with a washcloth on your fingertip. Carefully clean the folds of his ears and the creases in back of his ears.

Nose: Just as with eyes and ears, there is a housekeeping system in his nose. There are invisible hairs in the cells lining his nose. These keep materials such as mucus and dust on their surface moving down toward the front end of the nose. This material collects on the visible hairs near the opening. It tickles his nose and makes him sneeze or rub to eliminate foreign matter. This is a reason your baby sneezes so often. Do not dig into his nostrils with a cotton swab. His nose can be adequately cleaned by gently squeezing the nostrils with the washcloth at the time of cleansing his face. If there is foreign matter in the nostril that can be seen, remove it with a corner of the washcloth. Always hold your baby's head firmly in one hand so that he cannot squirm at the wrong moment and damage the lining membrane. *Never use oil of any kind in your baby's nose.*

Mouth: You can inspect his mouth by gently squeezing his cheeks together. His tongue and the insides of his cheeks are often coated with food material. Don't try to remove it. The natural irrigation of his eating and drinking will take care of this need.

Scalp: You may wish to shampoo his hair before you put him in the tub. Give him a fairly brisk shampoo every second or third day. Use the football carry to hold him either with face up or down over the water. Use your hand to lather his scalp with soap or shampoo. Don't worry about the fontanelle on the top of his head. As mentioned before, it is well-protected. After you have shampooed his scalp thoroughly, rinse it with a wet washcloth. Try not to get soap in his eyes. Then go on with the rest of his bath.

THE TUB BATH. If you are right-handed, pick up your baby so that he is supported on your left forearm and wrist, left hand under his left shoulder with the fingers of your left hand around his left arm, your thumb opposing them in front of his shoulder to give a secure hold. With your other hand, hold his legs together at the ankles, your thumb securing his right leg, your index finger separating his ankles, and your remaining fingers grasping his left leg. Then place him in the water. (See fig. 46.) Use a semi sitting position for your baby until he can sit alone.

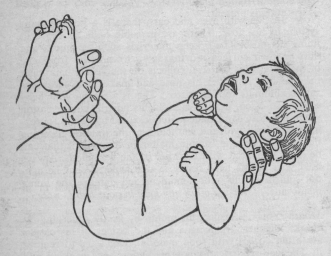

Fig. 46. The tub lift.

His bath proceeds from his head downward. Wrap a washcloth around your hand and wash his face with clear water or soap and water. Next, soap the front of his body with the washcloth. Pay particular attention to his body creases. Don't be concerned about the swollen breasts and genitals that are often found in new babies. The swelling will go away. Washing the palms of his hands may be a problem. If you grasp his right hand with your hand, his fist closes down on your finger. Automatically his left hand opens. At this point you can grab his open left hand and wash it before he knows what is happening. Reverse the process to wash his other hand. After you have thoroughly washed and rinsed the front of his body, turn him over, reversing the hold on his arm, or just bend him forward over your other hand. Some mothers use a gentle shower spray for rinsing. Bathinettes may have such attachments.

In girl babies the lips of the vulva should always be separated and washed with soap and water at bath time. Use a moist cotton ball and clean with a downward stroke from front to back. Don't allow soap to remain between the lips of the vulva. Don't attempt to remove completely the cheeselike smegma material found there. If you remove too much of this you take away the natural lubrication, and some irritation may develop. Vaseline may be applied if irritation is present.

If your son has not been circumcised, cleaning his genitals involves pulling the foreskin back from the head of the penis. His foreskin may be loose enough so that this is not difficult. Most babies at the time of birth have small, tight openings with adherent foreskin. This makes the pulling-back process difficult at first. In time his foreskin will stretch to free itself so that you will be able to pull it back as far as possible from the head of the penis. You may have to have Father help you at first with this pulling back. Many mothers have a difficult time making themselves do something that bothers their baby. If you shrink from doing this regularly, the foreskin will remain unstretched, and cleaning will be difficult. If irritating material is allowed to collect under the foreskin, irritation or infection can result. While it is retracted, clean the foreskin and the head or glans of the penis with soap and water. Don't try to take away all of the lubricating smegma. Be sure to rinse the soap off well. Do not leave his foreskin in the pulled-back position. It must be brought back down again into its normal covering position. If you leave it in the pulled-back position, the tightness of the foreskin may cut off circulation to the head of the penis. This causes the penis to swell, making it more difficult to bring the foreskin back into position.

If your baby has been circumcised, you will find that the sleeve of foreskin has been partially removed so that the head of his penis is exposed. The margins under the foreskin are easily cleansed, but leave some smegma in place. At first the head of the penis and the healing foreskin should be thoroughly covered with Vaseline or similar ointment, after soap and water cleansing and water rinse. Ointment may be used later whenever redness or irritation appears. A small gauze square with a good portion of Vaseline on it may be put over the penis like a cap or tent to avoid irritation. The diaper will hold it on.

The navel may appear red and moist after the dry umbilical cord has fallen off, but it is not painful. It may show some bloody ooze which is not serious. Clean the navel thoroughly with alcohol or antiseptic solution after the bath or whenever material appears to collect there. This is usually sufficient to keep it in a healthy state. After it has healed, a soap and water washing is all that is necessary. An abdominal binder or belly band is not used. It doesn't remain in position and serves no useful purpose. If there is any protrusion, your doctor can decide whether an adhesive strapping is necessary.

AFTER THE BATH. When you are ready to take him out of the water, use the same hold you used when you put him in. Lift him onto the warm, dry surface of the open bath towel spread out on the table pad. Dry him carefully all over after covering him with the bath towel. Don't rub him dry, pat him. Pay attention to his folds and creases. After he is dry, you can powder him lightly with powder, baking soda, or cornstarch. Avoid oil, especially in his body creases. Any irritated skin areas may require Vaseline or other bland, heavy ointment such as A-D ointment, Desitin, or Polysorb, or a hand lotion or simple cream. A heavy ointment is probably best for any irritated area on the buttocks or diaper area. Lotion or cream is best for irritated cheeks. After drying and inspecting him, dress him quickly. He may cry while being dressed and undressed.

Nails. If his fingernails need trimming, now may be a good time, or you may find that the job can be more easily done while he is asleep. Keep his fingernails trimmed short so that he can't scratch himself. Cut them straight across with blunt-tipped nail scissors or clippers. Don't cut down at the corners. The nail is soft and flaky, so be certain the scissors or clippers are sharp enough. If he is awake, let him grasp your index finger and place your thumb on the back of his hand. This will hold his fingers firmly in place while you trim. Watch for hangnails or the edge of the nail pulled down into the tissues. If you see this, apply antiseptic to these corners to treat the irritated tissues.

His toenails don't require very much care at first. Don't ever cut them too short.

You can use a toothpick to clean under the nails, if necessary.

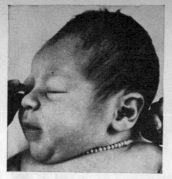

Plate 1. Newborn molding

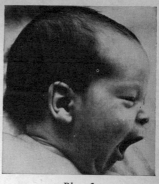

Plate 2.
Normal head at 1 month

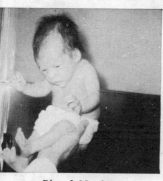

Plate 3. Newborn,
showing flexible spine

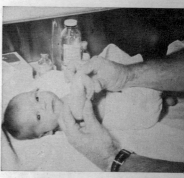

Plate 4. Newborn,
showing pliable joints

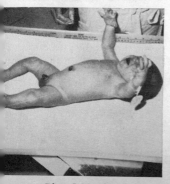

Plate 5. Newborn,
showing startle reflex

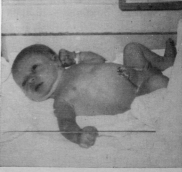

Plate 6.
Newborn, showing TNR

Stimulus

TRUNK-INCURVATION REFLEX

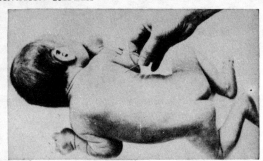

Plate 7.

MAGNET REFLEX

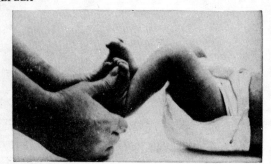

Plate 9.

CROSSED EXTENSION REFLEX

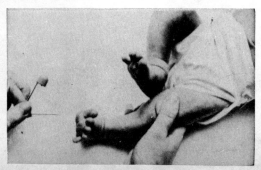

Plate 11.

Response

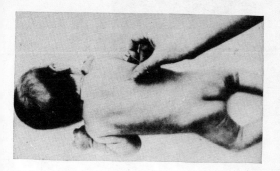

Plate 8.

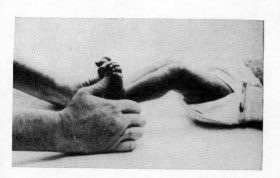

Plate 10.

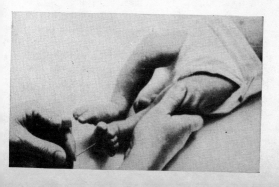

Plate 12.

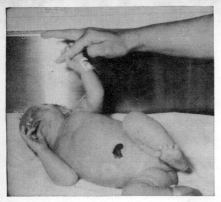

Plate 13.
Newborn grasp

Plate 14A-14J.
LEARNING TO WALK

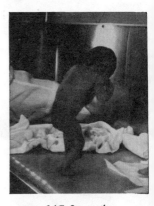

14A. Newborn

14B. 1 month

14C. 2 months

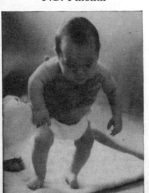

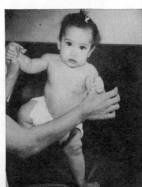

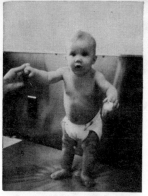

14D. 6 months

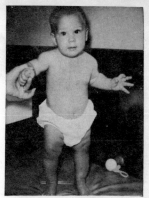

14E. 7 months

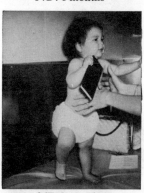

14F. 8 months

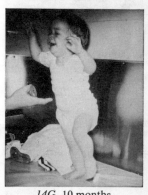

14G. 10 months

14H. 11 months

14J. 1 year

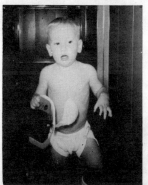

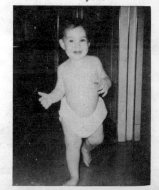

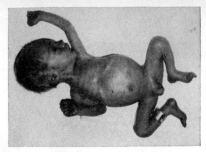

Plate 15.
A premature baby

Plate 16A-16C. MUSCLE TONE

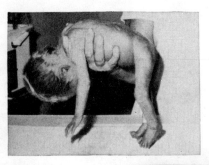

16A.
Premature newborn

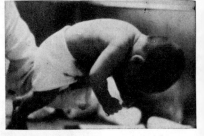

16B. Normal
baby at 1 month

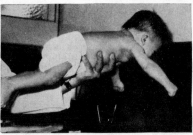

16C. Normal
baby at 3 months

Plate 17A-17M. FROM ABDOMEN TO ALL FOURS

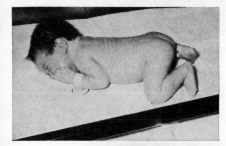

17A. Newborn

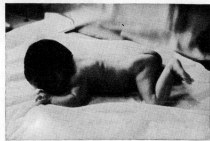

17B. 1 month

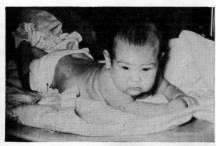

17C. 2 months

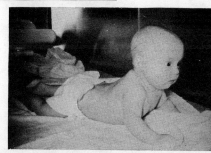

17D. 3 months

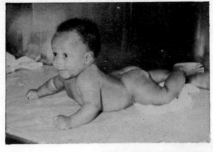

17E. 4 months

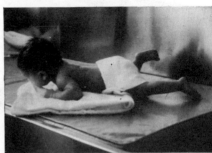

17F. 5 months

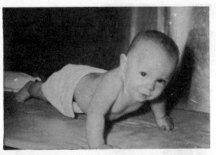

17G. 6 months

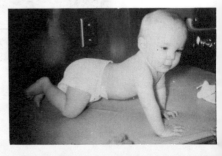

17H. 8 months

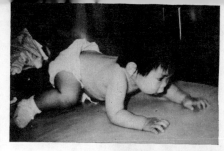

17J. 9 months

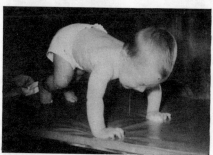

17K. 10 months

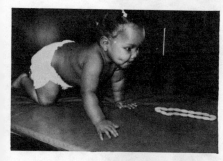

17L. 11 months

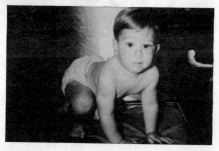

17M. 1 year

Plate 18A-18B. HEADLAG

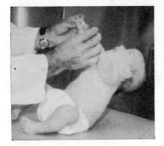

18A. 1 month

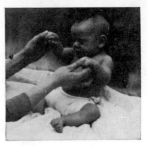

18B. 2 months

Plate 19A-19K. LEARNING TO SIT

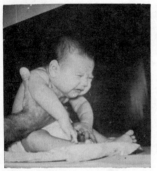

19A. Newborn

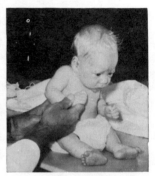

19B. 1 month

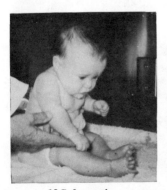

19C. 3 months

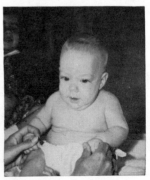

19D. 4 months

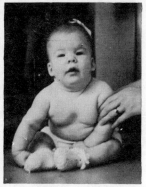

19E. 5 months

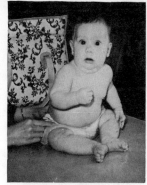

19F. 7 months

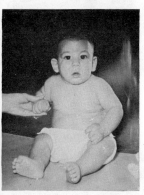

19G. 8 months

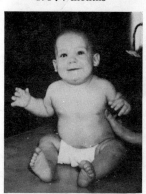

19H. 9 months

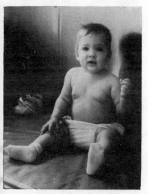

19J. 10 months

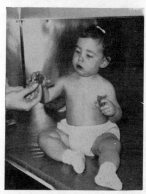

19K. 1 year

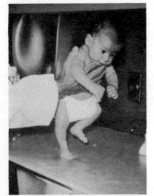

20A. Newborn

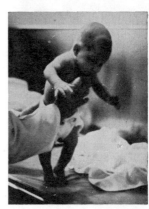

20B. 1 month

20C. 2 months

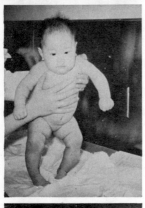

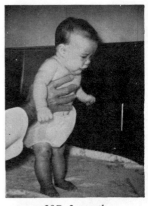

20D. 3 months

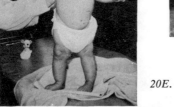

20E. 4 months

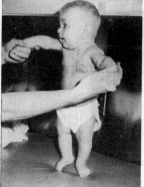

20F. 5 months

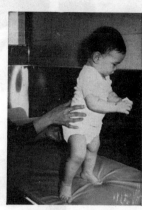

20G. 6 months

20H. 7 months

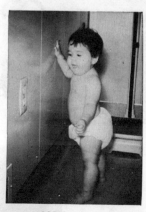

20J. 9 months

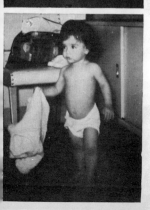

20K. 1 year

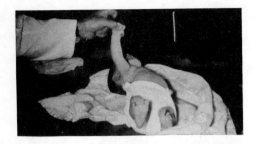

21A. Newborn

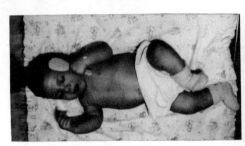

21B. Holding
at 1½ months

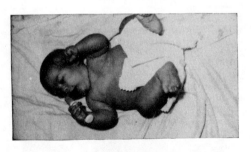

21C. Holding
and focusing
at 3 months

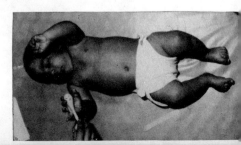

21D. Grasping
at 4 months

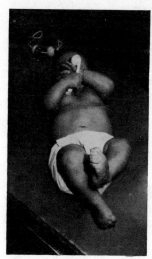

21E.
Midline holding at 4 months

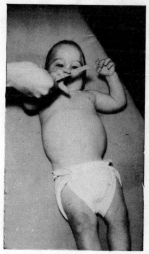

21F. Grasping at 5 months

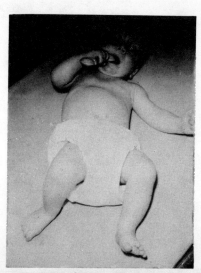

21G. Holding at 5 months

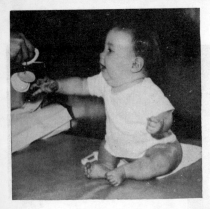

21H. Reaching from sitting at 6 months

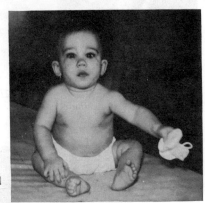

21J. 7 month's handhold

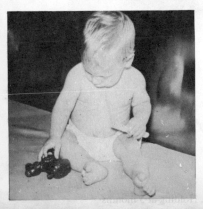

21K. 7 month's grasp

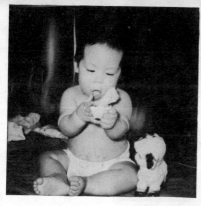

21L.
8 month's handgrasp

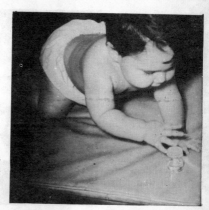

21M. Creeping with
one hand occupied
at 8 months

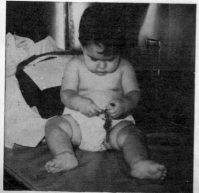

21N. One-hand hold
plus manipulation
at 9 months

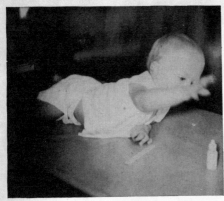

21 O. Creeping and reaching at 9 months

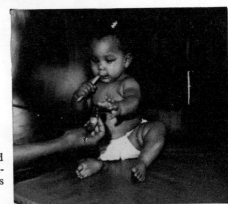

21P. One-hand hold while reaching at 10 months

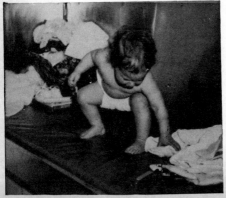

21Q. Squatting to facilitate reaching at 1 year

Plate 22A-22C. LEARNING TO DRINK FROM A CUP

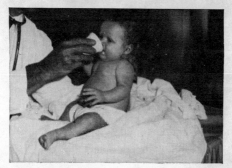

22A. 2 months

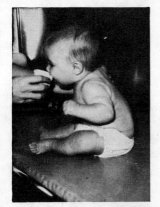

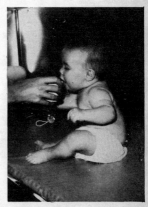

22B. 4 months

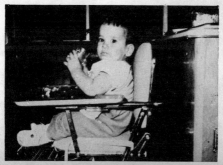

22C. 11 months

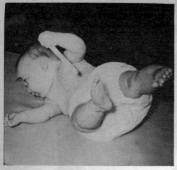

Plate 23.
Starting to roll over at 4 months

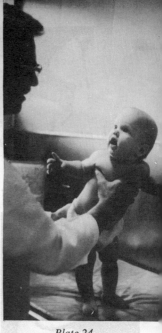

Plate 24.
Face to face with an adult

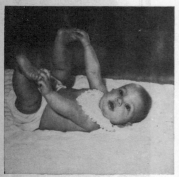

Plate 25. Toe play at 5 months

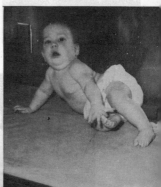

Plate 26. Shifting from sitting
to abdomen at 8 months

SPONGE BATH. This is essentially the soap and water bath I have described, but you don't put the baby in the water. The procedure is carried out on a table or on your lap. You will have to be more careful with this method to make certain that all of the soap is removed. You may want to use sponge baths first until you feel more self-confident. A sponge bath is also used when a child has a surgical wound or an open sore that must be kept dry. If your baby has fever or a cold, there is usually no need to use this type of bath. It is often more chilling and takes more time than a regular tub bath.

OIL BATH. This type of bath is sometimes used for the very small or ill infant. It should be given only if your doctor prescribes it. It is not as effective or relaxing as an overall soap-and-water bath. Use nonmedicated, nonperfumed mineral oil. Don't use too much. Warm the oil by placing the container in a pan of warm water. The oil can be poured directly into your hand as needed, or it can be placed in a small dish into which you dip your fingers. The oil is always applied with the fingers, never with a cotton swab. It is gently massaged into the skin. This also serves to stimulate the infant's circulation. The excess oil is then gently removed with a soft diaper or towel. Do not use cotton swabs or cellulose wipes. When you are finished, he should not feel slippery or greasy. His body creases must be clean.

SAFETY MEASURES AT BATH TIME. Some of these rules have been mentioned already, but they are important enough to bear repeating.

Always test the bath water first.

Never keep your infant in the tub while adding hot water to the bath.

Never leave the tub on a heater or stove while your baby is in it.

Always make certain that the tub, Bathinette, or table is firmly braced so that it cannot fall during the bath procedure. The table or Bathinette should be pushed well back to the wall so that your infant cannot fall off the far side.

Never leave your infant in the tub or on a table unattended. Do not trust a restraint at any time.

Do not use anything sharp around your infant, particularly around his ears and nose.

Always hold your baby firmly in the bath. Soap makes him slippery.

Watch your safety pins. Do not leave them open at any time unless they are stuck into a cake of soap. Place them well out of your infant's reach when you put them down. Do not use small safety pins (lingerie pins) at any time.

By the end of this first month your apprehension about giving a bath should be in the past. A full soap-and-water bath is now part of his daily routine. His umbilical cord is healed, but continue to keep the skin folds cleaned out well. The swollen breasts and genitals may still be there, but don't get too spic and span with them. His eyes may still show some discharge. If this is very great, check with your doctor.

What about the baby who screams all through the bath? Be sure that you are holding him comfortably and securely. Keep your voice and body relaxed. His crying may start when you undress him for the bath. In any case, ease along with him for a time—he will come to enjoy his bath.

Skin Care

As mentioned earlier, after his first bath in the hospital your baby may have shown a blotchy or red rash. This may be replaced by varying amounts of scaling or peeling of the skin for the first few weeks. His skin may look dry, wrinkled, and scaly. His hands and feet are especially bothered, but this appears to be almost a normal reaction of his skin to an air existence after he has lost his vernix.

His first stools can be rather irritating to his skin. He may show some irritation of the skin about his anus. As he ages and his feeding improves, this irritation will lessen.

A face rash like acne is the result of the hormone effect that causes his swollen breasts and genitals. His acne is due to distended, irritated oil glands. The small white heads are oil glands with retained secretions, which gradually empty out and disappear. Just keep his face clean; they'll disappear after a few weeks.

When he rests on one side of his face constantly, he may get some reddened irritation from the moisture of spit-up food. This drooling and rubbing against the sheet put his skin in contact with moisture and heat, which will bring out the irritation.

Cleaning and protecting your baby's skin is part of your

everyday care. You must protect his skin against chafing, irritation, and infection. Too often your faithful early regular care of his skin is neglected as he gets older. Skin problems are usually easier to prevent than they are to cure.

Too much warmth causes him to perspire and may in time produce a *heat rash*. This shows itself as tiny pink to red pimples, mainly in the skin creases. Sometimes his skin may become moist and oozing, especially in the skin creases, under the arms, and in the groin. This becomes more than just prickly heat. It is harder to clear up. Broken skin also exposes him to the risk of secondary skin infection. The likelihood of heat rash can be considerably lessened if you don't keep his room temperature too high or put too many clothes on him. Keep him cool and clean. Don't use waterproof pants—they hold heat as well as water. In hot weather, strip him down to his diaper, and sponge him down with lukewarm water if he is perspiring a lot. Give him an extra daily bath. When the temperature outdoors is over 80°F., he will need only a diaper. If the temperature is over 90°F., a thin cotton sleeveless shirt will absorb perspiration. He feels a little cooler as it evaporates.

Dusting your baby's skin with cornstarch or baking soda will soothe heat rash.

Diaper rash is a common concern of mothers. It can result from moisture in the diaper area, from too much warmth, from chemical irritation, from irritating breakdown products of urine, from airtight covering, from the diaper rubbing against the skin. Too often a severe rash is the result of relaxation of good diaper and baby care. The skin may just be reddened or irritated looking, or it may be so badly abused that it is thickened, cracked, scaling, and ulcerated in spots. Excessive heat is a common cause when coupled with a wet diaper. Urine itself doesn't irritate, but it serves as a good place for bacteria to grow. Bacteria also come from the bowel movement that soils his skin. Bacteria break urine down to ammonia, which gives the characteristic odor—and the all-too-characteristic diaper scald appears in the too hot, too wet area. Sometimes a fungus type of diaper rash comes, which can be very difficult for you to control. Other infections, like impetigo, can come along, but they usually respond quickly to local measures. Sometimes chemical irritants from bleaches, washing powders, or detergents can be at fault. The usual automatic washer and dryer are effective for good diaper care, but you will have to watch your cleaning agent.

But what do you do to treat diaper rash—and prevent it, too? As long as your baby wears diapers his skin must be regularly and carefully cleaned and protected. Change his soiled diapers without delay. If diaper rash is present, you may have to do this with his wet ones, too. Always clean the diaper area well when you change him. Keep his skin fresh and moist looking. Let your nose work here—his skin must smell clean and not like the dirty diaper you just took off.

Wipe away the bowel movement with the soiled diaper—remember, always wipe front to back. Use a soft washcloth, cleansing tissues, or cotton balls to remove the stool material from his skin. Don't just wipe the area in a smearing fashion to leave fecal material on his skin and then cover it with oil. Wash the diaper area with warm, soapy water. Pay attention to skin creases and folds. After rinsing the skin well, pat dry. Don't use oil at all. Use cornstarch or baking soda.

You can use ointments like Vaseline—or any of the heavier protective ointments available, many of which have a Vaseline base, such as A-D ointment or Desitin. Avoid medicated powders unless prescribed. If there is considerable irritation, leave his diaper off for periods during the day. Put him down bottom up. Expose him to the sun when you can. Don't use waterproof pants.

If you are not using a diaper service, launder his diapers properly. (See "Diaper Care," p. 249.)

If the above measures are not sufficient, consult with your pediatrician.

Seborrhea, or "cradle cap," is a common condition without a known cause. Some types of skin have more trouble with this. It appears as a scaling, greasy, crusting, reddened rash, primarily in the scalp but also in the eyebrows, cheeks, behind the ears, on shoulders and chest. Regular vigorous cleansing will keep it under control. It has to be treated regularly or it will come back. Don't use oil to treat it. After thorough daily or every-other-day shampooing, Vaseline, plain cold cream, or a good water-soluble ointment may be applied to soften the crusts. Use a washcloth or soft bristle brush to free the scales. Seborrhea is most noticeable during the first four months, lessens on the scalp after this, but can be bothersome on cheeks from moisture or heat.

A similar kind of rash can be a sensitivity reaction occurring on contact with foods, or with materials applied to the skin. Medicated baby oils, detergents, or any other material applied to the skin or scalp, particularly if there is already irritation, can produce this rash.

Eczema is a less common but more long-standing skin condition. Usually starting at three to four months, it is an itching, scaling, reddened rash that involves the entire skin thickness. You will have to try to discover what foods or outside irritants are at fault. Consult with your pediatrician as to procedures for diagnosis and medication.

Impetigo is a skin infection that appears on an irritated or broken skin surface. It appears anywhere on the body, but in your small baby most often in the diaper area. It starts as a small, reddened, blisterlike area, which breaks to crust over. The infection can spread from one broken area to another. You must consult with your doctor. Good skin care is necessary. The crusts must be removed and the underlying area scrubbed with soap and water. Your doctor will prescribe an antibiotic ointment for this.

Chafing, or intertrigo, results when two folds of skin rub together. The areas become reddened or macerated. You will often see this in the groin folds, the buttocks folds, or under the arms. Do not use oil or grease. Keep the area dry and avoid irritation.

DIAPERING AND DIAPER CARE

Look back to *Preparing for the Baby* for information on types of diapers and number needed.

DIAPERING. Make sure that enough of the diaper is where most of the wetness is going to be, in the front. Avoid too much bunching of the diaper between the baby's legs.

If the diaper is square, (see fig. 47), fold it in thirds to give a triple-thickness rectangle. Then fold the long end over, depending on your baby's size and size of diaper, to give you a pad of six layers of cloth at the end of the turned-back flap. This flap is placed on the inside. Put your baby on the diaper with the turned-back flap brought up between his legs to the front. The other end in back is brought around on either side to the front, even with the front fold. This gives your baby the most diaper in front for maximum absorption. Only three layers of the diaper are between his legs. The diaper ends are fastened at the sides with safety pins placed crosswise. The back fold of the diaper overlaps the front fold. A diaper liner may be use. This method is the same for boys or girls.

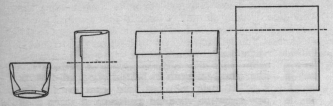

Fig. 47. Folding the square diaper.

If the diaper is rectangular (see fig. 48), it may be folded to give a center panel of extra thickness. This is called a panel fold. Use a 21" x 34" diaper and lay it out flat. Bring the right end to about 6 inches from the left end.

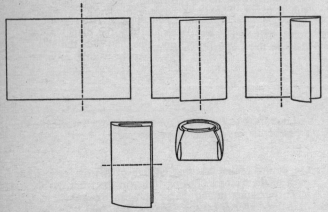

Fig. 48. Folding the rectangular diaper.

Turn the right end back on itself to about 3 inches from the fold. Bring the left end over even with the first fold on the right. This creates a diaper that with the first fold is 21" x 20". You end up with a diaper that is 10" x 21" with the panel about 6 inches wide in the center. It may be pinned on like a square diaper, but there is no flap.

A kite fold with the square diaper (see fig. 49) may be made by folding the two sides of the diaper to make a long V. Turn down the remaining flap above to form a triangle. Bring the point of the V up to the straight edge of the flap. This makes a neat diaper with a thick center panel. The *triangle fold* is similar.

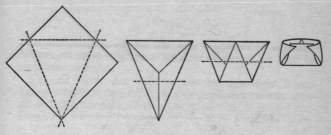

Fig. 49. The kite fold.

You should have your supplies ready before you put your baby on the table on his back. Place an opened paper bag handy for soiled clothing and diapers. After you remove his used diaper and wash and dry the diaper area, grasp his ankles, raise his legs and hips, and slide the clean diaper into place. (See fig. 50A.) Apply baking soda or cornstarch over the area liberally. Pay special attention to the creases.

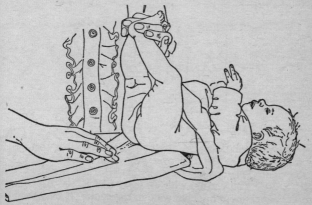

Fig. 50. Diapering. (A)

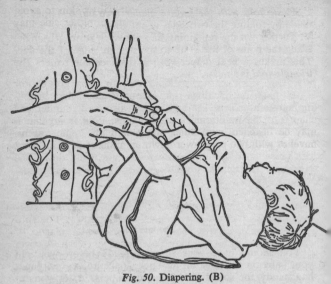

Fig. 50. Diapering. (B)

Bring the front part of the diaper up between his legs. The back edge of the diaper must be above his buttocks several inches higher than the front edge in order to snug down well about his waist. (See fig. 50B.) Pin the diaper at each side, catching both front and back folds. Keep a

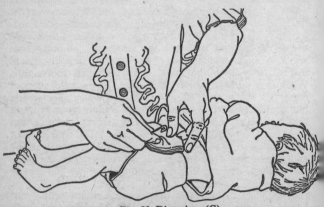

Fig. 50. Diapering. (C)

finger between the safety pin and your baby's skin to avoid sticking him. (See fig. 50C.) Two pins on either side may be needed. If you fit the diaper to him correctly, you won't have to pin the diaper to an undershirt. As you learn you will be able to snug the diaper into place so that it fits and stays up.

Change the fold of his diaper as your baby grows. For a new baby the rectangle fold seems to cause less bunching between his legs. As his stomach becomes rounder you change to the traditional triangle shape. Fold it so that it may be fastened with either one pin in the region of his navel or with two pins lower down on either side. This gives less fabric to bunch up between his legs. Fold down one corner of the triangle so that a pin is used over each hip.

DIAPER CARE. If you are not using a diaper service, the easy sanitary way to care for diapers is as follows: Put four quarts of water in a two-gallon covered enamel, plastic, or aluminum pail. The pail may be larger if you wish. A cover is essential. You may find it more convenient to have two pails, one for wet diapers, one for soiled diapers. Add two tablespoons of Borax, or one tablespoon of Zephiran (17 percent), or two tablespoons of Roccal (10 percent) to the water. These materials serve as mild deodorant and sterilizing agents, and aid in keeping the waste products soluble. Drop the wet diaper into the cold solution as soon as you remove it from your baby. Never dry and reuse it without adequate washing. Diapers soiled with bowel movement need a preliminary cleansing. Hold the diaper over the toilet bowl, shake off the feces, flush away the solid material (but hold on or you may lose the diaper), then drop the diaper into the pail with the antiseptic solution. Once a day wring the diapers out of the solution and dispose of the solution down the toilet. Wash the pail thoroughly. When it is time to wash the diapers, use a mild soap or detergent thoroughly dissolved in hot water. Never use bluing or strong soap, as these may irritate your baby in his diaper area. If you hand-wash the diapers, make certain they are thoroughly clean, then rinse them well two or three times. If you use an automatic washer, the washing and rinsing are done for you. If you don't have an automatic dryer, dry the diapers thoroughly either indoors or in any available sunlight.

When the diapers are dry, smooth them with your hands, fold them neatly, and store in a clean dry spot ready for use. Ironing diapers is not necessary, and makes them less absorbent. Make your diaper care as simple as you possibly can. It goes on for a long time.

Even if you use a diaper service, you should thoroughly rinse any soiled diaper before storing it for pickup.

CLOTHING

Check back to *Preparing for the Baby* for suggestions about kinds and amounts of clothing needed.

I have mentioned this before: Resist your natural inclination to overdress your baby! As long as the room temperature is 68°-70°, he will need only nightgown and diaper, sleeper and diaper, or, perhaps later, shirt and diaper. You may want to wrap him in a receiving blanket when you are carrying him about.

Don't wash his clothing with the family laundry. You can wash all his garments together. Use a mild laundry soap or detergent.

13.

The

Second Month

Your baby continues adjusting his inner tensions to his outside world. You will keep on spending a great deal of your time trying to help him do this adjusting. This month usually finds you less pushed by it all. You have learned some of the shortcuts, decided what is important, and discovered how to fit your life around your baby's rhythms. This means that you can breathe a little easier and pay attention to something beside baby care.

WEIGHT

Ranges: Boys 9.0–14.3   Average 10.9
           Girls 8.4–13.0   Average 10.7

HEIGHT

Ranges: Boys 21.0–23.9   Average 22.5
           Girls 20.9–23.5   Average 22.2

MOTOR DEVELOPMENT

Your baby will gain considerably more control of his muscles during this second month, although such control still won't be very obvious in most ways unless you look for it. You will notice that he seems more alert, that he responds to you with different facial expressions when you talk to him. All this is possible because he is getting more voluntary control over the muscles of his eyes, face, and neck. Although you won't notice any difference in the way he uses his arms and legs, you will notice more strength in them as he waves his arms, kicks, and pushes about.

REFLEXES

His reflexes are still very much in use, but some are fading out. He is most competent now in using his rooting and sucking reflexes when nursing. He is beginning to replace them with more conscious response in the use of his lips and mouth. His crossed-extension, trunk-curving, and magnet reflexes may still be there for you to see.

Let him grasp your finger to show his traction response by pulling gently on his arm. This response causes him to bend his elbow and pull his upper arm tight against his body. The reflex grasping you saw with this is disappearing. It will be replaced by his more controlled hand response. If you touch his hand on the thumb side of his palm he grasps to make a fist. His voluntary grasping will come only after his closed hands open and his eyes coordinate with his hands. His feet still show his toe grasping.

On his back his tonic-neck reflex (TNR) is still prominent. His arms may be flexed or bent more often than before. His startle, or Moro reflex, is fading. He tolerates much more than he did before without jumping or crying. His reflex walking is not so easily brought out after six weeks unless you have him positioned just right and he cooperates.

LYING, SITTING, STANDING, AND GETTING ABOUT

In his prone position he has come down off his knees now and is stretching out his legs. He is more assured and definite in his push-ups. He doesn't just lie there with his head to one side. It is now held in the midline and active. By the end of this month, he lifts his head 45° to 90° off the table to get his chin up. (See plate 17C.) He does this repeatedly, but he doesn't keep it up long. In his push-ups he may rest on his forearms with his elbows bent. His shoulders are beginning to share in his effort to get his chest up off the table.

On his back, your baby may act as if he wishes to be raised to a sitting position. If you try to pull him to a sitting position his head lag is less, but he still has a good deal of it. When you get him to the sitting position, his head is pretty wobbly when he tries to hold it up. (See plate 18B.)

He doesn't help you very much in your efforts to get him up to a standing position. (See plate 20C.)

On his abdomen he does manage to move about. The start of this is found in his swimming body movements in which he rhythmically swings his trunk back and forth and moves his arms and legs. He won't move far or fast this way until he can pull or push with his arms, dragging his abdomen and legs. A very active baby may already be using his legs at this point to help out in this first move toward crawling.

HANDS

By this time your baby may often put his thumb or finger or whole fist into his mouth. He doesn't know too well that he is doing it. If he sucks for fairly long periods of time, you are getting the message that he wants more to eat. He will suck before his meals when he is hungry. Make his meals adequate so he will be satisfied. If he sucks after his meals, this may be a settling-down time for him before sleep. (Look back to the section on "Rhythmic Patterns" for more on thumb-sucking.)

You may see him open his hands frequently now. He opens his hand to grasp at a rattle or a stick when his hand is touched. He holds it briefly, then drops it. (See plate 21B.)

EYES AND OTHER SENSE ORGANS

Your baby has stopped just staring blankly at a wall or your face. He makes rapid progress in the use of his eyes during his second month. He is able to focus his eyes better, though his eye nerves are not entirely formed yet. With his hands outstretched in front of his face, his eyes begin to see and recognize his hands. He can also look more steadily at an object. During this month he is able to make both eyes move together. He follows and watches a moving object and he can look from side to side, but not up and down yet. He is fascinated by bright colors, especially bright reds and blues. He turns his eyes to a fixed light but turns away from too bright a light. He blinks at a sudden light. He doesn't blink at any sudden approach toward his face. He begins to break into a big smile when he sees you directly in front of him or hears your familiar voice. By the end of the month he seems to recognize familiar daily objects.

By now the great majority of babies will have tears.

His hearing is becoming more directed as he halts his activity or fussing at any new noise about him. His hearing and seeing are tying in with his increasing use of his head and neck. He blinks his eyes at a loud sound. He turns his head and eyes at a sound, perhaps just pauses. Music or other rhythmic sounds may interest him. He may try out different sounds on himself.

EATING

As these months go along and I discuss what you should be feeding your baby you will find how much I stress his need for building materials. These building materials must be protein. Other items of his diet are fillers and must not replace the building materials. Only in this way can you give your baby a chance to put together a solid healthy body.

This past month your baby's diet consisted of the food groups of cereal, fruit, and meat mixed with breast or formula milk. Hopefully you were able to offer him enough of this solid mixture so that he was comfortably and adequately satisfied quickly and didn't require excessive amounts of milk afterward to fill him. Now you will move to expand and fulfill his diet needs so that you will be able to use items from all the basic food groups in these weeks ahead.

MENU

> cereal—1 portion
> fruit—1 portion
> meat–egg yolk 1 portion
> milk–milk solids–cheese 1–2 portions

Give these portions at each feeding. Give any amount he wishes as long as you keep the ratio or proportion the same. Continue to mix all of his food items into one concoction. It is easier for you to feed one mixture now than to bother with a dab of this and a spoonful of that. It is less wasteful too.

MENU COMMENTS

CEREAL. Rice, oat, or barley cereal continue to be the thickeners for the solid food portion of the meal. The fortified high protein infant cereals furnish vegetable protein in your baby's diet to complement the animal protein from the meat-eggs and the milk-milk solid-cheese groups.

MEAT. Continue to use at least one portion of meat to each feeding. If you can increase any amounts, meat and milk solids are the best to add. Beef, veal, lamb, pork, ham, and chicken are the usual meats available for your use. Any of these meats you have for your family can be used after pureeing in a blender. Season them lightly with iodized salt. Don't use the combination meat dinners offered in the line of prepared baby foods. Use plain meats.

EGG. Egg yolk is an excellent all-purpose iron-containing protein and has the highest rating. Wash the egg shell with soap and water first before you crack it. Separate the white and use the raw yolk to mix into your baby's other foods, as a portion for his meat group. You can hard-boil the egg to completely separate the yolk from the white if you wish. This should be done for a baby with an allergic family history.

FRUIT. Continue banana, apple, pear, pineapple, as fruit portions which may now include apricot, peach, plum, or prune. Keep in mind that some of these foods may cause you some temporary inconvenience with his loose stools.

MILK–MILK SOLIDS. Although breast milk is the most adequate of foods in the group, your diet has some influence on its adequacy. Very often it has inadequate iron and probably requires some supplementation by this time. This is done with the food groups you are adding to your baby's diet.

Continue to use the prepared infant formula as before. It is often better tolerated than evaporated milk at this time. Most of it will be going into the mix if you are feeding enough of the cereal mix. If he takes more than 2 ounces of his bottle or more than 10 minutes on breast after his solids, he probably needs more cereal mix. Some of you may wish to use evaporated milk but don't go to whole milk. Its butterfat content may bother your baby. The prepared infant formula has had butterfat replaced by vegetable oils. Your baby is able to hold just so much liquid volume of milk without over-filling and spitting back. A good way to avoid this is to start using milk solids added to the cereal mix. He gets the food value of milk without the filling effect of the fluid volume. Dry skim powdered milk with added vitamins A and D is available packaged in a carton. It is an inexpensive form of milk, easy to store and use. Start with a teaspoon in each feeding. Gradually increase this amount to 3 tablespoons in each meal mixture.

CHEESE. Another valuable milk solid is the cheese group which you start now too. Cottage cheese is the best of the cheese group to start with. Mash it and mix it thoroughly with the fruit before you add it to the other parts of the cereal mix. A blender solves this most easily. Cream cheese can be used but it is a little more difficult to mix. Yogurt is another substitute. Other cheeses are added later.

one portion = 3 tablespoons dry powdered skim milk
          = 3 ounces cottage cheese
          = 3 ounces yogurt

FRUIT JUICE. You may have offered water or fruit juice between feedings before this time. Now you start to offer fruit juice regularly between feedings from his cup or pitcher. Apple juice is a good one to start with. After this month you can start other juices such as orange, pineapple, grape, tomato, apricot. Add these gradually in the weeks ahead, but for now use apple juice. Dilute these juices with water when you first use them.

VITAMINS. Continue the use of the multiple-vitamin drops. Put the dosage in his cereal mix at one feeding.

BREAST-FEEDING

Continue breast-feeding as before after his cereal mix. The amount he will take will be very hard to guess. Just give him enough cereal mix first so that he is satisfied with 10 minutes of breast. A good nursing baby empties the breast adequately in 5–6 minutes. If he wants the second breast offer it, but try to increase the amount of cereal mix the next feeding.

Even this early your baby may begin to bite at your breast after he has nursed for a time. This may show his increasing dexterity but it is annoying. Perhaps if you stop your nursing when he has emptied the breast so that he doesn't mouth and such without eating, he will avoid this. He is using your breast as a pacifier, so stop it before it gets painful.

In his sucking you will see another developmental step. He is using his nursing reflexes less now. He fixes his eyes as he goes into a burst of sucking. He sucks in bursts or in a series of sucks . . . then something diverts him, he shifts his focus on something and stops sucking, then he sucks again. Apparently he needs to absorb one thing at a time. Any change—your shift in position, a loud noise, someone coming into the room—stops his sucking. This is another reason to keep his feeding time quiet and isolated.

You may feel that you want to wean your baby from breast at this time. By the end of this month about 4 out of 10 mothers have done so. From your baby's viewpoint another month fits in better with the scheme of things. But again, you may have a young fellow who just says in every way he can that he is done with this sort of thing. If he does, increase the cereal mix so that he is filled. Then he can take the cup for one to two ounces of formula afterwards. Try to make any such shift to cup or pitcher rather than to bottle.

BOTTLE-FEEDING

In your bottle-feeding he should take one to two ounces after he has had his cereal mix. If he takes more than this, try to increase the amounts of his solids so that most of the formula is used to mix with them. If he takes more than 2 ounces, or isn't going more than 4 hours between feedings, you are lagging on giving him enough cereal mix. Also, you are giving yourself more work.

WEANING

At this stage most babies are not ready to shift from bottle although some do shift off breast. Cup-feeding is started now to ready him for drinking from the cup when he starts to shift from the bottle. Don't wean from breast to bottle. Go directly to the cup. A pitcher may serve the purpose better. So-called special training cups aren't necessary.

Look back to "Eating" last month for comments on sterilization and cleanliness, leftover foods, use of prepared foods, day's mix, warm-cold foods.

Don't forget you can do a satisfactory job of food preparation with a blender. A blender is a great time-saver and money-saver too. Any foods you use for your own table can be used in your baby's diet and less expensively. But don't over-cook. If you cook the life out of your foods you make them less adequate as basic food items especially in respect to vitamins and minerals.

SPOON-FEEDING

By this time you have the knack of moving his food rapidly into his mouth with a spoon. You have learned something about your baby and his reflexes and make use of them at each feeding.

In his feeding pattern he is showing less of the pushing

out with his tongue. This retrusion reflex will be gone in another month. Now he can hold food in his mouth for a moment but he can't move solid food easily from front to back yet. So your successful feeding depends to a great extent on your adequate filling of his mouth. He shows his first signs of learning in his feeding now with his anticipatory sucking and mouthing when you get him ready for his feeding. Don't think you are making things easier for yourself if you are still putting his cereal mix all into the bottle. If you are, you must expect to have a little more trouble making the shift to spoon later.

CUP-FEEDING

If you didn't before, by now you give your baby fruit juice from a cup whenever he is awake between feedings and seems hungry. He can drink from a small glass or a pitcher just as well. Sit him up to drink but remember how he uses his mouth and tongue. You still see some pushing out of his tongue. When you touch his lips his tongue pushes out and arches up. Lay the cup edge on top of his tongue since he can't swallow without choking with his tongue in the cup. Since he is unable to control a single mouthful at a time, help him by tipping the glass to give him a little at a time. (See plate 23A.) You will have to practice a little in presenting it to him to learn how to do this. He knows how to swallow, so learn the rhythm of this. You will be messy at first but he may surprise you with how well he does. Cup-feeding prepares him for that shift from breast to cup when he is ready to wean in the months ahead. It also avoids the bottle if you are breast-feeding.

SCHEDULE

Four feedings at 7:00 A.M., 12:00 noon, 5:00–6:00 P.M., and 10:00–11:00 P.M.
   or
Three feedings at 7:00 A.M., 1:00 P.M., and 3:00 P.M.
Last month he probably dropped his night feeding so that you were giving him 5 feedings a day. As you increased his cereal mix during this month he lengthened the intervals between feedings to 5 hours and you found he was

on 4 feedings. If you have a big eater he may be trying to tell you that he wants to go 6 hours between feedings and eat just 3 times a day now. If your baby is an average eater he will shift to 3 meals some time during this coming month.

Encourage him to go longer. He is ready to start up a fairly regular schedule for himself if you will just go along with him. If your baby is hungry every 3 or 4 hours you aren't really giving him anywhere near enough food. Check his feeding schedule to see that he is satisfied.

By this time you will have lost your anxieties about feeding and can move large quantities easily into his mouth. If you are still having difficulty talk it over with your pediatrician and find out what you may be doing wrong. It is important to establish a good feeding relationship with your baby before any more weeks go by.

BETWEEN MEALS

You do not give him anything but juice between feedings at this time. If you give him milk to drink, you take away appetite for his next meal. This also upsets any menu planning and alters the balance of his diet. If he is hungry between feedings, give him fruit juice and let him wait. Then give him more food at his regular feeding time.

HOLDING

Again, hold him comfortably and securely at every feeding at this age. Your voice, your body contact, are things that count almost—almost, I said—as much as his food. Remember, the infant seat is not the place to feed him.

BOTTLE-PROPPING

Don't do it! Even with your cup-feeding you are not isolated or remote. You are there giving physical warmth, encircling support, and firm direction. Cuddling, talking, affectionate handling can only come from a warm giving human being, not a propped bottle.

Your own meal time should be kept separate from your baby's schedule. You will relax and have a comfortable meal after he is put somewhere else at that time. Don't start bringing him to the adult table even if it seems fun to have him around at this time. It doesn't remain fun!

BOWEL AND BLADDER FUNCTIONS

Your baby now produces his stools at slightly more regular intervals. Constipation is one of the things that is frequently talked about at this time. Constipation means many things to different mothers. It may mean that the baby strains at the stool, that the stool is hard and dry, that bowel movements occur infrequently, that the amount of stool is too little, etc. What may be needed is less concern with what happens at that end of his anatomy and a little more attention to what you are putting in at the other end. He needs more bulk—primarily meat and fruit—in his diet.

SLEEPING

Sleeping is still your baby's main occupation. He does sleep for longer periods at a time now—he stays awake for longer periods, too. His longest sleep period has reached about eight to eight and half hours. His P.M. fussing, colic, or whatever name you give it, has reached its peak in the six to eleven P.M. period and is probably lessening by now or soon will.

I am a firm believer in the principle that nighttime is for sleep. If your baby doesn't seem ready to give up his nighttime feeding by now, you may need to do something different in your care. If you haven't accepted my suggestion before, do so now: Get your baby out of your room and into his own!

EXERCISE AND PLAY

Fresh air, exercise, and sunshine all help to make your baby eat better, sleep better, and feel better, just as they do with adults. After four to six weeks, any healthy baby of average weight and development can be outdoors part of each day in good weather. You may have been too busy with new-baby routines to give your baby many outdoor airings before now.

Good weather doesn't only mean sunny days with balmy blue skies. Your baby can be out on a cold or overcast day if he is in a protected place. There is no advantage in having your small baby outdoors on a very cold winter day, a damp, windy day, or a day when there is smog or a strong dust-laden wind. Keep him indoors if he is ill.

To some extent, outdoor airings are guided by considering the outside temperature and your baby's weight. For the eight-pound baby, a temperature of 60°F. is perfectly safe for a daily airing. When he weighs ten pounds, he can be out on days with temperatures nearer to freezing. Temperatures below 50°F. are too rigorous for small babies. When he weighs twelve pounds, he can enjoy being outdoors in a sunny, protected place even when the temperature in the shade is slightly below freezing. Watch the thermometer. See that the sun shines on his carriage or playpen.

You can start his outdoor airings for twenty- or thirty-minute periods between 11 A.M. and 2 P.M. Increase the time gradually to two or three hours daily between 11 A.M. and 2 P.M.

Pick a sheltered outdoor spot where he can't be rained on, dropped on, or bothered by children or animals. "Exposing him" means to weather, not crowds of people. You may use a carriage, crib, or playpen, depending on your situation. Check him at regular intervals. He should not feel cold or sweaty. He usually sleeps peacefully. He may lie there comfortably with his eyes open, looking about.

Don't feel bad if you have to skip a daily airing sometimes. Air in the house may not smell quite as fresh, but it is usually perfectly healthy as long as there is adequate circulation and ventilation. Keep the baby's bedroom window open.

Some of you mothers have difficulty permitting your child enough outdoor time because of your own inclination to stay indoors. On the other hand, if you are the outdoor type yourself you may overdo the airing.

Sunlight is one of the real benefits your baby gets from his outdoor excursions. In the summer, you can start his outdoor sunbaths when he weighs about ten pounds. Pick a sheltered place. Strip him down to his bare skin and put him on a pad, in his playpen, carriage, or stroller. If the weather is too cold to expose his body outdoors, you can give him sunbaths indoors in the same fashion. Raise the window so the sunshine hits him directly. Sunlight coming through window glass is ineffective since the glass filters out all the esssential ultra-violet rays.

Start his sunbaths in the mid-morning or mid-afternoon in summer, between twelve noon and two P.M. in winter. Give him three minutes' exposure front and back. Increase this daily by one-minute intervals to fifteen or twenty minutes on each side. After this you may start dividing his total exposure time into two periods, particularly if the sun is very hot. Half an hour twice a day should be the maximum exposure time during this first year. If you have to skip a few days, start from the period of time you last used. If you missed longer than a few days, cut back and build up gradually. Do not leave him alone during his sunbaths in his baby months. You will need to cover him if the sun goes behind the clouds or other conditions change. When he is older you may be able to judge exposure time better.

If your baby is a blond or a redhead, use greater care. These skin tones don't tolerate much sunlight. They burn and do not tend to tan. They lack sufficient pigment in the skin to produce darkening or tanning. Your aim is to produce a moderate tan in a lighter-skinned baby. In the dark-skinned Oriental or Negro baby, sunbaths are just as necessary, but you have no good way to determine the exposure time by any change in skin tone or color. Do not exceed the time limits suggested above. Increase times gradually. You can burn any skin, no matter how much protective pigment it has in it. Excessive amounts of sun are not healthful.

Take definite precautions to protect your baby's eyes from the sun, particularly if he is on his back. Your older baby or child protects himself by closing his eyes, turning his head, bending his neck, or moving out of the sun. Your young baby tries to turn his head away from the glare, but this isn't safe enough. Arrange his crib, playpen, or carriage to avoid direct sunlight in his eyes. Your baby's eyes will not be injured by sunlight unless the rays enter directly into the back of his eye (the retina). If his eyes are closed and his face turned away from the sun, he will not be eyeburned. However he may be uncomfortable from the glare or heat. You must also be careful to protect him from insects in the summer.

You can continue the kinds of exercises described last month. Lengthen the time as he gets older. He will tell you when he has had enough by his lack of response or by getting cross at you. His clothing should either be removed or be loose enough to permit him full freedom of movement.

Much of his early exercise will be on his own. He should go into a playpen this month. (Look back to *Preparing for the Baby* for more on this.)

By now he may enjoy watching a mobile hung over his crib or playpen. See next month's "Exercise and Play" for more about toys.

AWARENESS AND SOCIAL RESPONSE

By the end of the second month he may give you a direct look of definite attention. This isn't accidental. It means he is learning by experience. He has connected you in his mind with contentment and relief from discomfort. He may also respond to the presence of other people. Although he still enjoys cuddling and motion, he is losing some of his concern with his insides and becoming aware of his outside world. He is discovering his hands. He swipes at objects with a closed-fist movement.

By now your baby has developed a true social smile. You may suddenly look at him as you are talking or caring for him, and there is a smile! He has very little control over it yet. He has very little memory. He is just starting to know there is anything outside himself. This new development is exciting, but he has a long way to go yet. Don't let this smiling business go to your head. It may be a blow to your ego, but he will smile at the front view of any human face, or a reasonable facsimile of one, for several months. You don't even have to be smiling to win his response. A side-face view or profile doesn't work, though.

ORAL COMMUNICATION

Your baby gurgles now and makes more noncrying noise. There may be some quality of musical rhythm to it. He makes single-word sounds like "ah," "eh," "uh." Babbling and cooing will begin now as a social response on his part. If you make cooing sounds, he may coo back. This is his first vocal expression of his good feelings.

Don't forget about the importance of talking and singing to him. When he is sleepy, use the lulling kind of talk. Anyone listening to you might wonder at your sanity, but don't be embarrassed. You can be happily silly with him and he loves it. Take your chance while you can. You only pass this way once with him.

IMMUNIZATIONS

Effective immunizing agents are available for whooping cough (pertussis), diphtheria, tetanus (lockjaw), poliomyelitis (infantile paralysis), smallpox (Variola), measles (rubeola), German measles (Rubella), and mumps. Your baby should be adequately protected against these diseases. Immunization against mumps and German measles may be given at one year of age.

There are also vaccines available for typhoid fever, typhus, yellow fever, and other illnesses. These are not needed except under special circumstances.

This month your doctor may start the immunizing injections or "shots" for whooping cough, diphtheria, and tetanus (D.P.T. shots). The second and third injections will be given at intervals of one or two months. Booster shots are given in the second year. The injections are mixtures of separate vaccines that give a better immune response in your baby than if each one were given separately. Combining them also reduces the number of times he has to get an injection.

These injections do not produce in your baby the diseases they are aimed against. They are materials composed of the ingredients or antigens specific for the infecting agent involved in the various infections. Giving this antigen stimulates your baby's immune defense mechanisms to manufacture an antibody or neutralizing agent specific for the disease. If he is later exposed to the infection, his body is prepared to manufacture large amounts of whooping cough, diphtheria, tetanus, or other specific neutralizers.

Whooping cough (pertussis) is a serious disease in infants, especially those under six months. Tetanus (lockjaw) protection is very important during childhood, since many minor skin breaks occur from various types of injury. Contamination of the wound can cause trouble. If basic protection by immunization is given early, a booster dose of vaccine will give protection should your baby later suffer a contaminated wound.

Diphtheria is no longer a dread disease, as a result of the widespread use of immunization.

Your doctor may defer immunization injections if your baby shows an acute infection.

The area of injection is usually high in the buttocks or lateral thigh. Measles injection is given in the upper arm. These injections do not leave scars, as the material is given under the skin (subcutaneously) or into the muscles (intramuscularly). Occasionally a hard lump develops under the skin at the site of the injection. This may be present for weeks or months. Leave it alone, as it will gradually be absorbed. Your baby may show very little reaction to the injection except for a brief period of crying at the time of the shot. Sometimes a baby is quite fussy and irritable later in the day. Remember that the shot is given high on his buttocks or leg, so don't pick him up to pat him. It won't comfort him to have his sore bottom patted. He may run some fever. You may use aspirin (acetylsalicylic acid) or an aspirin substitute (acetaminophen), such as Tempra drops or Tylenol drops, for relief. The usual dose for aspirin is 1 grain (65 mg.) per years of age. The aspirin-substitute drop dosage is 0.6 cc. Your doctor will indicate the amount to use. It is a help to give an initial dose as soon as you get home. The aspirin-substitute drops can be given in a little food, dropped into the mouth, or mixed with fruit juice. Baby aspirin or regular aspirin can be dissolved in a spoonful of water or juice. These may be repeated every three or four hours several times, if necessary. Any such reaction to the injection should be gone by the following day. If the fever continues beyond this time, it is probably unrelated to the injection. The area of the injection may be quite swollen, reddened, and tender. This subsides over a day or so. You need to do nothing to the area. If you are alarmed about the fever or swelling, check with your doctor.

This month your doctor may also start the oral polio (Sabin) vaccine. This vaccine—with all three polio strains combined, which reduces the number of doses needed—is given as a few drops placed in the mouth. It takes time to produce this lasting immunity. Four more doses—at four months, six months, eighteen months, and four to six years —will be given. This oral immunity is considered to be a lifetime affair.

BABY-CARE ROUTINES

BATH TIME

If your baby is still crying when he has a bath, it may mean that you are not yet handling him confidently and comfortably. However, many very young babies cry at bath time for no obvious cause. They quiet down gradually as the weeks go by. Make his bath time as rapid as possible. Have everything ready and get him back into his clothes quickly. This will usually help to solve the problem. Be sure that the room temperature is warm enough. This may help a little too.

SKIN CARE

Look back to last month for advice on the treatment of diaper rash, cradle cap, and other skin problems.

If you have been keeping your baby on his back too much, you may notice a bald spot developing on the back of his head. The bald spot will be covered by new hair in a few months if you get him off his back. Make sure that you are not leaving your baby too long in one position during the day. Give him a change of position and something different to look at occasionally.

Your baby's navel may push out with a little bump when he cries or strains. This isn't because the cord was badly tied, but because the umbilical opening is not yet closed. It gradually closes during the first months. If it is large, you can apply waterproof plastic tape to hold it back in place while it closes. Consult your pediatrician about this.

14.

The

Third Month

Your baby is less work now, especially if you have moved along with his feedings to three meals. He is more contented. This is the start of a pleasing period of his infancy, from your standpoint. He sleeps less frequently, but longer when he does, and is more alert and interested in his world. If Father hasn't shown too much interest before this, the new young personality may be quite intriguing to him from now on.

WEIGHT

Ranges: Boys 10.6–16.4 lbs. Average 12.6 lbs.
Girls 9.8–14.9 lbs. Average 12.4 lbs.

During these first three months you have seen a good deal of weight added to your baby. This is a gain in three months of five to six pounds for boys and four to five pounds for girls. This is as rapid a period of growth as he will ever show after his birth. (He did grow faster in your uterus.) From this time on he slows down considerably.

HEIGHT

Ranges: Boys 22.4–25.1 in. Average 23.8 in.
Girls 22.0–24.8 in. Average 23.4 in.

This is a gain of 3½ to 4 inches for boys and 3 to 3½ inches for girls in three months.

MOTOR DEVELOPMENT

He is better coordinated than he was last month. But this may lead to new difficulties, because he is trying to do so many new things with his developing equipment.

REFLEXES

Many of his reflexes are disappearing entirely now. Although he still tends to tongue thrust, this action is being replaced by more tongue control on his part. By the end of this period his grasping reflex is gone. Now he will only touch your hand, showing none of his former traction response. His tonic-neck reflex will be seen less frequently now for his whole body. It has served to give him a start on his eye-hand coordination by enabling him to catch a glimpse of his hand and focus his attention on it. Now he may hold his head to one side while his arms and legs work together. (See plate 21C.) With this more symmetrical position, his hands are directed toward his middle. His Moro reflex is mostly gone by now. His reflex walking has disappeared.

LYING, SITTING, STANDING, AND GETTING ABOUT

On his back he can't raise his head yet, but he holds his arms and legs symmetrically when he is active. He brings his legs up in the air to start some foot play. This will increase, but even now he can bring the soles of his feet together.

When he is prone, he will show you that his other muscles are stronger. He has developed more strength in his back muscles, arms, and legs. He lies flat on the table with his legs stretched out straight. He will raise his head several inches and hold it up for more than several minutes before he tires. He pushes himself up on his arms and brings his chest up, resting his weight on his forearms. (See plate 17D.) He can bring his legs up under him, but he more often pushes out with them. He may raise them from the table as he arches his back. He makes thrashing movements in which he uses both his arms and legs at once.

By this time he may show more definite preference for a front or back position.

When you sit him up now, you notice that his head comes up with his body instead of dropping back, although you will still see some head lag. (See plate 19C.) You know he is trying to straighten his body out when you feel him actively push backward against your hand. In his sitting position his back is still quite rounded. He will manage his head quite well, with much less sag or bobbing. You can call this true sitting. He looks ahead, but his head bobs about, out of control at times. He is making some effort to control his balance. When he is sitting, his legs are still flexed. He sets his head forward a little between his hunched shoulders.

When you pull him up to a standing position, he pushes out a little with his legs and makes a feeble attempt to get his buttocks up from the table. You have to place him in a standing position. He may push hard with his legs off and on and momentarily bear quite a bit of his own weight. (See plate 20D.) He does this by straightening out his knees. He flexes his toes when they come into contact with the floor. He may lift one foot, using the other for support, or he may just do a good deal of bouncing.

He may choose a favorite position for resting or sleeping. Awake he often appears to be making clutching or scratching movements. Thrashing movements are common. He may be difficult to feed because his arms and legs keep getting in the way.

The use of his swimming motion is still the way he gets about. He will hold a "flying" or "airplaning" position for several minutes, lying on his abdomen with his arms held out widely at his shoulders, his legs and head raised well off the bed. In this position he moves his arms and legs actively.

If your baby sat in your uterus with his toes pointed in, he may still show this pigeon-toed position. It may need correction.

HANDS

He is developing some control of his hands. He now holds them more open about half the time with fingers loosely curled. He is becoming aware of them as parts of himself. His own hand is one of the first things he grasps. Hand play is a favorite pastime for him at this time. He studies his hands intently as he tries to make them touch. He may spend quite a bit of time just looking at them as he waves them about. He acts as if having hands was the most interesting thing that had ever happened to anybody. He tries to move his hands together. He may get hold of his clothes and pull.

The old wives' tale that he will be cross-eyed if you dangle a toy in front of his face is disproved by this playing with his hands. If looking at something this way produced eye crossing, every child would be cross-eyed. Actually, anything that benefits his eye-and-hand coordination is to his advantage.

If you offer him something, he gets excited and eagerly makes arm and leg motions. His arm control isn't up to very accurate reaching yet. When he tries to reach for something, both arms come out jerkily. He reaches but misses. He has the intent, but not the control yet. He paws at things with his palms, not with his fingers. This is not prehension, or true grasping, yet. Such grasping starts on the little-finger side of his hand and goes finger by finger to his thumb side.

By this time, he may be able to put a thumb or finger into his mouth now and then in preference to his whole fist. Gradually he is starting to separate a thumb or finger from his fist. Until next month he may not get it far enough out of his fist to do much with it. If he sucked his thumb in your uterus he will already have rediscovered it. This mouthing is part of his developmental pattern. He needs to grasp and explore with both his mouth and hand. Some babies never get very interested in this kind of mouth learning, but use more hand learning.

EYES AND OTHER SENSE ORGANS

The bizarre eye movements of the newborn have gone through the stage of passing fixation to develop now into a coordinated looking at a fixed point. This is a big step in his eye use. His eyes follow you better. They begin to follow up and down. If you put your hand to one side, he will be able to follow it without losing track of it. This is a swing through 180° or a half circle. The ability to do this makes it possible for him to learn a great deal more about what goes on in his surroundings. Instead of appearing as vague, unconnected pictures, events around him are now perceived in smoother sequences—like a motion picture instead of individual still pictures. He stares at familiar objects and will change his attention to unfamiliar ones. He will recognize differences. You may have to attract his attention to something held in front of him, since he shows some delay in focusing on a toy not in his line of vision. As he tries to focus on a toy he may cross his eyes off and on. If you cover his face, he reacts to it.

Just as he turned toward a familiar voice or interesting sound, now he will search for the sound he hears with his eyes. He is quieted by your voice and listens to music.

TEETH

Drooling is more noticeable by now. He puts everything in his mouth, which means he will drool even more. He won't cut a tooth for at least another month. (Look ahead to *The Fourth Month*, "Teeth," for a fuller discussion of teeth and teething.)

EATING

The pattern of feeding I have been suggesting for your baby is roughly as follows: Cereal mix was started when he took 4 ounces or more of formula and wasn't satisfied for 3-3½ hours, or if on breast he went less than 3-3½ hours. Other foods were added to the cereal mix and the amounts increased to the point where he didn't want more than 1-2 ounces of formula or 10 minutes of breast after the solids. At 2 months he shifted to 5 hours between feedings with four feedings a day, then, between 2 and 3 months, to 6-hour intervals with three feedings. If you have been moving along with your feeding pattern as I have suggested, your baby will now be on a three-meal schedule, such as 7:00 A.M., 1:00 P.M., 7:00 P.M. or any 6-hour interval plan that fits your family pattern best. This means he is full, happy, and contented. His feeding will be given quickly with a few minutes following on the breast or bottle. Some of you, as old hands at feeding, will have your baby on the cup as he weans from bottle or breast. Try to keep the feeding intervals at six hours. If he is hungry between times, offer him as much juice as he wants from a cup and as often as he wants. If he doesn't care for a feeding give him juice in place of it.

You do not have to be too precise about his feeding times. If your baby is not going 4 hours or more between feedings quite regularly on his own, you are not filling him adequately. Your own attitude sets the feeding time to some extent too. You should try to keep your schedule quite flexible so you can vary it without upsetting your baby. He should be showing some ability to wait for food. A too-frequent feeding schedule is quite difficult to maintain. It does not give you the freedom you may sometimes require. If you need to vary the feedings an hour or two in either direction, you can adjust his feeding pattern for the entire day to accommodate this. Your baby will also be quite changeable from this age on as his activities and interests become more varied. Your aim is to come to some common ground with your baby on a reasonable schedule with sufficiently long intervals so that he comes to his feeding time hungry.

MENU

cereal	1 portion
fruit *or* vegetable	1 portion
(dark-green or deep-yellow)	
meat–egg yolk	2 portions
milk–milk solids–cheese	2 portions

MENU COMMENTS

Check above to see what constitutes a portion for each group. Give enough at each feeding to keep him satisfied for the 6-hour interval. If your baby eats less, then halve the portions but keep each group in the indicated relationship.

You may still prepare a whole day's feedings ahead of time if you wish to use your blender. Store the mix properly and take what you need at meal time. Maintain your cleanliness precautions in your food preparation, handling, storing, and use. They are necessary.

CEREAL. The portion at each meal may have to be increased to thicken the feeding if it is too runny to give easily by spoon. Use the prepared infant cereals rather than the adult cooked type.

MEAT–EGG. Now use 2 portions of any member of the meat-egg group in each feeding. The proteins of this group with the milk–milk solids–cheese are the building blocks for his good nutrition. Don't use the prepared meat dinners or similar combinations as meat. Use plain meats from jars, or blender those from the family table.

FRUIT. Look back to last month as to what this group may include. Fruits are excellent taste-improvers and make the meal more appealing, but don't overdo the portions at the expense of the proteins.

VEGETABLE (DARK-GREEN OR DEEP-YELLOW). At one feeding the vegetable group may be given in place of a fruit portion. In this group is the dark-green or leafy group of vegetables including asparagus, broccoli, Brussels sprouts, green beans, cabbage, chard, collard, spinach, endive, kale, lettuce, okra, green peas, green peppers and beet, dandelion, turnip greens. The deep-yellow vegetables include carrots, rutabagas, yellow turnips, and pumpkin or winter squash. You will find only some of these in the canned baby food so that you will have to prepare the others at home, cooking them properly and putting them through a blender. This is a valuable group of foods and should be used more widely than the fruits.

one portion = ½ cup cooked vegetable
1 jar strained vegetables

You may wish to wait to offer him the stronger tasting vegetables like cabbage, Brussels sprouts, rutabagas, turnips, or broccoli until he is older.

MILK—MILK SOLIDS—CHEESE. Continue to use the prepared milk formula to moisten the food mix. Evaporated milk with equal parts of water may be substituted now. Stay away from whole milk yet. Use cottage cheese or dry skim powdered milk in the food mix as milk solids. His need for solid foods with good protein and iron content is greater than his need for a large amount of liquid low-iron milk. Make up your milk portions from the cheese—milk solids to mix in the solid food mix. For instance, cottage cheese ½ portion (1½ ounces), dry skim powdered milk ½ portion (3 tablespoons), formula 1 portion (4 ounces with 2 ounces in mix, 2 ounces to drink) would be the 2 portions for a feeding. Give enough food mix at the start of the meal so that he takes two ounces or less from bottle or cup. Breast time is usually no more than 10 minutes.

BETWEEN MEALS. Any between-meal feedings should consist only of fruit juice. He may show some appetite change either this month or next. Don't get into 5 or 6 little snack meals a day or you will be in trouble. In addition to apple juice you can offer other available juices. Dilute them with equal amounts of water to start. Don't use the syrup of canned fruits. It is too sweet. You can use the unsweetened juice from any canned fruit. Orange, grapefruit, lemon, tangerine, and tomato juice are the Vitamin C-containing juices. Give them to him in his cup. In hot weather or illness urge water and diluted juices between feedings. Offer him juice any time between meals if he seems thirsty or hungry.

VITAMINS. Continue adequate dosage of his same multiple vitamin drops with or without fluoride.

BREAST-FEEDING

During this month at least half the babies who started breast-feeding will have weaned themselves, either because of mother's desire or need or baby's wish. Your breast-feeding·baby will be cutting down on the length of time spent and the amount taken if you are increasing the amount of his solids regularly. In the breast-fed baby this is preliminary to his weaning himself. By now, he may be growing indifferent to the breast. He may bite at the nipple, push away the breast, or mouth about without taking any milk. When you see such signs take his word for it. He is telling you he is ready to change. Be prepared to take advantage of his readiness to shift either now, or in the next month or so. You have already started cup-feeding. Just offer juice from the cup in place of the breast. In this way there is nothing abrupt about the change. Your baby shifts to cup and stops bottle or breast usually between three and six months, if you take advantage of his readiness. Permit him to move on into his next developmental level of accomplishment, making certain that you are not missing the leads he gives you because of your own preconceived ideas or needs which may have very little to do with your baby's development and maturing. Let me repeat, don't make the mistake of shifting to bottle from breast at this time. By having alternate methods of eating he depends on no one way to be fed. These should all be started in this first few months. If you wait until nine months or longer you can expect nothing but difficulty and resistance to change. The longer you wait, the more problems you create in his shifting from bottle or breast to cup.

BOTTLE-FEEDING

Between three and five months your baby may show less interest in his bottle. If he has shifted to three meals and is getting sufficient solids so that he has enough to eat he will take very little milk after his food. He doesn't want more. This is a good time to shift gradually to a cup. This may concern you if you are not realistic about the amount of milk he needs. Liquid milk will fill him so that he can't take sufficient solid foods . . . then you are in increasing difficulty. He will be hungry too soon. He needs his well-rounded diet first. If he doesn't want to take breast milk or the liquid formula, this should be accepted as his decision. Don't insist on his taking the bottle just because you have been told by someone that you "must get milk in." You don't have to push liquid milk if you are using your portions of skim powdered milk, evaporated milk, and cheese in his feeding. If he doesn't want the bottle, then offer milk from the cup after the solids. If this isn't acceptable, offer juice in his cup. Let him decide. The shift from the bottle can be quite sudden with some babies while others take longer.

Because of the false emphasis placed on bottle- or breast-feeding from a misreading of theories, parents have been concerned about weaning. Too-early weaning was supposed to produce emotional insecurity, thumb-sucking, neurotic over-dependence, etc. Yet there is nothing to support the view that the timing of weaning has any effect on the personality. Weaning should be considered as a natural process in the maturing of the young child. There has been no proof that a cup-fed baby or an early weaned baby thumb-sucks any differently than a breast- or bottle-fed baby.

For most babies fed as I am suggesting, weaning from bottle or breast to cup is a satisfying experience, not a frustration. He has accomplished another step in his maturing. He has mastered the control of his own drinking. He can gulp or sip, drink it all down, or take just a little at a time. Babies differ in their readiness but you must be ready for the cue. Lack of parent approval or support can be a real cause for slowdown in his shift to cup. Your attitude helps to determine how quickly and easily he will be able to do it, but the type of child your baby is determines the way in which he will handle any change or situation. Your baby may decide now to be a cup-user . . . or he may not decide for several months yet. So be positive. Work with his leads to guide you, not your preconceived ideas. The earlier your baby weans the more smoothly it is accomplished. By early I mean 3–6 months as opposed to one year. So just feed him enough before offering breast or bottle and he will take care of the weaning when he is ready.

SPOON-FEEDING

Spoon-feeding usually goes along very nicely now as he gains in his ability to cooperate with you. There is some change in his feeding pattern now. During these previous weeks you have seen his rooting and sucking reflexes as well as his tongue-thrusting. Until now his tongue-thrust has pushed out everything placed on the front half of the tongue. He can't swallow it until it gets to the back half of his tongue. As he develops control of his lips, cheeks, and tongue, he will be able to carry food from the front to the back of his tongue in a definite swallow. This month and next he develops this ability. The disappearance of this pushing-away reflex of his tongue allows your baby to handle solid foods on his own. From now on you can expect him to show more and more control over his eating pattern. The beginning of his hand-to-mouth cooperation and the increased activity of his arms and hands may cause him to get in your way when you are feeding him. He is not being deliberately difficult. He is just showing you his new ability. You can still determine the progress of the feeding sequence. There are "gobblers" and "dawdlers" each of whom can be helped to follow a more middle-of-the-road pattern. If your baby is taking very little milk from bottle or breast after feeding, don't worry. It shows that you are giving him enough solids. Many babies take milk poorly from a cup, so offer the cup with juice after the solids. The skim powdered milk and cheese in his solids furnishes him the milk solids without the extra volume of liquid.

CUP-FEEDING

Start his cup-feeding regularly now if you haven't before. Water and juices should be familiar drinking items by now. He may take none of it or gobble it down like a veteran. Offer the cup with water or juice an hour or more before a meal. In this way you won't interfere with his appetite. He may be starting to get a little hungry or thirsty and will be ready to take something at this time.

PLACE

He's still not too big to hold on your lap for feeding. I say this with some reservations since you may have to make some concessions to this if you are trying to hang on to a 15-pounder as you try to present him with food. If he wants to sit straight up now, then he needs to. The infant seat can be used if you sit it upright and anchor it securely. Or you may have to prop him up securely between pillows. Remember . . . you never leave your baby in any type of restraint or seat and go out of the room. Put him in a safe place first or take him with you. This in-between stage of sitting sometimes makes feeding time a problem. Don't use the infant seat in a half-reclining position. When you do use this type of semi-independent feeding position, don't forget that your voice, your face, and hands have uses in maintaining contact with him.

Bottle propping, either on a pillow or folded blanket or by use of a commercial bottle holder, should not be done under any circumstances. I believe it is a harmful, even dangerous, practice. During the first few months feeding times are some of the best times for you to hold him close to you. A propped-bottle gives him no chance to stop or rest. There is no one around to allow him to pause and let him catch his breath. He may have to eat very quickly and gulp too much air.

EATING WITH THE FAMILY

I mentioned before about your baby and bringing him to the adult dining table. The best advice I can give you is still "Don't do it!" Breakfast time, especially, can be a hectic time for many households. Try to arrange his meal at a separate time, either before or after the mad morning rush. Your baby is really too young to appreciate social meals. He certainly isn't ready to conform to any of your patterns of behavior yet.

APPETITE

At this stage, the pattern of a baby's appetite often changes. Which brings up, either this month or next month, a situation which you may misunderstand.

You may find yourself the mother of a young fellow who is trying to tell you to ease off on the feeding business. He will protest even to the point of regurgitating his feedings if you are pushing him too hard. This is the time to realize that you are no longer dealing with a baby who operates by reflex. He has begun to have some ideas of his own. Now is the time to understand that your job is to prepare his food—he is the one who has the responsibility of eating it. This slow-down may not happen until next month. It may not happen at all. But don't be surprised if it does happen. And don't make the mistake of cutting way back on his food. Offer him his food three times a day. Give him as much as you can when he eats, but don't expect him to eat every meal as eagerly as he did last month. He may skip one meal a day. If he doesn't care for his solids, give him fruit juice from his cup and let him go until the next meal.

Don't get into an argument with your baby. You may be tempted to urge him to continue the easy eating sequence of the early months, but this isn't always possible because of changes in his appetite. It is all right to be firm in your feeding but not harsh and overbearing. He will only fight back. Try to be consistent, firm, and appreciative of his needs.

I hope that you haven't been so inconsistent as to give your baby a few sucks of bottle or breast, then a few spoonfuls of food, then a few sucks of bottle or breast. You do have the responsibility for setting a pattern for him to follow and limits to go with it. The main trouble with this sort of off-and-on business is that you never let your baby settle down to feeding of either kind. He doesn't know what to expect. The method of feeding described above is so unpredictable that it cannot fail to produce a tense, jittery, and constantly hungry child.

BOWEL AND BLADDER FUNCTIONS

His bowel habits will probably be about the same as last month. The number of movements in a day and the number of days without one are not important. You will seldom find any real regularity in his bowel movements yet. As long as the consistency of the stool remains moist and your baby's health is good, you need to pay attention only to his feeding, not to his elimination.

A medicated suppository may sometimes be prescribed by your doctor when your baby needs to absorb a medicine and he cannot take it by mouth. A plain glycerin or soap suppository can be used to stimulate a bowel movement. A thermometer or a rubber finger cover would do as well. Use a suppository only if it is ordered for special reasons.

Regular use of a suppository, thermometer, etc. to produce a bowel movement will set up an unfortunate habit pattern for your baby. (Look ahead to the section on *Sick-Baby Care* for instructions on how to use suppositories.)

No baby is ready for toilet training at this point, or at any point during this first year. Until he can exert some control over the lower bowel and has some idea of what it is all about, you'd better forget about toilet training.

SLEEPING

You should have him in a six-year-old crib by the end of this month or soon after. He is outgrowing his bassinet, car bed, or one-year-old crib. In another month they may be dangerous. (Check back to *Preparing for the Baby* for more information about cribs.)

At three months your baby has put together his short periods of sleep into one continuous period in the night. His sleep is deeper and sounder. You will hear less hiccuping, grunting, and sneezing. He develops a day-night pattern or cycle. During this three-month period there has been rapid maturing in his ability to sustain a prolonged period of sleep. His longest period of sleep now ranges from eight to ten hours. His ability to sleep is matched, if less strikingly, by his ability to sustain longer periods of wakefulness. Those changes in his sleep pattern match other aspects of his behavior showing development in his nervous system. They are independent of any of your efforts at training.

He may wake up early in the morning. Leave him alone. If he is truly hungry, give him fruit juice and try to feed him more at mealtimes. Night feedings should be things of the past by now.

With the average young fellow, P.M. fussing has now decreased a great deal. He is finding other ways to discharge his tensions. His digestive system is working better and he is responding more to his surroundings. He may be replacing his crying periods with social activities, such as hand watching, babbling, or pushing about. A baby who has found his hands early is also able to use hand- or finger-sucking as a replacement for fussing.

If you are still in trouble with protracted evening crying, you will need to look for possible causes in your baby's surroundings. Perhaps his sleeping facilities are unsatisfactory. He may still be in your bedroom. His eating patterns may be erratic. His diet may be inadequate or improper. Your household may be in a continual turmoil. Parental oversolicitousness may be to blame. A few nights of letting the baby cry it out may help more than any medication. A child who is fussing nightly is usually not an ill child. A baby who has not done this till now and suddenly starts sounding off at night may be ill.

EXERCISE AND PLAY

Give your baby sunbaths as regularly as the weather permits. See last month's "Exercise and Play" for instructions on increasing the time of exposure.

His exercise is more active now. Continue the kinds of exercise and play suggested before. His playtime should be a regular part of his day. Both father and mother should join in, perhaps at different times. This is important to him from this age on.

A father often expresses his love and interest in his baby by active physical play, such as tossing the baby in the air. This can be quite safe (although it frequently terrifies the mother) if the baby is handled securely, and not too roughly or suddenly or for too long. Babies generally enjoy this kind of activity in their first six months. Later it may frighten them.

You will get a big response when you kiss your baby on the abdomen or nuzzle him there. You can produce a real belly laugh, the tummy-shaking type of out-loud laughing. But watch out. An occasional tickle on the tummy, which provokes an easy giggle or laugh, is fine. The continued pushing, demanding type of tickling, which produces convulsive laughter and makes the baby try to push the adult away, is not. Don't let your enthusiasm carry you away.

Even though your baby may seem quite helpless, there are several toys he may enjoy in his third month. While he can't reach out and pick up a toy yet, he does enjoy holding a noise-maker like a rattle or a bell. Even if he drops it very quickly, he will enjoy the sound it makes. At this age, or even as early as his second month, he is busy using his eyes.

He will enjoy having some brightly colored moving objects to watch. A store-bought cradle gym or a homemade equivalent can be strung across his playpen or his crib, high enough so that he can watch the moving parts. Mobiles interest your baby. Buy one, or make one yourself out of paper or plastic, and hang it from the ceiling over his crib. The combination of movement and colors fascinates a small baby. You can provide him with plastic rattle, a balloon, squeeze toys or stuffed toys, or anything that is brightly colored or makes interesting sounds. Be sure to tie it securely with a short string to the playpen or crib.

In choosing toys for your baby, bear in mind that his first toys must be large enough for him to handle easily. At first he will just look at the toy. Later he will push at it to make it move or make a noise. Finally he will grab it. As he grows older he will feel it, mouth it, suck on it, or bite it. All of his toys must be of the kind that can safely be put into his mouth. They should be washable with no sharp points or corners and large enough not to be swallowed. Parts such as wheels, bells, whistles, glass or plastic eyes, buttons, or pins can be pulled off and swallowed. Toys should be washed often. Good-quality rubber, plastic, or smooth hardwood toys with rounded edges are excellent. Painted articles are unsafe unless you are sure that the paint contains no lead. Do not use toys filled with liquid. No baby should have too many toys at one time. And keep them simple. Clothespins or spools on a short string, a rubber doll, a cradle gym, small plastic blocks, foam-rubber animals, will probably please him more in the coming months than any expensive toy. Give him time to explore one toy thoroughly before giving him another.

Consider certain things before you buy. Read labels carefully. Make sure the toy is color-safe and play-safe and that there is nothing in it that might be injurious to your baby. Many toy labels state the age group for which the toy is best suited, so it is wise to check for this. Be sure that look-toys, listen-toys, or push-and-pull toys can be attached securely to crib, carriage, or playpen. As your baby grows and holds toys, any bath toy should be sized to handle easily.

Try to find articles that give him a chance to use new skills. As he grows older and his use of his hands improves, he will enjoy a variety of simple lug-around, switch-around, build-up, and take-apart-put-together toys. He will need toys with which he can learn to do things. These toys are designed with particular age groups in mind. These do-something toys not only help eye-hand coordination, but also help to develop your baby's imagination. You will enjoy watching your baby learn countless skills through play. Examples of other good toys: a few blocks, a cup and spoon, a pie pan, a box with a cover to take off and put on easily, a large ball covered with different textured materials, a string of large wooden or plastic beads, a cloth or plastic picture book with large colored pictures of animals or common household objects.

Give him new toys one at a time. Keep a fresh supply put away to use when a spot of boredom threatens. Don't make the mistake of supervising his play too closely at any age. You may think you have many valuable lessons you can teach your child. But you are asking for dependence in your child if he looks to you constantly for things to do and how to do them. This doesn't mean you can't enter into his games occasionally. Just make sure he has plenty of chances to do things on his own.

By this time the playpen should be used regularly. You will begin to see from now on why I prescribed a playpen strong enough to withstand jumping or shaking by your young Hercules. It should be movable enough to use out-of-doors as well as indoors, and to take with you when you go visiting.

By now he should be using his childproof room, too. (Look back to the section on *Preparing for the Baby* for details on making his room safe so that he can roam in it.) He won't move about much at first, but as the months go by he will gradually learn that this is his area and begin to explore it.

Help him to learn the functions of his various pieces of furniture and areas. His crib is for sleeping; his playpen and room are for playing; his stroller is for outdoor excursions; his car bed is for auto rides. His infant seat, jumper chair, swing seat, sling seat, are all for short-term use. He isn't quite ready for a high chair.

AWARENESS AND SOCIAL RESPONSE

His intellectual understanding has brought him to the point where he recognizes his social world. He wants to be around people. He turns to watch you or to check on a sound. He gets all excited when you offer him something. He knows when you are getting ready to feed him, and opens his mouth for food. Quite a different fellow from that little guy in the nursery who looked off into that great void of nothingness at first!

Perhaps last month your baby seemed to show his happy feelings by smiling, but this month you aren't in any doubt. His smile tells you that he feels good. This doesn't mean he can't pucker up and cry, but both crying and smiling tell you something about how he feels. He isn't just hungry or full anymore—he is feeling other things, too. Crying may be used more as a social action than as an indicator of inner tensions. He is learning more and more how to cope with frustration in ways other than crying. He shows his happiness with his whole body—he wiggles his arms, legs and body, and pants with excitement.

His smiling is now responsive. This is said to be one of the most important developmental steps in your infant's recognition of objects. He reaches this stage of his maturity as a result of his experiences with people and the accompanying stimulation he receives. He is smiling a great deal now. He will smile broadly at you in response to your talking and smiling.

During this third month you will notice in other ways how much more responsive your baby is to you. His eyes follow you better, as he turns his head toward the sound of your voice.

About now you may realize that you have a much more reasonable baby than you had before. He is beginning to cry less, and he will wait a few minutes for food and attention. Your arrival can divert his attention so that he holds off even longer.

You are important to your baby, as you will have discovered by now. This is the reason I have emphasized the mother's importance as a first figure for her baby. He needs a single clear-cut image he can relate to and get something back from. Your household may be noisy and tumultuous most of the time with other children, the TV, the vacuum cleaner. But he tunes out all these distractions for the most part and focuses on you or your substitute. Someone must be constant in his world and not a will-of-the-wisp that comes and goes.

ORAL COMMUNICATION

In response to your smiling, your baby not only smiles and coos but also tries to make babbling sounds. This alternates with a rather fixed, studying gaze. He doesn't understand the meaning of specific words as yet, but he is beginning to recognize the feeling with which you say any word to him. This is why your baby may sometimes respond to the way you feel and react accordingly. By this time he may start to use different kinds of crying for pain and hunger. He extends his cry now to include two syllables that vary the pitch. To the vowel sounds he has used he adds the suggestion of consonant sounds "m" and "ng" so that you may hear "aah" or "ngaah." By the end of this month you may even hear k, g, d, or b with his vowel sounds. He responds to your cooing by repeating his own old and practiced sounds. Sometimes you stop his vocalizing when you join in.

BABY-CARE ROUTINES

SKIN CARE

You may have some problems with his skin care by this time. He may be sleeping longer, so that he isn't changed as often.

You may have had several episodes of diaper rash or possibly of heat rash. (Check back to *First Month* for advice on treatment.)

He may be drooling so heavily now that his chin, cheeks, and neck are broken out all the time. This type of drooling rash is essentially irritation. The reddened areas must be kept clean without heavy rubbing. Use ointments such as cold cream or Vaseline.

CLOTHING

His clothing remains much as before. You will be using nightgowns and pajamas less now, and coveralls and play-suits more. By now he should be in his playpen a good bit of the time. You may want to protect his feet with booties or socks, or use outfits with attached feet.

15.

The
Fourth Month

By and large the fourth to eighth months of your baby's first year are relatively restful ones. He is more fun to have around. He is up to something new in his learning every day. At the same time, he can't move too far too fast or get into things by crawling or climbing. You can relax a little. The only thing that may really bother you is that he isn't eating as well. By next month his appetite will improve.

WEIGHT

Ranges: Boys 11.8–17.8 lbs.   Average 14.3 lbs.
           Girls 10.8–16.6 lbs.   Average 13.3 lbs.

HEIGHT

Ranges: Boys 23.2–26.0 in.   Average 24.6 in.
           Girls 22.7–25.6 in.   Average 24.2 in.

MOTOR DEVELOPMENT

Your baby shows a great deal of improvement in his coordination this month. He loves exercise. Since he is now awake for longer periods, he has more time for practicing his developing physical skills.

REFLEXES

His reflex grasping and traction response have disappeared. He is acquiring more complicated ways of reacting. You can produce his hand response by contact with his fingers or hand. Now he will turn his hand toward any object touching his hand. He does this fairly well by four months. This is just a turning of his hand without any real reaching movement as yet. His tonic-neck reflex is being replaced by a change in his control. It will still be his position of rest on his back.

LYING, SITTING, STANDING, AND GETTING ABOUT

When your baby is lying on his abdomen, he can lift his head up at a 90° angle and get his chest 2 or 3 inches off the mattress. He holds his head well and high, looking straight ahead steadily for a longer time. (See plate 17E.) He does let it fall back finally, then lifts it again. This shows his neck muscles are stronger. His legs will flex while he is doing this.

He also has improved at what I have called airplaning. With his arms out and raised, legs stretched out straight and raised, and back arched, he puts his full weight on his abdomen. Maybe the parachute jumper in a free fall is a better picture. He will also support his weight on his arms or hands, but then he can't get his hands together in front of him to use. He can't hold his head up long enough for much hand play without his hand support, although he is at the point of using only one hand for support to free the other. When he turns his head back and forth, he manages to do so quite steadily.

When he is on his back, he is quite relaxed at times, with his knees bent and his feet flat on the table. He even waves his feet about to bring one foot down on the other knee or leg. He holds his body more symmetrically. He moves his head freely from side to side as his interest changes. If you have kept him on his stomach most of the time, he may object to an on-the-back position. He would prefer to sit up, either held or propped up. He wants to see.

He is replacing his tonic-neck reflex with a neck-righting reflex, which is really the start of his rolling-over mechanism. This righting response is composed of a series of reflexes, which develop along his body length from head to buttocks. Turning his head now affects the rest of his body. (See plate 23.) He turns his face and head to one side toward his back, arches his back by raising one shoulder to turn his trunk and pelvis in the same direction. His arms and legs are curved toward the abdomen. He may even manage enough push to turn onto his side, but not usually enough to go over onto his back. But he is trying. He likes to change position, and he really struggles at it.

With support, he is able to sit much straighter. (See plate 19D.) Although there is still some back-rounding, curving is in the low back now. He holds his head fairly erect without wobble, but his control isn't complete. If you nudge him, his head wavers or falls forward before he gets control again. With your full support, he can sit up for ten or fifteen minutes or more without tiring. He likes to get up into this position. He will grasp your fingers strongly and with help will pull up to a sitting position with very little head lag. He holds himself ready to make an effort when you start to help him. This is exciting to him. His eyes may widen, his breathing may quicken, even his pulse may increase. He has definite control of his head and neck muscles, but he still needs some support for his trunk. He holds his head quite steadily but still a little forward. When he tries to pay attention to other things, he will still bob his head around. He jerks himself back into his sitting position to try to hold steady and straight.

When you bring him from a sitting to a standing position, you will see some signs of his extension phase. This is the start of his pushing against gravity to finally stand erect. He now has an urge to push upward with his legs when his feet are against any hard surface. He tries to raise his buttocks from the table. He can't hold the position, but drops back down. His pushing up is quite limited, but he is practicing for his next step. This shows development in his lower legs. When you hold him up on his feet, he pushes out with his legs to try to support himself. He holds his knees straight to lock them so that he can hold his weight. He holds his head up more erectly. He seems more interested in holding his weight up than in stepping out. (See plate 20E.) If you have played bouncing with him, he will show less desire to hold the standing position.

Crawling and creeping seem to be nearer. He is much stronger now. There is improvement in the control of the muscles that support his arms and legs. His general body activity continues to be a sinuous wriggling or pushing type of motion.

HANDS

One of the most noticeable changes this month is in the interest and ability he will show in using his hands. He begins reaching out to grasp objects and bring them to his mouth. (See plate 21D.)

His hand and arm movements are now related to the position of his head and eyes. His hands are fisted far less of the time. He can use his thumbs a little, but not much yet. On his back, his hands come together in play. His aim is poor, and he overshoots and misses quite often, but he keeps on trying. If he sees a toy in front of him, he may look at his hands and the toy as if to say, "I want to get it, but I don't know how." He holds it with his eyes even if he can't reach it with his hands. He is still good-natured about this. He doesn't show much frustration as yet. If he does get his hands on something, he will hold it and look at it, then bring it to his mouth. If he drops a toy he can't pick it up.

You can see now how he is getting his hands into a position for use. They started out flexed up on his body and not usable, then went out to the sides of his body for support, and are now coming back together so that he will learn to grasp and manipulate things.

He begins to deliberately and consciously put his hands or objects into his mouth. In fact, everything goes into his mouth from now on. He tries to handle anything near him. In these weeks ahead he will gradually be able to come toward an object with his hands, touch it, grasp it, handle it, and then bring it to his mouth to complete his identification of it. He feels and grasps at the edges of furniture. Police the area where he is. Safety pins and buttons get popped into his mouth very quickly even now.

He spends a good deal of time just admiring his hands, turning them this way and that. He brings them together to touch in front of him. He fingers his fingers. He is trying to find out about them.

EYES AND OTHER SENSE ORGANS

By this month his eyes are fully developed. They are as perfect now as they ever will be from the standpoint of development. However, certain areas of them are not yet fully organized and functioning. From this time on his development in seeing is up to his brain. His nervous-system pathways for associating the signals from his body and through his senses are developing to the point where his seeing and his arm-muscle control will get together to give him the ability to reach a toy by next month. His vision is usually farsighted until he is six or seven months old. He is focusing fairly well now since his eyes are beginning to move together more. His cross-eyed look is disappearing, but you still see it off and on.

He likes to look around at his surroundings. Perhaps he can even identify some familiar shapes. He looks at his own hand or he looks at a toy. He turns his head to follow any object moving from his sight, like a ball rolling across the table. He looks for a lost toy. An adult face is still his most interest-holding object. (See plate 24.) He may turn his head and make some response to a familiar voice or face. He may show fright at strange objects, people, or voices. He is recognizing differences now. He is not only looking with his eyes, but he has some memories stored up to use. He is starting to associate these memories with present objects or events. He begins to learn to do something about them when he sees them. He is becoming perceptive. You may see him look at you, then at an object, and then back at you again. When he is propped up he may look around busily trying to see what goes on—or he may just sit and play with his hands.

If your baby's eyes show crossing *a good deal of the time*, you should check this more closely. You can watch for a few months, but have an oculist check them by six months if you find definite crossing. Make certain that what you think is eye crossing isn't just the result of the broad nose bridge and heavy skin fold at the corner of his eye.

Look at the direction of the pupils. Do they move together, or is one off on its own while the other looks at you? If you hold a light in front of him, the light reflection will be in the same place on both eyes. You may cover the good performing eye with an eye patch to make the turned, or "lazy," eye perform until you can have your eye-man advise you as to care.

TEETH

Your baby will develop two sets of teeth during his life. His first set is called his primary or deciduous set. This consists of twenty teeth, ten in each jaw. His second or permanent set consists of thirty-two teeth, sixteen in each jaw. Moving from the center of each jaw backward, his first teeth are named central incisors, lateral incisors, canine or cuspid, first molar and second molar. The same name system is used for his second teeth, except that the five teeth behind his canines are, successively, first and second premolars or bicuspids and first, second, and third molars.

His twenty first teeth usually show up in his mouth between four months and three years. The first tooth to break through appears between four to twelve months, with the average at seven months. You may have the rare baby born with a tooth or two—or the equally rare one who has nothing in his mouth until sixteen months.

There are many individual variations in the order in which your child's teeth appear. The wide possible variations don't indicate abnormality or disease. Usually the first teeth to appear are the two lower central incisors, followed by the four upper central and lateral incisors. Some lag occurs after these, but then the two lower lateral incisors come, followed by the four first molars, the four canines, and finally the four second molars.

At one year your youngster usually will have six teeth—often the two lower central and four upper incisors—but he may have none or twenty and still be quite normal. He may complete all of his first teeth by one year or not until three years. The average is two and a half years. Individuals vary widely in the order in which the teeth erupt, especially with incisors and canines.

There is no relationship between the time of your baby's teething and his intelligence or general development.

As you can see from the above synopsis, this month is about the earliest you can expect to see a tooth if your baby is average.

Before the eruption of a tooth you may sometimes see a soft lump over the tooth. This is the tooth sac, the enamel organ, which sits over the tooth. It may fill with blood and rupture as the tooth comes through. Lancing the gums should never be done. You damage this enamel organ and may cause trouble with the tooth later.

Teething is not always comfortable. If your baby is uncomfortable, give him some help. Let him chew on something hard, like a rubber bone. Rub his gums vigorously with your clean finger. He needs something to clamp down and bite on. He will also want to chew on his own fingers or thumb.

Aspirin is usually enough of an analgesic to give him. If aspirin does not help, you should check for some other cause of trouble. Never apply aspirin or anything else to his gums.

Drooling starts at about six weeks in most babies and has no *direct* relationship to teething. Your baby may drool a little more when he is teething because he keeps his mouth open and his tongue working over the gums. Loss of appetite, coughing, and loose stools are rather indefinite symptoms and difficult to associate directly with teething.

Your child may teethe from four months to two and a half or three years with his first teeth—which makes a nice long period during which you can blame almost any situation on this natural event. Generally unsatisfactory health or behavior should not be blamed on teething. Teething is not a cause of illness. *Teething does not cause a fever.* Convulsions, fever, diarrhea, brain effusions, squints, bronchitis, and rash have all been blamed on teething at one time or another. There is no relationship.

Several major factors influence the appearance of tooth decay. The mother's diet, medications, and state of health during pregnancy have a place here. A baby's diet that contains a lot of refined sugars is always poor. Soft drinks and sweets set the stage for decay.

Fluorides in the diet are a must. As noted before, use a vitamin drop with fluoride added if your water supply is not fluoridated. But don't expect fluorides to stop decay in the face of bad diet habits.

EATING

So far, your baby's diet has included the cereal, fruit, meat–egg, milk–milk solids–cheese, and vegetable (dark-green, deep-yellow) food groups. These are basic food groups which supply many nourishing substances, protein, minerals, vitamins, fats, and carbohydrates. Most of these foods contain more than one nutrient but no single food furnishes all the necessary food materials in proper proportion. For this reason, you should make every effort to widen your choice of foods in any one group. Don't use the same foods in any one group all the time. Part of the fun of diet construction is thinking up new combinations in the months ahead. Pay attention to what you are doing so that you always keep a good pattern of protein with meat, eggs, fish, poultry, and milk solids. Protein with its essential amino acids is absolutely necessary for your baby's body function, growth, and development. It satisfies hunger longer than other foods. It also assures a good general mineral and vitamin intake. Vegetables and fruits also give a variety of minerals and vitamins and are fillers. Bread–cereal groups supplement the animal protein of meat, egg, milk solids, and cheese along with vegetable protein. Fats give zest to a meal but are also appetite-satisfiers. So let's look at your diet for this month.

MENU

Morning	cereal	1 portion
	meat and/or egg	2 portions
	fruit	1 portion
	milk solids–cheese	1 portion
	milk	1 portion
Mid-Day	cereal	1 portion
	meat and/or egg	2 portions
	fruit *or*	
	vegetable (dark-green or deep-yellow)	1 portion
	milk solids–cheese	1 portion
	milk	1 portion
	(fat–oil)	

Evening	cereal	1 portion
	meat and/or egg	2 portions
	fruit *or*	
	vegetable (dark-green or deep-yellow)	1 portion
	milk solids–cheese	1 portion
	milk	1 portion
	(fat–oil)	

MENU COMMENTS

With the variation in size and weight among babies (from 11 pounds to 18 pounds) yours may wish anywhere from half these portions to twice as much. Keep the rates between these foods as indicated. If you use less, try to increase the amounts of the meat–egg and milk solid–cheese groups if he wishes more.

SCHEDULE. If your baby has had enough food to keep him comfortable he has been on 3 meals a day for at least this past month. If he is trying to keep 4 meals going, give him 3 regular meals 6 hours apart, then let him go as long as he will at night. When he wakens, offer him juice or water from a cup and not a full feeding. In a way, you are following the modified self-demand schedule I've talked about in the first month. You are setting reasonable limits and paying attention to his reasonable cues and choices.

GIVING FOODS SEPARATELY. Up to this time you have fed his foods mixed together and the same ones at each meal. Now you will begin three different meals a day, giving foods separately or in various combinations. This encourages him to develop a variety of taste experiences. He will become quite discriminating about his foods from now on. Before this time the matter of variety in taste and color didn't make much difference. You used his swallowing reflex to spoon in a large amount of the food mix. Now you try for variety in each of your food groups. Don't use the same foods day after day just because he likes them. He needs to find out that he likes other foods, too.

It is my suggestion that this month you start to make the change from puréed or homogenized foods by thickening or coarsening his foods gradually over these next months. As you make this shift he comes to coarser table foods between 6 and 8 months, not later. Your infant won't mind a little coarser food mixed in with his sieved food. He may gum it around, but will down it without much trouble as long as there is no great issue made of it. He doesn't need teeth for this. If you wait until he has chewing teeth, several years may elapse. On the other hand, he may have biting teeth by this time.

Your baby may object to the commercially prepared junior (chopped) foods and yet take to table foods quite readily. You can duplicate junior foods by chopping or grinding family table food. Start with junior or table foods mashed with a fork. Meats can be fine ground. Add scrambled eggs, cooked vegetables, stewed fruits, and diced and finely cut-up meat. Get as large a variety of foods in his diet as you can. This breaks up the monotony. Strangeness can be exciting as well as a cause for suspicion.

Your baby may show a variable reaction to lumps in his food. You may have to nudge him a little to accept coarser food. Perhaps mixing table food with his puréed baby food will help. Gagging on lumps is not uncommon while he is learning to handle food in the back of his throat. Avoid encouraging this as a learned pattern of reaction. If he wants to gag back food, you may have to stop the meal at this point and make him hungrier for his next feeding. His appetite is so much better a persuader than all your smiles and coaxings . . . make use of it!

Cereals and fruits are continued as before.

MEAT-EGG. This group is unchanged except that now you may use whole egg. The yolk is still the important part. Use the egg cooked or raw, mixing it with the other foods. Clean the shell before opening. If there is any question of allergy, hard boil the egg and separate the white. Use only the hard-boiled yolk.

VEGETABLE. This dark-green, deep-yellow group is continued and the variety enlarged as you can. Now that you have separated his food you want him to find the taste and texture differences in foods. You may wish to add a little margarine (vegetable oil) to the vegetables you prepare at home. You have already discovered that vegetable changes the color and texture of his stool. Tomatoes, spinach, beets, or other vegetables may cause a contact rash on the face. Vaseline or bland ointment will help this. You don't need to avoid the food unless the reaction is severe or causes some other problem.

MILK—MILK SOLIDS—CHEESE. Continue to use prepared formula or evaporated milk to mix into his solid food to make it moist enough to feed him. You may use this undiluted for mixing if you wish. He won't be taking as much milk after his solid feedings if you have increased his foods as he needs. This means that you will have to use the milk solids—cheese group in substitute amounts to get adequate milk protein in his diet.

BETWEEN MEALS. Between-meal snacks or feedings are still definitely out. If he doesn't eat a meal, don't give him something to take its place between then and the next feeding. Give fruit juice liberally but not within an hour of his next feeding.

VITAMINS. Continue his multiple vitamin drops, with or without fluoride, in appropriate dosage. Use them mixed in his food in the first portion you know he will eat.

For food handling, care, and storage, utensil care, warm-cold food, blender use, or similar subjects, look back to *The First Month* and *Breast-Feeding and Bottle-Feeding*.

BREAST-FEEDING

Your feeding pattern on breast may continue about as described last month. With your baby's possible eating change, the next section on weaning may be appropriate.

WEANING. If your nursing baby acts indifferent after any feeding, offer cup with 2 ounces of either juice or milk in it. If he doesn't want to drink, then let him go. He will be hungry for the next feeding. As he refuses the breast more frequently, he takes the cup oftener. The juice he takes well but not milk. Take advantage of this change but don't go to the bottle for feeding. In this gradual weaning process that I have suggested your breasts accommodate to the reduced stimulation. Rarely will any special care be necessary, since the breasts go through a gradual drying-up process.

If you are a breast-feeding mother you must watch from this time on for your baby's readiness to be weaned. As noted last month, he may already have given you such indications. He tries to tell you that he is ready for his next step. He may tell you in very clear terms when he chews hard or bites you. Or he may be kinder and just try to push the nipple away. He may let go of the nipple and look at you or play with his hands and look away. Pay attention to him, and don't feel that you are depriving him of anything. You will deprive him of his right to grow up if you insist he continue on breast.

With many bottle-fed babies this same readiness to shift to cup may be evident now and in the coming months. Some babies just want that ounce or so of milk from the bottle after the solids a little longer in order to call it a meal. You can often substitute juice from a glass or cup just as readily.

Some babies want to go a month or two longer before they shift entirely to cup. The time of weaning depends on your readiness and your baby's. The decision is partly baby's. Is he satisfied? Partly yours. Is it convenient and easier? In shifting from bottle or breast to cup a great deal depends on what you have done in your feedings before this. If you have followed my suggestions by this time your baby will not want much milk after a feeding. If you are uncertain and shift back and forth, your baby will be confused and cause you some difficulty. However, you can be assured that he will eat if he is hungry. No starvation will occur. If you continue on bottle or breast make certain you are not ignoring his signals, that you are not encouraging a dependency he is ready to give up.

Your attitude determines the ease, rapidity, and success with which this shift is accomplished. You may be made uncomfortable by your baby's shift to his next stage of development. This is usually expressed as "He is a baby such a short time!" or "He is only a baby!"

The average baby slackens off on the amount of food he takes at about three or four months of age. He will take enough to satisfy hunger. He may need very little to do this. This is an ideal time to start the substitution of cup for breast or bottle. Choose the meal that he takes most poorly to offer his milk from a cup. This is usually the mid-day meal.

Give his milk in a cup after his solid feeding, in place of breast or bottle. If he doesn't want it, offer him juice instead. If he is full, take his word for it. Leave him alone. After another week or more, replace his morning breast- or bottle-feeding by a cup-feeding. After another week or more do the same at his evening meal. This can be carried out in any other order that seems best for you both.

Your baby may show great variations. He may have ups and downs in his acceptance of weaning. Don't get discouraged. No matter what you do you'll get your child off the bottle or breast eventually. That much you know. He will probably do it for you. Your job is to set up a pattern in which he can perform easily and comfortably to make this shift. You must pay attention to his readiness.

Try to make the shift so little noticed that he continues to eat and enjoy it. Avoid a sense of urgency. Avoid appearing harsh and demanding or he will resist you. It is important that your loving attitude does not change during this time of transition. Your anxiety about making the change may give you away. It can cue him as to how he should act —either "good" or "bad."

If you will notice, you are not forcing a change in his feeding habits, as I have outlined it. You are taking advantage of certain changes in types of activity. You offer food. You have made the cup available. You have let the bottle or breast become less important as a source of food as the weeks have gone by.

Don't go backward in your training. You can be flexible in your handling of his acceptance or refusal of the change until you have made the change. Then keep the pattern. In other words, if he refuses the cup at first, the breast or bottle is offered. Once you have stopped breast or bottle and he refuses a cup, then let him alone. Don't offer a bottle or try to start the breast-feeding all over again. This isn't flexibility. This is vacillation . . . and confusing to your baby.

When you do not take advantage of readiness on the part of your baby, you may set up an unpleasant pattern. If you continue breast or bottle, you will very often have trouble changing later. Before you realize it, he is using the bottle as a pacifier. Later he will be resentful and frustrated no matter how skillfully you encourage him to give it up. The bottle has become his symbol of security.

In order to help your child develop, you try now and again to encourage him to accept the next more grownup thing to do. One time it may be something in connection with his feeding. Another time it may be some aspect of his social behavior or his motor development. You try to prepare him for his next period of readiness. His cup-drinking is a new skill. He will swing into it gradually since he learns a skill by doing it. At first he swallows automatically. Then he begins to discover how to drink, which is active participation, not a reflex matter. This is a learning process, so you must expect him to make mistakes. As long as you don't consider his errors serious and over-react to them, he will take them in his stride. Don't thrust the new experience on him suddenly. He will be suspicious. You need to help him to independence. On the other hand, you may find that he is way ahead of you. He may shift to cup suddenly and completely, almost as though he were waiting for you to get out of his way.

You may have some concern that your baby is not getting enough milk. I have tried to point out the relative place of milk. You will recall also that extra milk solids are added to the feeding.

I don't want to belabor the point about weaning but let me stress once more the importance of noting your baby's signs of readiness to give up breast or bottle now or in coming months. Be prepared to offer him confident support in making the shift.

SPOON-FEEDING

His tongue-thrusting is now gone for the most part. He has more ability to hold food in his mouth and control it with his tongue. He moves it backward into his throat to swallow. He has a grasp and release position to his tongue now. He is in control and not controlled by his reflexes. He manages his own food. You no longer manage for him. He takes and handles his solid foods quite well, but perhaps he doesn't eat as much. He does follow a more erratic appetite pattern this month.

He may also be quite a nuisance when you are trying to feed him by waving his hands about. He makes some kind of grab at your hand or spoon. You may have to devise some way of keeping his hands occupied or restrained.

During his first three months you were able to urge your baby to eat automatically. When he starts to show signs of maturing to the point of putting his hands voluntarily to his mouth, then you can assume that he is able to make decisions about his eating. At this point you must be careful. You cannot urge or force him without expecting his resistance or his coming back at you in some way. He may take a feeding under stress and then spit it up.

Get firmly in your mind your responsibility as far as feeding is concerned now and in the coming months. You need only to make suitable food available three times a day and present it in a pleasant manner in comfortable surroundings. Your responsibility ends there. You can't take the responsibility for mouthing, swallowing, and digesting such food. This is your baby's job. This is the most difficult lesson for a mother to learn at this point. You have been encouraged to feed your baby as much as possible in the early weeks. In your eyes this may have seemed like a tremendous amount compared to his size. Now you must shift gears. It is the common American failing to feel guilty if your child does not take three square meals a day. You feel you are not an "adequate" mother if anything is refused.

But your child has his responsibility too. You must be willing to let him take it. It will do him no great harm to miss a meal, if you don't upset the apple cart by your attitude, or substitute milk for his solids, or feed him between meals. If you have offered him his food and he has taken a fair amount or practically nothing, don't worry! If you offer the cup and he takes a sip and is done, let him go! He will be hungry for the next meal or the next one after that. He should be offered juice between times.

CUP-FEEDING

You see a definite developmental change now in his use of the cup. (See plate 22B.) He can approximate his lips to the edge of his cup. His cup-feeding is often quicker than either bottle or breast now. He is still a tongue-thruster now and again so you will have to watch his mechanics of feeding or you may get a surprise. Proper positioning of his cup on his lips and tongue will help. A pitcher with a spout may fit better into the curve of his tongue.

APPETITE

If you didn't see a shift in his appetite and eating last month you may very well see it now, although some babies go right on eating three big meals a day. If you are aware of his changing patterns of eating, you won't be concerned at some of the shifts he is showing in his demands and refusals. Like many babies at this time, he is just not as hungry. He may begin to wait for his other meals without fussing. He may not seem interested even when food is presented. He may act hungry and fuss at you a little. When you start to feed him he is all done. He will sometimes need gentle persuasion or mild coaxing to overcome some passing resistance. He may fuss at you all during the feeding. Go ahead and feed as long as you don't let the process develop into a fight. If there is just too much scolding and rebellion on his part, stop right there. Give him a little fruit juice in a cup and let him wait until his next meal. A skipped meal doesn't indicate starvation. Such meal refusal is very common at this age. He just wants to eat twice, maybe even once a day.

If you try to urge his former three meals you will be met by quite vigorous and noisy refusal. You may push him to the point of vomiting back the food. If your anxiety pushes you to urge his food unreasonably and excessively, you're setting him up to be a noneater, a resister.

By next month your baby, like most, will go back to eating three meals daily with good appetite.

If he is on a reduced appetite swing, this isn't a good time to try to introduce anything very new or different in his foods. If your baby is the type who doesn't slacken off in his eating, go ahead with your new taste and texture sensations.

HIGH CHAIR

If you have a very active fellow, you will find now that a high chair helps at feeding time. Trying to hold him in your arms or on your lap gets to be quite a gymnastic event. Wedge him back into the corner of the high chair. Bring the tray back into position, slide his left arm under the tray so he can't get it in the way. Once the tray is down, he can't pull his arm back well enough to get it out from under the tray. Then let him grasp the finger or thumb of your left hand with his right hand while you feed him. This way, his hands will be out of your way. If you are left-handed you will have to reverse this process.

You will still be personally involved in the feeding, which avoids one of the objections to bottle propping. Not much change in your feeding routine is needed. Privacy, quietness with a relaxed take-it-or-leave-it attitude on your part, set the stage for his eating time. This certainly is no time to get involved in any family dinner table situation. He may eat so erratically, involve you so much in the process, and behave so differently that he makes meal time a strenuous affair.

BOWEL AND BLADDER FUNCTIONS

At this time your baby probably has one or two bowel movements a day, usually after a meal or in his late afternoon waking period. He may skip a day, depending on how much and what he is eating.

Some vegetables can change the color and texture of your baby's stools. Indigestible vegetable fibers are passed with the colors still present. This doesn't mean anything is wrong. If they produce excess mucus in the stool or a very liquid, irritating stool, slow down on these foods. Use some of the others.

He urinates less frequently, but the volume each time is greater. Your usual four-month baby isn't bothered about wet diapers.

SLEEPING

He should definitely be in a six-year-old crib by this time. Bassinet, one-year-old crib, or car bed are all too confining and too dangerous. He needs room.

His total sleeping time during the fourth and fifth months will average fourteen to fifteen hours. Nap times occupy about three and a half hours in two periods. His longest period of sleep is about ten and a half hours.

His sleep pattern at this time is changing. There is a state of readjustment here in which he tends to have a later morning waking hour. Bedtime comes earlier to answer his need for an earlier sleeping hour. This is a fairly common shift in his sleep pattern.

He no longer wakes up simply to eat. He is a much bigger boy than that. He is able to wait for food. He often talks to himself for a period when he wakes before he shows any particular interest in food.

He may have difficulty in letting go and dropping off to sleep. He is so busy with other things.

He should be adapting easily to the family pattern of living if you've been conditioning him to it. He is now over his P.M. fussing, unless he has come to depend on your floor-walking, singing, or rocking. You will be much happier with him if you let him settle down on his own. Give him a few minutes of gentle talk or patting before you leave. If you have set up a poor pattern, you will have to start a regular schedule. Put him down. Turn a deaf ear to his crying. The first night he may cry three hours, the next two, the third night a half hour, and then only briefly each night afterward—if you remain consistent!

His active play periods precede and follow his naps. Waking introduces a period of intense activity and experimentation. In the late afternoon he may have a period of wakefulness and fretfulness. He wants to play.

At four months he usually does not fall asleep at the end of his feeding. He talks to himself and plays with his hands for a while. Crying may precede his sleep, although this does not always occur before every nap.

EXERCISE AND PLAY

Sunbaths and exercise are continued as before.

From now on he will enjoy playing with small toys more and more. Don't get a lot. He doesn't need many. Dole out only one at a time so that he will pay attention to each one longer. He may know his own familiar toys and recognize a new one. Movement and color in a bright toy or a mobile still get his attention. In his play he gets excited, breathes heavily, and works hard. He waves his arms and moves his body when he sees it. He enjoys mouthing and handling things. On his back he grabs at a toy dangling over him. After four months of age he begins to use his fingers separately. Gradually in these next months your baby's hands turn from paws to hands. He practices his new ability by scratching. Keep his fingernails short so he won't splinter them in the process. Give him a variety of surfaces on which he can practice. He scratches on his high-chair tray, on his playpen pad, his sheets, or on his mattress pad.

He will begin now, or in the coming months, to enjoy playing with a rubber bone or animal, a plastic rattle, suction-cup toys, a set of measuring spoons, a cloth-covered stuffed animal or doll, a soft rubber ball or a wooly, brightly colored ball, a piece of carpeting or heavy fabric. Give him a chance to feel and test, to get the idea of various degrees of hardness and softness. (Look back to last month's "Exercise and Play" for more about toys.)

He may increasingly appreciate rhythm and music. Rhythm, rocking, and playing are all parts of his experimental process. You should encourage them.

AWARENESS AND SOCIAL RESPONSE

He is improving on what he started last month and what he will continue next month. When he sees something he knows he does an allover wiggle. He pants, his eyes widen, he moves his arms and legs, and even laughs out loud when he sees you, his meal, or his toy. When you sit him up he stares at everyone and everything. He isn't unhappy, just curious. He looks over a strange place and a new voice or face. This is not true of all infants at this age. Some are late bloomers socially.

He may be spending a good deal of time now with his fingers, fist, or thumb in his mouth. I hope that you will beam at him and say "Good for you. You are growing up." (Look back to "Rhythmic Patterns" for more about thumbsucking.)

Although he is getting interested in other things, a human face is still the most interesting object to him. Now he prefers mother to all other people. He watches you closely, smiles, and "talks." He may scold you if you break off contact and move out of his sight. His reaction is much more rapid and certain now. He knows you. He has some idea of what you do for him. When he sees you getting food ready, he knows he will eat soon. He recognizes his spoon and dish as soon as he sees them.

He is expanding his interest to include father and the other children in your family. A baby will give attention to any well-defined human face, in the flesh, in sculpture, or in a color picture. But he smiles three times as often at a familiar face. He will not respond to a grotesque or distorted depiction of a human face. The reason he gets along better with father and the other kids now is that, even though he doesn't associate them with the giving of food, he can accept another type of relationship. He is joining the family group as a responsive member.

Your infant may begin to initiate social contact as well as responding to social stimulation. He isn't selective in bestowing his smiles. He charms his family and friends. This is the age when individual differences among babies really begin to show up, however. His personality becomes more defined.

His increased desire for socializing may come in relation to his feedings. Such a demand for social attention is especially strong toward the end of the day, usually in the four to six P.M. period. He will enjoy being shifted around from his bed to his playpen or other play area. He particularly likes his playpen. He likes to have people talk to him, pay attention to him, sing to him. Very shortly he is going to enjoy being talked to so much that he may cry when people leave.

ORAL COMMUNICATION

You will be aware that your baby has more control over the muscles of his face by the way his facial expressions change when you talk to him. By this time he uses his face more to express a little of what he feels. He is also getting some control of his tongue and throat. His beginning social cooing of last month is now a responsive babbling in answer to your talking to him. He adds loud shouts to his cooing. He isn't angry or upset. He has discovered how to make a loud noise and he has fun doing it. By the end of this month he is laughing out loud. He will also make sounds and squeals that indicate pleasure or discomfort.

His previous vocal play showed the beginning of repetitive noise-making last month. His old vowel sounds, used with varying pitch, show more signs of the addition of consonant sounds. You may hear a fairly close imitation of m, k, g, t, b, ng, tied to the vowels. As he practices these, more often when he is alone, he changes the pitch sometimes quite dramatically. He seems to be doing this for his own pleasure.

He may get quite fancy with bubbles and a raspberry or Bronx cheer sound as he learns to blow with his lips closed. He usually will try this with a mouthful of cereal. You and he find the results quite interesting indeed.

IMMUNIZATIONS

This visit to the doctor's office will be the time for your baby's second D.P.T. injection and his second dose of oral polio vaccine drops.

BABY-CARE ROUTINES

BATH TIME

Bathing is now a much more active process. He may like to lie on his stomach in shallow water and splash. He splashes with his hands when he is sitting up in the tub. He usually has a good time—and so do you!

16.

The

Fifth Month

If you handled your baby's eating slowdown comfortably last month, he's probably back to eating well again. He continues to be a lot of fun in his attempts to learn what to do with his body and how to get along with people.

WEIGHT

Ranges: Boys 12.9–19.3 lbs. Average 15.0 lbs.
Girls 11.8–19.3 lbs. Average 14.2 lbs.

HEIGHT

Ranges: Boys 24.0–26.9 in. Average 25.2 in.
Girls 23.4–26.4 in. Average 25.0 in.

MOTOR DEVELOPMENT

You will see more signs of intent in many of his actions, though some of his activity is still rather automatic. Most of his primary reflexes are being submerged now by his growing muscular control and nervous-system progress.

REFLEXES

You will still see his rooting reflex when he is asleep and his sucking response when you stimulate his lips. He startles only with definite provocation. His hand response is changing. When you touch his palm now, you don't get the finger curling as before. You can show this if you stroke the thumb-side of his hand when his palm is up—he turns his hand over. He still will curl his toes in a grasping motion when you stroke the sole of his foot. This plantar grasp will remain for most of his first year. His TNR may have disappeared this month to be taken over by his own voluntary control.

LYING, SITTING, STANDING, AND GETTING ABOUT

On his abdomen he is becoming more agile and accurate. He can support himself easily on his arms to get his chest and upper abdomen off the table. (See plate 17F.) He controls his head and shoulders well and can look about the room and shift his weight easily. His legs are becoming useful to him.

On his back he is starting to raise his head from the table to look around. He plays with an overhead toy and makes social sounds at it. He can reach it with fairly good aim. He now plays with his feet much as he played with his hands the past two months. (See plate 25.) He can swing his feet up to his mouth with good aim and may suck his toes in preference to his fingers. They are great playthings, and he talks to them like good companions. When he sits, he leans forward less. With your support he sits well, with a straight back. (See plate 19E.) His infant seat is no longer safe, since he keeps trying to sit up straight and may flip over.

When you stand him up, he shows you that he is learning how to work against gravity to stand erect. He holds his head in line with his body quite well. He almost succeeds in standing if his feet are braced. He holds his legs out straight and rather stiffly, but control is still lacking. (See plate 20F.) You are still the one who does most of the work.

He will roll from his front to his back now. He has increased his control over his arm, shoulder, and trunk muscles. He raises his head and shoulder, arches his back and twists, then gives his body a kick or push with his legs—and over he goes. He doesn't really understand what he does to produce this result. He just keeps trying it. When he starts to flip, he has no idea what will happen or where he will land.

He pushes with his legs to pivot about. But he can't get his abdomen much up off the floor yet.

HANDS

For some time you saw your baby reach and touch a toy with his eyes—now you are seeing him do this voluntarily with his hands. On his back he can reach out with both hands to bring them upward toward an object dangling in front of him. (See plate 21F.) He surrounds it and finally grasps it. He will reach only a short distance, since he doesn't raise himself up much.

On his abdomen he reaches out in front of him to scratch at a bunched-up sheet or a table-top. When he tries to reach for a toy, both hands get involved. He can only get hold of large objects. He often bats at the toys since he has to hold himself up at the same time. He may let go with his arms and plop down so he can free both hands to get at the toy.

When he is sitting, he scratches at the table to test it. Then he will reach out rather erratically to try to corral a toy that isn't too far away. He often still overshoots his mark, but he tries until he finally gets it. When he makes contact, his hand closes down on it. He likes the sound of crumpling paper or any noise he can make with a toy. He works with both hands when he goes after the toy, but he uses only one hand to grasp it now. His aim isn't always good, but he'll make another pass at it if he misses. If you hand him a toy, he will take it and hold it fairly well. He holds onto his cup with both hands—but don't trust him. He grabs anything and everything within his reach, and everything still goes into his mouth.

His grab is full-handed. His fingers are spread straight out until he touches the toy. Then he closes his hand, using all his fingers at the same time as if his hand were a mitten.

He won't learn the more efficient method of picking up something until later, although you may see the start of some finger-to-thumb movement.

EYES AND OTHER SENSE ORGANS

He is much more efficient in using his eyes and ears. His eyes begin to work together for his binocular vision. When he responds to the sound of a voice or bell, he may not always turn in the correct direction. He turns about in his search to locate a voice. He listens to music, TV, or the radio, and seems to respond. He looks at a small object in front of him and reaches out to try to touch it. His eyes cooperate in his beginning efforts at thumb-finger grasping and manipulation that is coming. He can look easily side to side and up and down.

TEETH

Most babies don't have any teeth as yet. Some may have gotten one last month or this month.

EATING

Each meal your baby has is now different. His diet is looking more like an adult diet in its basic structure. This month you will add more of the fillers and increase the variety of foods, but don't neglect the basic groups of meat-egg and milk-milk solids-cheese. Keep his diet varied and flexible so that he eats well without any "have-to" attitude on your part. There is certainly no place in the eating plan suggested for your baby that calls for the clean-plate idea. Finishing everything on his dish is not character-building at this age any more than licking the plate clean is later. Try to make foods taste good to him as well as good for him.

MENU

Morning		
	cereal	1 portion
	meat and/or egg	2 portions
	fruit	1 portion
	milk solids—cheese	1 portion
	milk	1 portion
	(fat—oil)	

Mid-day		
	cereal	1 portion
	meat and/or egg	2 portions
	vegetable	1 portion
	fruit	1 portion
	milk solids—cheese	1 portion
	milk	1 portion
	(fat—oil)	

Evening		
	cereal	1 portion
	meat and/or egg	2 portions
	vegetable	1 portion
	fruit—simple dessert	1 portion
	milk solids—cheese	1 portion
	milk	1 portion
	(fat—oil)	

MENU COMMENTS

This past month you used the food groups separately or in varying combinations with each different meal. This gave you a chance to use new foods in different combinations with familiar foods or to give them separately. Continue to follow the proportions indicated for each of the food groups.

APPETITE

Your baby will probably be back to happily eating three meals a day by now. There are some babies who are quite contented to remain on two good meals a day with the mid-day meal a token affair. As long as you offer his food three times a day and allow him to decide you will have no trouble. You may run into a lot of negativism in this period so that an erratic eating pattern can be seen off and on.

Again, don't offer milk in place of his solid feeding. Give him juice from his cup and offer his food at his next regular feeding time. Go ahead and try your new foods and new combinations. As long as you present them repeatedly without pushing, he will get the idea.

SCHEDULE

Continue a regular three-meal schedule with meals about six hours apart. Seven A.M., 1:00 P.M., and 7:00 P.M. is a suggested pattern for the average household. Any schedule that fits your family needs is satisfactory. He probably will have a one-half hour swing either way if you need to vary the time.

CONSISTENCY

Continue the gradual coarsening of his foods. If you didn't begin to make this change last month, begin now. If the shift from puréed to coarser foods is made gradually over these next months your baby will be ready for bite-size pieces of table foods by eight months. Your baby may already quite willingly accept rougher textures without difficulty.

CEREAL. Continue with the prepared infant cereals and, except for breakfast feeding, use them as thickeners for the other foods.

FRUIT. Cooked fruits are usually favorite food items. The trouble is that you may stay with one or two favorites and not offer him others to increase his experience and broaden his taste. Use them mixed in some other food like cottage cheese. You may find that a spoonful of fruit offered between a spoonful of meat and one of vegetable keeps the meal moving along.

MEAT–EGG. Use two portions of this group in each feeding. In this period of rapid growth and change your baby needs a high protein intake. Try to include organ tissue like liver, heart, or tongue. Rotate the meats so that a good variety is obtained. Egg may be used as one portion from the group at one or two meals.

VEGETABLE (DARK-GREEN OR DEEP-YELLOW). Use the jars of baby food vegetables which are not mixtures. If you can prepare your own, you have a choice of asparagus, carrots, all kinds of leaf greens, pumpkin, squash, peas, and green beans, as starters. Include one portion of these foods at two meals daily.

OTHER VEGETABLES. There is a group of vegetables other than the dark-green, deep-yellow vegetables indicated at 3 months. For the present, these other vegetables include white potatoes, beets, cauliflower, celery, chicory, cucumbers, egg plant, escarole, lima beans, mushrooms, onions, parsnips, summer squash, tomatoes. These are filler foods that help round out your baby's diet in these months ahead. Once a day certain vegetables in this grouping may be given in place of a dark-green, deep-yellow vegetable portion, but your emphasis should remain on the dark-green, deep-yellow group.

$$1 \text{ portion} = \frac{1}{2} \text{ cup cooked vegetable}$$
$$= 1 \text{ cup raw vegetable}$$

MILK. Continue to use 1 portion of the prepared infant formula to moisten his food mix with 2 ounces for drinking afterward (or breast-feeding). Diluted evaporated milk may be substituted now. Either of these is replaced by whole pasteurized milk at the end of the year, unless your pediatrician advises otherwise.

At each meal make up the second portion of milk with the cheese or milk solid group mixed with some of the other foods.

SIMPLE DESSERT. The dessert group is introduced now as a substitute for one fruit portion. Don't substitute such desserts for fruit too frequently. Milk-egg puddings, junkets, and custards are the best choices. Add powdered skim milk to them if you want to increase the milk-solid content.

1 portion = ½ cup cooked fruit
= 2 ounces ice cream
= 2 ounces custard
= ½ cup plain gelatin dessert
= 2 ounces plain milk pudding
= ½ jar baby dessert

At no place in the diet have you added sugar to foods. Keep it that way. When you realize that 50 calories are taken up by 1 tablespoon of sugar you can see that the diet would be sadly lopsided if you had to make up many of his calories this way. Don't sweeten foods to get your baby to take them.

FAT–OIL. Regularly include the fat–oil group in his menu now. Add the portion to vegetable, to meat, or to any other food item. His diet has been kept low in butterfats with the use of the dry skim powdered milk and adjusted special formula. The fat to be introduced will be a vegetable oil. Vegetable-oil margarine or a vegetable oil are suggested as a source of added fat–oil.

1 portion = 1 teaspoon of margarine
= 1 teaspoon butter
= 1 teaspoon of salad oil

BETWEEN MEALS. Again let me warn about between-meal offerings other than fruit juice. You may have to wake him sometimes between feedings to offer juice. Continue to try for more variety in juices and be sure that you are offering regularly some of the Vitamin C-containing juices like orange, grapefruit, tangerine, or tomato.

VITAMINS. Continue his multiple-vitamin drops in appropriate dosage mixed in his food.

Don't forget in all this food talk that cleanliness is still the watchword for any utensils you use. Sterilization has been limited to nipples for these months.

BREAST-FEEDING

Your baby may be one of the one in four still taking some breast-feeding. This is often down to one feeding a day and may be almost a token feeding. Just make certain that he is getting his solid food in sufficient amounts to be satisfied and offer breast after the meal. If he is not interested, offer a cup of juice. If he wants to nurse briefly and be put down, this is fine. Take his word for it when he is not interested.

Don't hesitate to shift to an offer of the cup in place of the breast or bottle. (Look back to last month for a discussion of weaning.)

SPOON-FEEDING

Most of the time your baby is easy to feed. He seems contented and conversational. He appreciates your food preparation. However, his waving hands may get in the way while you are feeding him with the spoon. He may be trying to get his hands on his food, or his fingers on his spoon. In self defense you will have to limit him. You can't feed much with his help. You may have to work out some system at the high chair to get around this.

CUP-FEEDING

Cup-feeding goes along quite well. He may be trying to hold the cup, at least he grabs at it with both hands. Encourage him to hang on, but be sure you control it, or both of you may get wet. Give evaporated milk after his solid foods in a cup. Sometimes it is better to use fruit juice after a feeding and use evaporated milk or skim powdered milk in his food as the source of his milk solids.

HIGH CHAIR

Keep your feeding place quiet and comfortable with few distractions. Privacy is still important. Eating time gives you a chance to make quiet contact with your baby. It can be hectic if you feel pressured or under some other strain. It is his social time with you. He needs your undivided attention.

If he wasn't ready last month your baby may be ready by now to use a high chair.

As discussed before, his high chair is not a good playpen. Don't use it for that. At mealtimes, use the strap and tray so that he will be well secured. Your baby can wiggle around and fall out if you leave him unattended. A chair that can be converted to a low chair later will be quite useful.

EATING WITH THE FAMILY

Although your baby may be quite sociable, the family dinner table is still too much for him now and for many months to come. You save yourself no time if you sit there and try to feed him while you eat. Try to feed him before or after your own meal. This should give you a quiet time of your own with your husband. If you want to bring him to the table at dessert time, this may work out. Each family will have to decide what is best. A good question to ask is how much interference is the baby at the table? Is he distracting and annoying so that the adults cannot enjoy their meal?

BOWEL AND BLADDER FUNCTIONS

There probably have been no great changes in your baby's bowel and bladder routine or in the type of bowel movements he has.

SLEEPING

His sleeping patterns are similar to last month's. He should be sleeping through the night without any difficulty. Some babies may wake up and talk to themselves.

EXERCISE AND PLAY

During this fifth month your baby's play with toys is largely one of investigation. He spends most of his time feeling them, tasting them, chewing them—in other words, finding out about them. He can grab a toy, even hold it quite well, but he may drop it just as soon as something else catches his attention. He may object when a toy is taken away from him. At this age, his interest in toys doesn't last very long. He can be diverted easily by you or other people.

AWARENESS AND SOCIAL RESPONSE

Anything new delights your baby—but not always anyone. While he shows a marked interest in those whom he sees daily, he may begin this month or the next to act shy with strangers. This shows his increasing ability to distinguish between the familiar and the unfamiliar. However, since your baby has a short memory, someone he hasn't seen for a few weeks—even his father—may again be a stranger. He may stare steadily at the stranger, as if he is sizing him up. If the view doesn't reassure him, the baby may act distressed and fearful. If a stranger approaches too closely, or reaches out to pick him up, the baby may give him a tearful reception.

It's better not to let a stranger pick up your baby right away—even if the stranger is grandma! Anyone the baby sees as an outsider should stay away from him for a while after he comes into the room. You should reassure the baby by staying close. Talk and act unconcerned until your baby has a chance to complete his inspection and go on about his play. Then the stranger can approach.

It is sometimes hard for visitors—especially grandparents—to understand what they see as the baby's rejection of them. They must realize that this is just another step in his development. Your baby may skip this phase entirely, but if you see it, don't force people on him. At his own speed he will come to accept many people on his own terms.

His interest in himself is quite exploratory. He puts everything into his mouth. He may be doing a good deal of thumb-sucking. He is discovering himself as an individual. He will play alone for a bit. He talks to himself when alone. His smiling is about as before, but his crying has lessened considerably and become much more purposeful.

ORAL COMMUNICATION

Your baby may not be doing very much yet with speech sounds involving the tongue and lips. More often, he is experimenting with throat sounds that express his feelings. His squeals and shouts may indicate joy or anger. He has developed several sounds he uses with people. He watches your face as you make sounds for him, then he practices, usually when he is alone. The vowel with consonant combinations are coming clearer so that you may hear "ah goo" but real vowel-consonant syllables are yet to come. His greater performance may be in the variations of pitch so that he gets a musical sound to his babbling, using mainly vowel sounds over and over.

IMMUNIZATIONS

If you are planning to travel to any of the countries in the world in which smallpox is endemic, your baby will be given his smallpox vaccination sometime in the next six months. This vaccine is made with a virus similar to the smallpox virus, but far less virulent. A single drop of the vaccine is placed on the skin and introduced into the topmost layer of the skin with a few superficial needle pricks. The vaccine stays in the upper skin layer and doesn't go through it. The vaccination reaction is actually a localized infection. In about three to seven days a small red spot appears, blisters, and then crusts over. The area about this can become quite reddened and swollen.

There is no special care necessary for the smallpox vaccination. It should not be covered tightly. I usually give the vaccination high on the baby's buttocks. He can't reach it. It is a safe spot. No scar will show when he is dressed. Some doctors prefer other areas. You may bathe your baby in the usual fashion. Light cleansing of the area with soap and water will not do any damage. It may take several weeks for the scab or crust to come off on its own. Don't let your baby—or anyone else—touch the vaccination.

Any reaction your baby may have to the smallpox vaccination will come within the week after the actual vaccination. This may last one or two days, during which he may be fussy, look uncomfortable, and run a fever. The vaccination area will look quite swollen and inflamed for a matter of 2 to 3 inches around the vaccination. If the vaccination was given in the buttocks, sometimes a light streak of red runs around his side to the swollen gland in the groin on that side. Give him aspirin every four hours as necessary for fever or discomfort. If the fever lasts longer than two days, some other condition may exist. You may want to check with your doctor.

If no reaction occurs at all at the site of the vaccination, for some reason the vaccine didn't get into the top layer of skin. In other words, the vaccine didn't get where it was supposed to, so that it will have to be repeated. If your baby has a good vaccination "take," with a local reaction evident during the ten days following the vaccination, he will not need to be vaccinated again for a three-year period. It is not necessary to have a large scar to indicate a good immunity.

Your doctor will postpone the smallpox vaccination if your baby shows eczema, impetigo, or any form of dermatitis in the diaper area. His skin must be clear in the sense that there is no area of broken skin. If there is another child in your home with active eczema or severe dermatitis, the same restriction will hold true.

BABY-CARE ROUTINE

BATH TIME

His bath continues to be an active process and probably is an integral part of his play pattern. He may enjoy some bright floating plastic toys. He increasingly enjoys lying on his abdomen in a small amount of water, where he can splash and carry on.

CLOTHING

There is no great change in types of clothing at this time.

17.

The
Sixth Month

This halfway mark in your baby's first year is a good place to remind you again not to try to push your baby into any of the development patterns I describe. He may not be ready. If he isn't prepared to try, don't attempt to force him. All you'll succeed in doing is making yourself unhappy. If he is going ahead in one area and standing still in another, he is quite usual. If you really feel your baby is falling too far out of line with what the majority of babies his age are doing, talk with your pediatrician about it. You may not be reading your baby's growth map correctly. But do ask your questions—don't worry and keep it to yourself.

WEIGHT

Ranges: Boys 14.0–20.8 lbs.   Average 16.7 lbs.
            Girls 12.7–20.0 lbs.   Average 16.0 lbs.

As you can see from the month-to-month weight ranges, variations in weight are often quite extreme from one baby to another. This is not only because one baby is thin and another plump. It is also because of differences in body types. The light, delicate bone structure of one baby will not carry the weight characteristic of the heavier-boned broad body of another. This light-boned Dresden-doll type of baby is just as healthy as the heavyweight wrestler type.

This is the reason I caution you about looking too much at weight values and forgetting to look at your child. Compare your baby with himself as he goes along rather than with other children. It is his progressive rate of growth that is important.

His rate of weight increase has slowed down since his first three months, but it is still fairly rapid. During these second three months boys have gained three and a half to four and a half pounds, girls three to five pounds.

Not all babies will conform to the old saying that birth weight is doubled by six months and tripled by one year, but they will usually show regular increases. Your baby's weight should not remain stationary for longer than a month. No baby loses weight unless there is a problem of some kind.

HEIGHT

Ranges: Boys 24.8–27.7 in. Average 26.1 in.
Girls 24.0–27.1 in. Average 25.7 in.

During these second three months, boys have grown 2½ inches, girls 1½ to 2 inches.

MOTOR DEVELOPMENT

You can't fail to be impressed by the energy of your offspring. He puts himself through a real workout every chance he gets. He tires quickly so he has to rest—but then he is back at it again. Several skills are coming into view all at once. His body is more compact, more powerful, and under better control. His ability to shift his position is increasing. He has more skill and purpose in handling his body parts. He gets more done when he moves. He is at the beginning of a whole new set of skills, although he doesn't have any of them yet. He still has much practice ahead. He is at a good behavior level from your standpoint. His abilities about equal what he is trying to do, so he isn't pushing himself beyond his capacities. This will happen in the months ahead, and he will then show increasing frustration.

REFLEXES

His reflex activity is not easy to demonstrate any longer. His Moro reflex has disappeared. At rest he may take up his tonic-neck reflex fencing position but you see his neck-righting reflex quite definitely replacing this. You can demonstrate this when you turn his head to one side and he turns his shoulders, trunk, and pelvis to follow it.

LYING, SITTING, STANDING, AND GETTING ABOUT

On his abdomen he is increasingly adept at pushing himself straight up on his arms to hold his weight on his hands. He now handles himself well in this position, holding his head and chest high. (See plate 17G.) He is very confident of himself now. He can swing his head about and look wherever he wishes. He arches his back and elevates his arms and legs high in the air to do his "airplaning." Both of his arms come out from under his chest easily. He puts his weight on one arm as he reaches to grab something with his other hand.

On his back he may play contentedly for some time. He uses his hands in front of him for play. Although he can bend his legs easily at the knees to make his feet available for play or mouthing, he is more interested in other activities. He holds his legs straight out to raise them. He kicks actively. He's able to raise his head up from the table to look down at his feet.

Rolling is now one of his favorite pastimes, although he still does not understand just what he is doing. He rolls easily from front to back. From back to front is harder for him, but he can sometimes do it. If he has learned how to roll both ways, he will have accomplished his first full-body maneuver. This takes strength and good coordination. You will have to watch him carefully, since he can roll off a couch or table.

You can see his improved control of his head when you give him your fingers to pull him up to sitting. He holds out his hands when he sees your fingers coming. There is no head lag now, and he raises his head easily from the table in anticipation of your pull-up. But when you give him your fingers, he doesn't always slip into sitting. He may hold his legs straight out, trying to push upward. He gets his bottom off the table. He wants to stand—and you will be impressed with how much he wants to do this. He may wear you out with his demand for this kind of exercise before he wears himself out. He is coming forward more on his legs to be more vertical. It isn't really a straight-up standing yet, but he does love it.

Some babies don't care for this kind of thing at all, and are quite content just to sit. They may not do anything like this for another three or four months.

If you hold your baby upright under his arms, he may push down and try to bounce. In fact, this can be such a game he won't let you quit without a fuss. He doesn't really stand, but you can get him to hang onto the side of his crib or playpen briefly. Then suddenly he sags at the hip and knee to let go and fall. He doesn't realize that his letting go was the cause of the fall.

There is an old wives' tale that a baby will become bow-legged if he is allowed to stand or walk too soon. He won't do either until he is ready to, and when he does, it won't be because anyone made him. So don't interfere with his attempts to stand or walk; he needs the exercise to strengthen his legs and to learn how to use them.

He may not really be sitting too well yet, but he pushes himself up to lean on his hands. (See plate 19F.) If you support him he will manage quite well. He can even sit alone briefly, but he wobbles and falls over. You can prop him up to sit for quite a time before he gets tired, but you may have to be a little watchful here. Prop him up well so that he doesn't tire too quickly. His enthusiasm exceeds his ability. If he sits with his shoulders drooped forward, his back in an extreme curve, his chest slumped down on his abdomen, he is not really ready for sitting alone. Nor will he sit any sooner if you push him. If he isn't ready it is because he doesn't have the muscle control or strength. If you try to teach him you will only end up with a tired baby. As I have stated repeatedly, he can do only what he is ready for—not what you think he is ready for. When he starts to fuss, slump badly, or act uncomfortable, get him down into his familiar prone position. Sitting seems to be necessary for some babies before they crawl or creep. It may parallel crawling. Some babies skip it entirely until later.

HANDS

Your baby's hands are becoming much more useful to him as he increases his ability to sit up and free them for use. He has good control and has a compelling need to use his hands. He reaches out for what he wants with both hands. He may shift to using a one-handed approach more often, since he no longer has to surround an object to get it. He transfers something from one hand to the other and back and forth. He may be able to hold an object in each hand. If you offer him a toy, he will drop what he has to take it. He reaches for something, grabs it, and brings it to himself, examines it, mouths it, perhaps bangs it, and passes it back and forth from one hand to the other. He just has to have something to hold or to hold onto, such as the side of his crib or playpen. No matter what his position—back, front, sitting, or standing—he hangs onto anything for dear life. He still grabs an object with a mittenlike grasp, but he does hang on. He presses it against his palm—up to now more on the little-finger side. In the coming weeks he will begin to shift to hold the object against the base of his thumb, but you don't see much use of a thumb-and-finger movement yet. He may pick up a toy he has dropped, but if he has to reach for it he may go to something handier. He grabs at a moving toy and tries to put it in his mouth. (See plate 21H.) When he is sitting, he looks for a toy that has fallen from his high chair or from your lap. He likes to play with his toes, fingering them and wiggling his foot.

EYES AND OTHER SENSE ORGANS

His eyes now show pupil-size change with an increasing ability to accommodate and converge. He looks with both eyes and fixes, but his gaze wanders off easily. At four months I talked about crossed or lazy eyes. If you still see this turned eye, now is the time to check with your oculist as to what is to be done.

His eyes may have settled down to a definite color, or you may be in doubt for another six months or more. His awareness of what he sees is more definite and specific. He may be able to recognize differences in geometric forms 1½ to 3 inches in size. He will look hard at something without becoming distracted. He has a preference for bright reds and yellows. He follows up his looking with his hand exploration. When he holds something in his whole hand, he looks at it. He shows evidence of his eye-hand cooperation. If he drops something he may look for it. He begins true blinking. His eyes can follow from side to side and up and down without head turning.

His palmar grasp reflex is gone but his foot still grasps at your finger when you stroke the sole of his foot.

Before this time your baby would stop what he was doing, act alert, and turn to search for the source when he heard a noise, such as a bell ringing. Now he may turn his head quite accurately in the proper direction of the noise.

TEETH

By this time most babies will show signs either of two teeth coming through, two teeth outlined in the lower gum to come through later, or four outlined above and two below.

EATING

If your baby is like most you have been able to move along with him so that at his half year mark he eats three times daily, eats his food separately or in different mixtures, drinks well from a cup with or without the use of breast or bottle. He is now ready to get into the business of using more adult table food, food prepared for adults. The food groups in his diet are not different but variety and coarseness will increase, with each meal different in some way. Continue to search for variety in tastes and textures. Your small baby may be a good eater, but he won't necessarily be a big eater. He doesn't need to be. He doesn't require as much food as the baby half again as big as he is.

MENU

Morning	cereal	1 portion
	meat and/or egg	2 portions
	fruit	1 portion
	milk solids–cheese	1 portion
	milk	1 portion
	(fat or oil)	
Mid-Day	cereal–cereal substitute	1 portion
	meat and/or egg	2 portions
	vegetable	1 portion
	fruit	1 portion
	milk solids	1 portion
	milk	1 portion
	(fat or oil)	
Evening	cereal–cereal substitute	1 portion
	meat and/or egg	2 portions
	vegetable	1 portion
	fruit or simple dessert	1 portion
	milk solids–cheese	1 portion
	milk	1 portion
	(fat or oil)	

SCHEDULE. Keep the six-hour interval between his three feedings but start his day with some regard for the family routines. He may wait very comfortably for you to get his meal ready especially if you give him something to amuse him and occupy his hands.

CONSISTENCY. Continue your program of coarsening his foods. If he uses the prepared junior foods you will still have to mash them. With your home-prepared foods, coarse grinding, fine chopping, or mashing may be sufficient. He may have a little difficulty accepting this change but you still have time to make the shift gradually. Your baby may already have accepted rougher textures without difficulty.

APPETITE. A very active, busy, on-the-go fellow may present a problem for you. He is hungry but he can't slow down long enough for you to give him as much as he needs. If you have a leisurely baby, you won't have to try so hard.

He will placidly wade through his meal as he gazes around and "talks" between bites.

Try to use variety in each food group so that your baby has an opportunity to taste new foods. He knows differences and newness, he has likes and dislikes, but he can be quite flexible in his acceptance. He has a good memory for his foodstuffs. Try to rotate your presentation of foods during a meal although he may want to eat all of one thing before he starts another. If you see this, offer his proteins first when he is hungriest.

CEREAL. Continue prepared infant cereal at the morning feeding. At the other two feedings cereal may be replaced with one of the cereal substitutes.

Cereal Substitutes. There is a group of foods that you can use now in place of cereal at either of two meals in the day's menu. These will later be alternated with the bread group. They include white potato, corn (hominy), beans (kidney, lima, navy, wax, dried, baked), dried peas (split peas, cow peas), rice, spaghetti, noodles, parsnips, sweet potatoes, yams. Some of them are more suitable for later months after he is taking bite-size foods. He may surprise you even now in the ease with which he accepts some of them. White potato is the commonest example of this group. Your baby may object to its mealy feel in his mouth, but he may come to enjoy it, too.

    1 portion = ½ cup beans–dried peas
             = ½ cup spaghetti–noodles (cooked)
             = ⅔ cup parsnips
             = ½ cup rice (cooked)
             = ¼ cup sweet potatoes–yams
             = ½ cup white potato

By now he may get his hands around a piece of zwieback or toast well enough to hang on and try to get it to his mouth. Everything he gets a grip on has to go to his mouth. He may not do too much with it as far as eating is concerned, but it is good finger-feeding exercise. Don't count this as food until he is able to actually get some of it swallowed. This may not be for several more months.

MEAT–EGG. Try to keep variety in your meat choices. He needs the taste and texture differences as well as the basic protein content. You may begin to prepare his eggs in different ways, boiled, coddled, poached, or scrambled. Eggs mixed with powdered skim milk as an egg-nog can be a nice change to use with his cereal or to drink.

FRUIT. Use cooked fruits of all kinds, feeding them separately or mixed with some less well-liked food group. Change the consistency gradually to coarser mashed, then to chopped over the next several months.

MILK–MILK SOLIDS–CHEESE. This milk–milk solids–cheese group continues to be important in your diet construction. Don't forget in these months ahead that liquid milk is filling and may replace other basic food items if you offer it inappropriately. Continue to keep one portion of skim powdered milk in each meal as a basic unit and make up the second portion with cheese and evaporated milk.

VEGETABLE (DARK-GREEN OR DEEP-YELLOW). Include a portion of the dark-green, deep-yellow vegetable group at two meals each day. Start to introduce some of the stronger tasting ones now when you are preparing them for the rest of the family. This group requires a little more experimenting with when you first introduce it to your baby. Except for fruit, there is a greater difference in color, taste, and texture in this group than any other. Start with small amounts and increase to full portion.

OTHER VEGETABLES. The other vegetable group (non-green–yellow) mentioned last month may be used as a substitute now and again at one meal for the above group of green–yellow vegetables. Look ahead to *The Eighth Month* to read how to prepare your vegetables.

FAT–OIL. Continue adding a margarine or butter portion to each meal.

DESSERT. Use this group in place of one fruit portion. Don't give them in place of the basic food elements in his diet. The fruit group is really better to use than the Jell-o, gelatin, milk–egg custard, milk pudding, or ice cream desserts. Try to add skim powdered milk to these desserts whenever you can to increase the milk-solid content. But no chocolate!

And again about sweets. Avoid them! Don't sweeten any food just to get him to take it. If you start using sweets as bribes or rewards you set up a poor eating habit and are not being honest with him. He should eat because he is hungry, not bribed or fooled.

Just to remind you of the portions of the basic food groups:

Cereal	1 portion =	½ cup (8 tablespoons) dry prepared
	=	½ cup cooked
Fruit	1 portion =	½ small banana
		½ cup cooked fruit sauce
		1 jar baby fruit
Meat	1 portion =	1 egg
	=	1 ounce (2″ x 1½″ x ½″) lean meat
	=	2 ounces (½ jar) strained meat
Milk	1 portion =	½ cup (4 ounces) diluted formula (evaporated milk)
	=	4 ounces breast (10 minutes)
Milk Solids	1 portion =	3 tablespoons dry powdered skim milk
	=	3 ounces cottage cheese
	=	3 ounces yogurt

BETWEEN MEALS. Continue to offer a variety of fruit juices freely between meals. He may need the extra fluids. Pay some attention to the Vitamin C content of what you offer.

VITAMINS. Continue multiple-vitamin drops in appropriate dosage in his food.

BREAST-FEEDING

By this month eight out of ten breast-fed babies will have shifted from breast to cup without any great difficulty. This is part of the natural development in the preparation process for taking coarser food which he will be ready to mouth, chew, and swallow on his own. As you follow his cues, you may find that juice from the cup after his full solid food meal may be all he wishes. He may not care for milk. Patience is needed with any shift in feeding. Your reluctance to give up breast-feeding may be the interfering factor here, not his difficulty in changing. Is he trying to tell you he is done with this business? Are you insisting that he continue when he insists that he is finished?

BOTTLE-FEEDING

Just as with weaning from the breast, you may be having difficulty with yourself rather than with your baby. Try to avoid feeling sorry for him since he doesn't need your pity. He deserves your admiration as he goes step by step along his path of development. You will have to be prepared for a certain amount of comment from those around you. Many people feel that a bottle must be continued indefinitely. Others are concerned about the need for milk. Others about the digestibility of solid foods, and so it goes. In his diet you are emphasizing proteins, the tissue builders. He shifts to the cup as he is ready to handle the mouth activity himself.

SPOON-FEEDING

His spoon-feeding goes along smoothly for the most part. He is over his third or fourth month slow-down. He handles food easily in his mouth. His lips and tongue are under good control. He even begins definite chewing now. Although he doesn't have chewing teeth, he can gum his food quite nicely.

CUP-FEEDING

His cup-feeding goes along easily. He can place his lips on the cup fairly accurately. He drinks easily, if perhaps messily, from his cup when you hold it for him. He tries to get his hands on the cup to help hold it.

HIGH CHAIR

Once he can sit up for himself he should be in a high chair regularly. As indicated before, make certain that it has a wide, steady base, so that he can't tip it over. Use a safety strap to prevent him from standing up or sliding out. Place the high chair far enough away from stove, table, draperies, or any other article he can grab.

EATING WITH FAMILY

If you wish to include your baby at the family meal do this for dessert time, after he has eaten. He can sit in his high chair and hold a piece of zwieback. Don't include him for your entire meal. There is too much excitement. He won't eat well, and neither will you.

BOWEL AND BLADDER FUNCTIONS

You may be receiving a good deal of advice by now about the importance of toilet training your child. How this pernicious idea was instituted is hard to determine. As a result of a good deal of false propaganda, faulty memories, and misunderstanding of child behavior, you may be pressured into trying to train your baby now. You will be training yourself, not him. You can train yourself to jump at every change of his expression. You pop him on the toilet seat and catch his automatically expelled product. But he doesn't cooperate in your maneuvers, and your temporary success often won't last. You only produce difficulties for yourself and your baby later by pushing toilet training now.

SLEEPING

From six to twelve months your baby has a total sleeping time of fourteen to sixteen hours. His total nap time by this month is about three hours. His longest period of sleep remains about eleven and a half hours.

Your baby has probably settled down to two fairly long naps daily, one in the morning and one in the afternoon. At this age his morning nap is the longest.

As your baby reaches this more active stage he may resist going to sleep at night, even though he's tired. He loves to be with people. He is eager to keep moving about. Keep his schedule regular. You have to be the decision maker.

There is very little you can do about his urge to keep moving. If he is at the point where he is learning to sit and stand, he fights against being laid flat. He is like a toy that bobs upright whenever it's pushed over. When you put him to bed, try letting him assume whatever position he wants. This may be either sitting up or standing hanging onto the side of the crib. Sooner or later he will topple over and go to sleep. You can cover him up then. It's the lying down, not the sleeping itself, that bothers him so. His reluctance to see you go may also account for some of the problem.

If he calls out after you've left his room, call back to him to assure him that you are nearby. Don't make this a game, though. And remember—don't go back into his room unless you sense real urgency. The fretful cry of a sleepy baby may be just his way of whining himself to sleep.

You may find your baby waking during the night to cry. This is not because he is hungry. Possibly it's because he is alone and wants company. Often it's because he wants to stay busy and active. He may not fuss, but he stays awake for a while. He talks to himself. He plays with his hands. Don't go in if he sounds happy. If he cries, give him a few minutes to make up his mind. He may decide to go back to sleep again. Wait until you know he means it. If you go in and he stops crying, you know he wants to be sociable. Check to see that he isn't in trouble, talk to him, pat him, and then leave, and don't go back. Don't take him to bed with you—it's a hard habit to break and it's also dangerous.

If your baby is still in your room, you have really asked for this trouble.

EXERCISE AND PLAY

Your baby loves to romp now. He enjoys being lifted up in the air, gently rolled and tumbled.

His stroller for airings and shopping trips and his car seat for car rides are important in his life. Just be certain to use an adequate safety harness with each. A carriage or stroller is a necessity by now. A stroller is more useful than a carriage. When he tires of sitting, you can convert the stroller into a flat bed for him.

AWARENESS AND SOCIAL RESPONSE

Your baby takes real pride and pleasure in his skills. You can see it in his delighted expression when he pulls up to sitting or does that quick roll-over.

By now you may find yourself making excuses when he really tears into a good crying jag in the pediatrician's office —"He hasn't had his nap," or, "He is pretty tired." This kind of excuse covers your embarrassment at a good display of temper. This can't be called a temper tantrum, but he is letting everyone know he doesn't have things the way he wants them. He has no other way yet of dealing with a situation that doesn't suit him. You will see more of this frustration crying as he tries to do more and more things.

In these first six months he has been very dependent on you, his mother. You gave him his first gratifications. Now he begins to change as he finds the outside world. He is so active that he does no listening or stopping to look. He grabs out to the world without any discrimination. But he is able to amuse himself for longer periods without your help. He begins to shift his interest from animate objects like people to inanimate ones like toys. He needs neutral objects to deal with, which don't have the emotional charge of people—he needs to manipulate them on his own. But this means he will be presented with frustrations and he will have to begin to cope with them.

He now shows fear, disgust, anger, distress, loneliness, excitement, and delight in his emotional equipment. Loud noises may frighten him.

This month you may definitely see signs of concern about strangers. Look back to last month's "Awareness and Social Response" for suggestions about dealing with this.

Your infant now initiates more social contact for himself. He looks up expectantly when people enter the room.

When he is left alone, or when a toy is taken away, he may object noisily, but he gets over losing his toy faster than he gets over the disappearance of a person.

His self-knowledge continues. He continues to explore and to be interested in himself as an object. He exploits all the possibilities of his play material, too. His hand-to-hand transfer, banging, and putting things to his mouth are all types of self-activity that aid in his learning. He may start to smile at his own image in the mirror.

ORAL COMMUNICATION

Just as his sociability is more noticeable, so is his awareness of your language. He begins to make some sort of vocal social response. He may babble two or more distinct sounds, perhaps several well-defined syllables. He babbles to a person. He blows bubbles. He may imitate you when you stick out your tongue or cough. He shows his eagerness with his voice. He says by his tone variations whether he is pleased or unhappy. He laughs and shouts. He makes a number of imitative sounds. You may be startled to hear some that sound like your words. His repetitive babbling has a marked rhythm to it that is quite noticeable. You will hear a nasal tone in what he is saying. He may have some beginning tip-of-tongue sounds too, like d, t, n.

You may find that he uses a special sound to call you or greet you with in the morning. If you don't answer after several tries, he will fall back on crying. These are his first true word sounds or verbalizations. When he uses a sound that you believe is a word, your enthusiastic response makes him use it again. Eventually it will become a word with meaning to him—such as "bye-bye," "da-da," "ma-ma"—because you have given it a meaning by your response.

You must keep in mind that your baby is becoming increasingly aware of differences in the tone of your voice. He knows whether you are happy, disapproving, angry, or in a hurry. He knows the difference between friendly and angry talking, but his response depends on other things that go with it—like gestures or physical contact. He may begin to recognize some of the word sounds you use.

IMMUNIZATIONS

At this time your baby should receive the third D.P.T. injection and the third dose of oral polio vaccine.

BABY-CARE ROUTINES

Bath Time

By this time your baby's bath time has become so routine that you may be forgetting some of your regular bath procedures. So remember: A daily brushing and a shampoo every second or third day will keep his scalp in good condition. Short fingernails are a must now, with all his hand use going on. Be sure to keep his diaper area, body creases, and the spaces between his fingers and toes clean and dry.

Clothing

When you dress your baby you may notice that he seems to anticipate some of the things you are trying to do. He may try to fool with his shoes and pull off some article of clothing.

18.

The
Seventh Month

Your baby may not look much different from last month, but you feel some personality changes are taking place. His heightening awareness tells you that he is getting experience and memory. This is in part the result of the tremendous increase in the size of his brain during these past months.

WEIGHT

Ranges: Boys 14.9–22.0 lbs.   Average 17.8 lbs.
            Girls 13.5–21.4 lbs.   Average 17.1 lbs.

HEIGHT

Ranges: Boys 25.2–28.4 in.   Average 26.7 in.
            Girls 24.6–27.8 in.   Average 26.4 in.

MOTOR DEVELOPMENT

This is usually still a good month for your baby and for you. He continues to pause a bit to catch up with all that he has been trying to learn to do. He still isn't pushing himself beyond his capacity. When he tries something and succeeds, he seems pleased with himself and satisfied. He doesn't scold himself when he doesn't manage the job. He just tries again—usually pleasantly.

But this little period of things in balance may already be disappearing. The urge of his growth and development push him along now or very shortly into new frustrations and tensions. The pleasant harmony of these days gives way to fussing, feuding, and fighting. This month may be the conclusion of his attempts to raise himself up and sit. Next he has to get on to new struggles in learning how to get about.

The age when your baby sits up, stands, and creeps is very unpredictable. Most babies will get to their head-eye-arm control at almost the same time. From here on the various skills of locomotion come at different ages for different children. His body type and the type of baby he is influence this timing more than his age. I will just have to continue to talk averages to you.

Your baby's muscle strength is an important factor in his ability to perform some physical acts. Prematurity, inadequate diet, or illness may give him poor muscle tone so that he is slowed down in his activity. His performance will be poor because he lacks the strength to sit alone, push about, stand with help, or do any of the things he wants to do—but is unable to do. This is the reason I stress again and again your baby's diet and its proper content.

REFLEXES

His rooting reflex is gone. Most of his little-baby reflexes have disappeared. He continues to show a righting reflex in which he tries to get upright. His previous automatic grasping response loses some of its simplicity as he tries to develop control. Now if you stroke the little-finger side of his hand he will turn his hand downward. If you stroke the thumb side of his palm he turns his hand palm up. If you stroke his hand he makes groping movements with it as he searches for the touching object.

LYING, SITTING, STANDING, AND GETTING ABOUT

When he is on his back he can lift his legs off the floor and hold them up for long periods, raising his head at the same time. Now he moves his feet up and down much of the time rather than sucking on his toes. He may pivot about, pushing his legs unevenly to squirm along.

When he is on his abdomen, he is better able to hold his weight on one hand as he reaches or plays with the other. If he is interested in some hand play, he gets into a frog position with his legs spread out, the soles of his feet together. He continues to roll over a great deal. He is probably rolling from back to front by now.

He wants to do pull-ups over and over again. If you give him your fingers to hold, he pulls up to a standing position. He now does a pretty good job of holding his legs straight with his knees stiff. (See plate 20H.) He can support a large portion of his own weight for a longer period. He hangs onto the side of his crib or playpen. Some babies may even try to pull themselves up to standing position—or lower themselves to a sitting one.

Your baby definitely has better control of his trunk muscles, with improved arm and leg coordination. His head is in a line with his trunk and his arms and legs are carried straighter. When you hold him up to stand, he still does a lot of up and down bouncing, with some stamping of his feet. His bouncing doesn't carry much weight-bearing with it. He expects you to hold him up. You do get the impression that he can do more than this, so encourage him to bear his own weight. He is putting together the mechanisms for posture control and motion control. He is trying to learn control of his body position. The mechanisms that control his posture are all learned faster than those controlling his walking movements. Good standing can come in another month.

In talking about sitting, I must warn you again about the wide differences in babies. By seven months your baby may be able to sit alone quite well on a hard surface. (See plate 19G.) His back muscles are strong enough so that he doesn't weave back and forth to finally topple over. But don't be alarmed if your baby doesn't do this. He may not sit alone until nine or ten months. He may be a creeper and not a sitter. Some babies stand with support and try to walk before they manage to sit well.

He can be put in some type of chair, such as a swing or a walker, for a brief play period now. Try to give him a change of position at fairly frequent intervals. He may get tired unless he can shift about. It is better not to prop him for too long a period. Get him back in his playpen on his abdomen. If he isn't ready yet, he is much better off on his abdomen, making whatever motions he wishes at his own speed. His back muscles may be strong enough, but his desire to use them may not be. Most babies will sit alone well sometime between seven and ten months.

Your baby has been a modest example of perpetual motion for some time. He is now directing his efforts at the acquiring of locomotion. This doesn't come all at once. The first attempts he makes may make you laugh. He works so hard that he may resemble a crab more than anything else. He pushes about on his abdomen but often just manages to move sideways. This doesn't mean he doesn't get around. He can cover a lot of territory just by rolling, kicking, or squirming about on his tummy. You may see him scoot along on his abdomen pushing with his feet while he holds something in his hand or reaches for something. It is usually another month before he gets his abdomen up to creep. If he does creep now, that is, move on all fours, he may go backward before he learns to go forward. Sometimes he hitches along sideways, half sitting and half leaning. He may get up on his hands and knees and rock back and forth. This may develop later into his walking on hands and feet like a bear.

Some babies never crawl (that is, move by dragging the whole body along the floor) at all but go from sitting to standing and walking. Babies who prefer sleeping on their backs often sit alone well before they try to crawl much. They sit and bounce up and down, or hitch along in a sitting position to fall forward on their hands in a creeping position.

HANDS

He no longer has to use his hands to hold himself up. They are free to use for exploring his world. He can reach out and grasp an offered toy with one hand. He handles it, turns it about to see and examine it. When he holds an object in one hand, he can use the other to touch something else. (See plate 21K.) He passes the toy back and forth from one hand to the other quite easily. This is a very important point in his development. One-handedness means he has increased his freedom to explore and decreased his dependency. He doesn't show any particular preference for either hand. You may feel that he seems to prefer his left hand. Usually his supposed left-handedness comes from your right-handedness. You face him in feeding and other activities—and come at him from his left with your right hand. Check and see. Actually he uses both hands quite well, so don't interfere.

He has used his mouth and eyes to investigate objects. Now his hands are coming into more use for this purpose. Although his eyes are still more valuable to him at this point, his hands are learning rapidly. His mouth, eyes, and hands are a three-point system he uses to develop his knowledge of the world. He has been using his hands centered on his middle. With his one-handedness he is able to move out to either side in his activities. Now he will approach an object with his eyes and hands, with some sense of distance.

His hands show improvement in the way his fingers are used. He still grasps and holds a toy in his palm, but he operates his hands more delicately. He holds an object primarily on the thumb side of his palm, with his second and third fingers pressing it against his thumb. He can pick up a small toy, but not a crumb-sized object. With a crumb he uses his whole hand, squashing down on it to try to rake it toward him with his whole arm.

EYES AND OTHER SENSE ORGANS

His eye control and behavior are still well ahead of any other part of his development. You will see definite signs of his eye-and-hand coordination. In his first six months he looked at his world in general. Now his world is background and he is increasingly interested in single objects. This exploring of his world with his eyes and hands is giving him a multitude of impressions and experiences which he stores up for future use.

He is beginning to bring his other senses more into his everyday living. He enjoys rhythm. Tasting, smelling, and feeling are all essential ingredients in his appreciation of his world. He may not always put them all together properly, but he is using them.

TEETH

The average baby has his first tooth, usually a lower central incisor. Some babies may have a couple of teeth by now —or six—or none. Your baby can gum his food quite effectively without teeth. He can do a very good chewing job on some quite coarsely textured foods if you give him a chance. Chewing teeth don't appear for some time. Even his front incisor teeth don't help him chew much. They are for biting.

An erupting tooth may make your baby chew hard, act touchy about his mouth, perhaps become fussy and restless, sleep less well, or eat erratically. As mentioned before, rubbing his gums with your finger or giving him a hard rubber toy to chew on may help.

Once teething has started, you must avoid improperly regulated bottle-feedings. If you are still bottle-feeding on a self-demand schedule and let your baby suck on his bottle for very long periods, you are subjecting him to possible overexposure to milk curds in his mouth. Damage to his teeth can result from the breakdown of milk curds. They form acids in his mouth to damage tooth enamel.

EATING

This period in your baby's eating is most interesting, not because of food changes but because he is changing so rapidly and so much in his participation in the eating process. Adapt his diet to his abilities as he is able to handle foods increasingly well.

APPETITE

This usually is still a period of good appetite. He is so active during the day that he has a chance to exercise himself into a good hunger pattern. Even now you have to pay some attention to the attractiveness of the food you serve. Keep the amounts or portions of food small. He will eat these quickly, be ready for more, and enjoy a feeling of success when he takes more. Small portions also allow for variations in the amount he takes at different meals, so that you don't have a lot of food left over after a meal. Be a little cautious when you offer a new food. He has a tendency to gag at this time which may be hard for you to understand, or tolerate. He is beginning to chew. He also begins to discover that he has some control in his mouth and throat that he didn't have before. Sometimes the least difference in food consistency provokes his gag reaction. Don't overreact to it! Just go on and feed, or stop and wait until his next feeding. You are still in the process of increasing the coarseness of his foods so that you are ready to use table foods, diced, cubed, or coarse mashed, when he is ready to finger-feed.

SCHEDULE. A three-meal schedule with five and one-half to six hour intervals still works best for most babies. The hours of the meals should be determined by the family needs and can be quite variable from day to day. The baby is able to wait now since he can anticipate what is coming and accept some change.

CEREAL. Continue to use the prepared infant cereal for his morning feeding as a balanced vegetable protein source. Breads as a food source are still in the future until his chewing and holding are better.

You have undoubtedly tried toast by this time. Zwieback, toast, or teething biscuits will give him a chance to practice his hand-to-mouth skills, after his meal is finished.

At one of the other meals a cereal substitute, described last month, may be used for the cereal group.

MEAT–EGG. Choose his meats for variety in taste and texture. One or more eggs a day may be used, cooked with powdered skim milk as was suggested last month. Continue to wash the egg shell before opening it.

FRUIT. The fruit group is still apple, apricot, banana, peach, pear, pineapple, plum, prune, or tomato. Larger pieces of fruits are used as your baby's skill increases with his finger-feeding. Over these past months your effort has been to give coarser and coarser foods until in another month you will be using table food diced or cubed. You may use chopped junior foods in jars, canned fruits, or soft raw fruit. In place of the fruit group at one meal offer a simple dessert, not highly sweetened, at the end of the meal.

MILK—MILK SOLIDS—CHEESE. The milk—milk solids—cheese group is the one you may have trouble with now that meals are different and your baby is older. Use two portions in each meal. It is more difficult to get adequate amounts of formula or evaporated milk in each meal. Depend on your more concentrated milk solids.

One portion = 4 ounces diluted evaporated milk
= 3 tablespoons skim powdered milk
= ¾ ounce cream cheese
= 3 ounces cottage cheese
= 3 ounces yogurt

Continue to use evaporated milk, or prepared infant formula, undiluted or diluted with equal amounts of water, to mix into his solid food where possible. Mix in the 3 tablespoons of dry skim powdered milk with other solids where you can. Never give liquid milk in place of food. Offer two ounces of evaporated milk or reconstituted skim powdered milk from his cup after his meal.

VEGETABLE (DARK-GREEN—DEEP-YELLOW). Cooked vegetables are good foods to use diced or cubed for his early finger use in getting food to his mouth. He may not do much yet but mess with them. Accustom him to the wide differences in the vegetables. Use the junior chopped vegetables if you don't prepare them yourself. No raw vegetables yet. Look ahead to *The Eighth Month* to read how to prepare vegetables. Look back to *The Fifth Month* for the members of this group available to use. Other vegetables (not dark-green or deep-yellow) may be used now and again as one of the vegetable portions at one meal.

FAT—OIL. Continue to add a margarine or butter portion to each meal. A liquid vegetable oil can be used.

DESSERT. This substitute for fruit at one meal a day can be offered at the end of his meal after he has taken his basic food groups. You will notice that breads, cakes, pies, are not included in his diet.

You must remember what you are trying to do with food. It is so easy to get into the habit of using it to get your own way. Try to keep food as an answer to hunger, not as a means of persuading your child to "be a good boy."

BETWEEN MEALS. Between-meal snacks can be a problem at this time. Your child may get quite hungry with all his moving about. If you give him something other than fruit juice, try to make it a food with protein value and not too much filling effect so that it won't ruin his appetite for the next meal.

His fruit juices have been and will be his dietary source of Vitamin C until he starts using raw fruits containing Vitamin C. Always offer juices once or twice between meals to make certain your baby is not thirsty. One portion should be one of the Vitamin C-containing group.

VITAMINS. Continue to give his regular multiple-vitamin drops in his food. These are a regular supplement for his diet.

BREAST-FEEDING

If your baby is still on breast, he is the one in ten who still is. Nursing at this time is getting to be more and more a termination point of eating. Very often it is taken for just a few minutes and your baby is finished. Some babies may use only one breast-feeding a day. Others may continue a night-time or bedtime nursing, especially if rocking is part of the bedtime ritual you have set up. As long as you're not bitten harshly or refused this may go on as long as both of you are comfortable with it. I hope you don't ignore your baby's needs because of your own wishes. Look back to "Eating" in *The Fourth Month* for reminders about weaning.

SPOON-FEEDING

You will see a kind of eager participation now. He sets his mouth to receive the spoon and reaches for it with his head. He manages the spoon quite well, perhaps trying to suck the food off. This is done on his own and as he wishes. However he isn't ready to manipulate the spoon on his own yet, although he may be eager to get his hands on it. As you feed him he may grab the spoon or your hand.

CUP-FEEDING

He and his cup are good friends. He demands it but sometimes more for curiosity than drinking. He takes water or juice easily and well. He doesn't care much for milk. He may take only a few swallows at a time. He seems to be experimenting with it rather than depending on it as his source of food. This is the reason I suggest the addition of dry skim milk solids to his food rather than depending on any liquid milk. When you offer him the cup he may try to bring his hands up to hold it too. (See plate 22.) He puckers his lips and hits the rim of his cup with fairly good aim. You must keep the cup in place while he drinks. His control isn't good enough to handle more than a mouthful at a time. When he is done he quickly pulls back and away. So be prepared.

FINGER-FEEDING

There is a wide difference in babies about finger-feeding at this time. He will give you a little clue if you watch how he grabs his toys. If he still grabs as if his hand was a mitten, without taking the object between his thumb and fingers, he is not quite ready for much finger-feeding. This doesn't say that he can't grasp a piece of toast when you offer it and smear it all over his face and high-chair tray. It does say that he can't reach out yet and pick up a piece of cheese or fruit and get it to his mouth with any accuracy. This is the first step in his efforts to feed himself. Encourage him when you see him try and stay out of his way, but be ready to move in comfortably and take over his actual feeding. He may still be trying to get that piece of fruit in his fingers as you load the food into his mouth, chasing it all over his high-chair tray as he automatically opens his mouth for the next spoonful. In some ways this is a good stage of eating development unless he gets angry about his inability to get his fingers working.

HIGH CHAIR

He is much too active now and probably too big to hold at feeding time. He wants to see. His high chair gives him a commanding view of all that goes on. The chair back, arms, and tray give him steadying support so that he is free to use his hands. He must not be able to slide out or stand up. Never place his chair too near anything he can grab. Just because you don't hold him on your lap any more doesn't mean that you have retired from the scene. In all of his feedings you are still actively engaged in the whole process of his eating. Your face, your voice, your physical presence, are all very much involved and necessary, so use them to good advantage. He will need you even as he gets more grown-up in his eating. Although self-feeding is in the future for him you are laying the groundwork now for his finger-feeding.

Get him to understand by your actions that he is in his high chair to eat, not to play, or just mess around. Don't play games. When he starts to twist or squirm away from your attempts to get food into him, take his word for it. Stop! If he blows his food, even in play, stop. Eating is to get food. Don't let it deteriorate into a contest, a game, or a battle. If he isn't hungry at one meal he will be at the next.

Perhaps you need to be reminded about play too. Don't get too active or stimulating in your play with him just before or after a meal. He needs a brief slow-down or quiet time before he eats. Over-exercise him on a full stomach and he may demonstrate his gag reflex on you. After he has eaten get him down to quiet play or put him in bed for a rest or sleep.

He is not yet a good companion at the family dinner table. Let him eat at his own time with his own food in his own chair and place.

BOWEL AND BLADDER FUNCTIONS

By now your baby may be down to a single bowel movement each day, but he can still skip a day or two or have two or three movements a day. Morning is his usual production time, although it can be any time of the day or night.

He urinates in great quantities. He may stay dry for a couple of hours before he floods his diaper.

SLEEPING

Your baby may wake up early in the morning, or he may sleep comfortably late. If yours is the night-waking type, he is likely to play or talk to himself and then drop back to sleep on his own—especially if you have been following the suggestions I made about this activity last month.

You may be concerned that with all this nighttime activity he will get uncovered and catch cold. If you dress him in a sufficiently warm sleeping suit he won't be in any trouble. He doesn't catch cold this way. You just look silly getting up half a dozen times a night to cover him. Usually you just end up annoying him. So don't harass him and don't harness him. Tying a child in bed is always a dangerous practice. He must have freedom to move. Once you have settled him down for the night you can leave him alone. By this time you should be able to distinguish between the cry of hurt and the cry of a fretful or angry baby.

Naps usually continue to be two in number and total about three hours a day. But don't depend on it. He may have his own ideas. The three-hour estimate doesn't include the little catnaps he may take between periods of play. He may wake just long enough to eat a big breakfast and then retire for a long mid-morning snooze. If you don't give him enough sleep you will have a very tired, impossible creature to deal with late in the day. He won't eat well at dinner and then he'll be hungry during the night with more fussing. So keep adequate nap times going.

Your baby is now well into the second half of his first year. He has settled down into a regular pattern of living and you have a good idea of what sort of baby he is. But you are discovering that sleeping is not always going smoothly. What are some of the things you look at?

You can let a baby under a year decide how much sleep he needs—if you pay careful attention to what he tells you. I have no magic formula for the precise amount of sleep an individual baby needs. He can show you plainly enough when he is tired and sleepy, although with some stubborn babies you do have to watch closely for fatigue.

You know he is getting enough sleep if he seems reasonably happy, active, and alert, is eating satisfactorily and gaining weight, and does not appear to get too sleepy or tired. If he is whining, cross, irritable in his play, rubbing his eyes and acting out of sorts, you get the message—he needs more rest and a quieter life.

There is nothing sacred about sleep schedules. They can be varied to meet the family pattern. Your baby can adjust to your family patterns if you let him know them. You ease him along into whatever schedule seems easiest for you. If he misses a nap one day or stays up late one night, you give him a chance to make up for it the next day. Since most babies are quite flexible, you can use this relaxed approach satisfactorily.

But not all parents can handle this relaxed approach well. I have discussed the oversolicitous kind of parents who pick up their baby whenever he makes a sound and never allow him to settle down on his own. There are also parents who constantly invade their baby's privacy in the name of fun. He has settled down for the night peacefully. Suddenly someone decides that it will be fun to play with him. Up he gets, asleep or not, to "play." If this becomes a regular affair, they are training him to get up to play at irregular times. If he is expected to get up and show off whenever visitors come, you can expect him to respond as you might anticipate. He shows irregular sleep patterns, disturbed settling down, and all the rest of it.

There are some new parents who are so enthusiastic about their baby that they insist on his constant presence. He sits in his infant seat at the dinner table. He shifts to the bedroom while they get ready for the night or the morning. He sits in the living room to be included in the family conversation. He is being trained to constant stimulation and involvement. This isn't to say that he shouldn't be included in family fun at times—but there are limits.

If you are so socially minded that you gad about night after night, or every afternoon, and keep your baby out late, awake or sleeping irregularly, tired from too much stimulation or handling, you will have to expect trouble. He will be fussy, unhappy, apathetic, and will end up sleeping poorly. He doesn't know what is expected of him. And he may be too tired to drop into a natural sleep pattern. This doesn't mean that you can never take him along on your social outings. But if you go out a lot, leave him at home, or get home early enough so that he can go to sleep in his own crib.

Many of these situations start innocently enough, but after some months conditions change. Now the parents don't want the same kind of behavior from the baby they asked for earlier. But the baby has learned to expect a certain sequence of events. His parents want him to go to sleep now—but he hasn't had this explained to him. His parents are certain to get noise and arguments from him.

If you've allowed such poor sleep patterns to develop, start at once to establish consistent bedtime routines. Set up a regular time for naps and bedtime, keeping your family schedule in mind. Don't worry about his protests when you put him to bed and leave the room. He isn't afraid. He is mad. He'll adjust if you leave him alone.

Your child may be one of those babies who has a hard time fitting into any regular pattern. This difficulty arises in all of his areas of living and developing, not just his sleep routines. With such a baby it is particularly important not to become erratic and inconsistent in your approach. He needs your patient, firm, consistent handling—not your worry about possible frustrations and emotional damage.

In the later months of the first year, many babies want a favorite object like a blanket or a doll in bed with them. Give him his favorite toy, but don't stack the crib with toys. He is in bed to sleep—not to play.

You may be surprised at the intensity of his attachment to a favorite object. Encourage him to use several similar objects. That way you may be able to get a disreputable-looking blanket or dirty stuffed animal away from him long enough to wash it.

Don't get into the habit of always having mother put him to bed. Perhaps alternating this task on a regular basis is best—or maybe this can be father's job as the baby gets older and into the period of separation anxiety, when he doesn't want mother to leave his room.

EXERCISE AND PLAY

You certainly won't need to set aside a period of his day for exercises now. You will more likely have to set aside a slowdown time. He exercises constantly when he is awake. He does need to get outdoors daily as much as possible. Don't forget his sunbaths.

Playing now takes up a large part of his waking time. As he plays with things he learns how to manage and coordinate his body parts. He still shouldn't have too many toys at any one time. Keep them simple and the type that he can manipulate and use in his learning of muscular control.

As his finger control improves, give him a big spoon, a plastic can, a large pot, or blocks. (Look back to "Exercise and Play," in *The Third Month* and in *The Fourth Month*, for more about toys.)

Be sure that you plan your time so that you can play with him for brief periods. As you become more of a person to your baby you see that he responds to your clowning. You never realize how funny you really can be until you hear his chuckle and see him grin at your antics—and they don't have to be much. A funny sound, your marching fingers across the floor and up his leg, a breezy tune, just your laugh, any of these get a response. But don't expect it every time—and not time after time. He may just watch you very soberly and not be amused at all. Don't be discouraged—no one is funny all the time.

This may be a good time to start a deliberate peek-a-boo routine. You need to help your baby to understand that things—and people—can disappear and then reappear. You can start this as a game, having a toy or your own face appearing and disappearing behind a chair, a door, or a blanket. When he is playing in his room, tap on the door and pop into the doorway . . . when he looks, pull back . . . tap again and reappear. Get the idea started that you are there—go away—then come back.

AWARENESS AND SOCIAL RESPONSE

Your baby is increasing his ability to recognize differences among people, to differentiate among members of the family. He is demonstrating more awareness of himself as an individual, too, as he separates out other individuals. He will reach out and touch his image in the mirror if you hold him close enough to attract his attention. He smiles in response to his image, but he may not look at any other figure in the mirror.

In previous months your baby discovered his hands and

feet. Now he is exploring his other body parts. Some parents are disturbed when their baby finds his genitals. This is just part of his finding out about himself. He knows nothing about the social taboos about this sort of thing. You can diaper him to block this exploration process if you want—but no grabbing his hand away, no shaming, "no-no," slapping, spanking, or other signs of disapproval. You only confuse him. At this age, he doesn't know what you are talking about. Later you can do your education about what the differences are between private and public behavior—but certainly not at this time or in this way. Your attitude will be important. Treat it in the way I have suggested for thumb-sucking—as a natural event. Put his diaper on and protect him from busybodies who feel this is some of his original sin sticking out.

Thumb-sucking from now on can be considered a comforter as well as a source of exploration. You will see your baby use it when he is tired or frustrated.

He may like noise, a sudden appearance or movement—but not in big doses or in strange places. He is intrigued by new things—as long as they don't come at him too hard. He may show some fright at doorbells, sounds on TV and radio, the flushing of the toilet, the vacuum cleaner, or other usual household noises. If you treat these as normal events, he will come to accept them matter-of-factly after a while. Don't push the frightening thing at him.

His uneasiness with strangers may well be increasing too.

ORAL COMMUNICATION

He tries out many sounds as the basis for his learning to talk. He makes sounds when he notices the readying process for going outdoors or to bed. He babbles and squeals when he is trying to be friendly or just talking to himself. He stops all this to look—to stare—and then to cry—if you are a stranger. He talks happily to a toy. On the other hand, if he has been busy getting control of his trunk and hands, he may not be doing too much inventing in this department.

He listens to his own talk now. He may enthusiastically try the same sound for several days—you may think continuously—and then drop it for something else. But he is perfecting his equipment and his control. He has been trying quite a few mouth exercises in these past months—like blowing bubbles when you are trying to feed him. Now he makes vowel sounds in series, like "ah-ah-ah" or "oh-oh-oh." These developed out of the gurgling, growling high squeals of not too long ago. He still does these, but his babbling now hits one of these vowel sounds and starts him off repeating it. This is lallation—repeating the same sound in polysyllables. His babbling, squealing, and vowel repeating get some added dissyllables. By now he has added consonants d, t, n, w to his vowel talk, but he is not easily persuaded to repeat any sound for you. Imitation is not his thing at this time. He is more concerned with his own world, although he may respond to your gestures and voice.

When he cries, it is often a "mum-mum-mum" sound. These sounds may sometimes sound like definite words, but he doesn't know it. He may also be copying voice tones. Single-syllable sounds like "ba," "ka," and "da" are heard. As he has experimented with his voice production in these last months he has gradually brought his voice forward in his mouth. These were vowel sounds as he used the middle of his throat. Now his tongue or palate is involved in making "da-da-da" sounds.

IMMUNIZATIONS

By this time your baby will have had immunizations for whooping cough, diphtheria, tetanus, poliomyelitis. These can be caught up with now if they have been missed.

I hope you are not a parent who has neglected to have these preventive measures taken—whether out of ignorance, religious scruples, or procrastination. You wouldn't sit calmly by while your child played with a burning match or started to swallow poison, or ran out in front of a car. Yet there are many conscientious parents who neglect to have their children immunized against diseases that can weaken, cripple, or kill. Perhaps you believe that all those shots aren't really needed, or you don't want your child to be hurt, or you think those diseases aren't present anymore, or are just "ordinary childhood diseases." If so, I hope you will change your tactics and get protection for your child

BABY-CARE ROUTINES

BATH TIME

You may be using a full-size bathtub by now and finding it hard on your knees. If you're using the family tub, put a mat or towel on the bottom so he won't slip. He will do very well on his abdomen in a few inches of water. He splashes with great enthusiasm with both hands and feet. Nothing is safe near him. Keep him occupied while you go at the cleaning-up process. Approach him from the rear with a washcloth, washing from behind.

19.

The

Eighth Month

This month has its pleasant aspects in spite of your baby's continual activity. He is so responsive—so delighted at so many things. You don't feel so foolish now when you talk and make with the funny faces—you have an audience. He is a good playmate if you don't tire him out too much. He is confusing, too, since he can so quickly shift to tears of frustration as he tries to do, but is not ready for, a new skill.

WEIGHT

Ranges:	Boys 15.8–23.2 lbs.	Average 18.9 lbs.
	Girls 14.3–22.8 lbs.	Average 18.2 lbs.

HEIGHT

Ranges:	Boys 26.0–29.1 in.	Average 27.4 in.
	Girls 25.1–28.5 in.	Average 27.0 in.

MOTOR DEVELOPMENT

During these past months I have been describing your baby's developing use of his big muscles. He has been learning to hold up his head, turn, roll, and, in general, gain control over these sets of big muscles. Now he shifts some of his emphasis to learning control over the small muscles, particularly of his hands. He has eye muscle control, but it must be coordinated with his more skilled hand performance.

REFLEXES

About the only easily visible reflex action you will still see is his neck-righting reflex. He continues to show some hand response when he turns his hand upward or downward, depending on which side of the palm you stroke. He also continues to grope toward your stroking finger.

LYING, SITTING, STANDING, AND GETTING ABOUT

Although he can raise his head and hold it up quite well when he is on his back, he won't do it very often. Why? Well, he just isn't on his back very often anymore. He is sometimes content for a short time to play with a toy while he's on his back, but very soon he rolls over and gets active again.

On his abdomen he continues to move very actively, pivoting about. He may cross one arm over the other to make a circling swing, or he may not be up to this yet. The one thing you can depend on is that he will move.

It is in his sitting ability that you see the greatest development. Your average baby is a full-blown sitter now, with a straight back holding him erect if he is on a hard surface. (See plate 19H.) His trunk-muscle control is better, so that he may be able to lean forward to reach for something and come back up without falling over. Or he may just sit erect and suck his finger while he looks around, holding a toy in his hand. Your more active baby may even get so confident that he shifts from sitting onto his abdomen with-

out too much flopping about. (See plate 26.) This shows
how far he has come in coordinating his trunk control with
his arm and leg control. He may also be able to get from
these positions back to his sitting position.

His rolling is by now definitely a more coordinated
whole-body exercise. He may use a series of roll-overs as
his way to get about.

When you give him your fingers to pull up, there is no
more of the heavy-bottomed, weak-kneed coming up to a
stand. He comes up in a fairly smooth, continuous motion,
with his legs pushed out straight. If he comes up with a
half-bent knee, he pushes it out straight as he gets upright.
This is an active process on his part now, and not just your
doing. He stands fairly straight, but not quite in a truly two-
legged posture as yet. Your average baby is doing a fairly
good job on his own of pulling himself up, holding onto
his crib or playpen sides, or onto furniture.

He steps out a little, particularly if you can get him to
hold some of his own weight on his legs. (See plate 14F.)
This is walking of a sort. In another month he will try more
definitely to stand straight and step out. You may have an
early starter who has been stepping out since six months,
but the average fellow doesn't do this for another month.

Many babies are getting about on all fours in some
fashion. Most will be doing so by another month.

HANDS

Now when your young fellow sees something, he reaches
out and grasps it easily. Up to this time he reached with an
unsteady, partially bent arm, with his fingers spread out
and up to grab at something with his full hand. Now his
arm is extended and quite steady. (See plate 22M.) He
holds his hand with his palm turned in for the first time.
With this new position, he is ready to use his thumb and
finger in a pincherlike grasp. (See plate 21L.) This is a big
step forward. He picks up and handles large toys quite
easily. He pulls the toy strongly to him if he can reach it.
He is also ready to try with smaller things, using his thumb-
finger grasp. He tries repeatedly to reach a toy that is out
of his reach. He is able to hold an object in each hand
without losing them for a fairly long period of time. He
may prefer one toy at a time, but he can handle two—

maybe to discard one in preference for the other. He now can make a deliberate choice. He has started to use his thumb and forefinger together! This grasping develops progressively from his fifth finger step by step to his index finger, until he uses all his fingers. He still tries to pick up any small object by raking it to him with his thumb and second and third fingers without much arm movement, but this will gradually change.

Eyes and Other Sense Organs

He has a mature macula now, which gives him accurate central vision. He could distinguish forms and color differences at birth, but this ability is now refined with his matured vision. He can spot a toy or object across the room. He may be able to get to it if he is learning his lessons well enough to use his brand of crawling. He has the ability to see and recognize an object, control his body muscles, and go to something. This intricate association between eye, mind, and hand will be seen more and more in your baby. As he matures he will increasingly use his hand as an extension of his brain, not only to identify but to create. The intimate relationship between hand and eye is extremely important in all this.

TEETH

At this eight-month level your baby may have no teeth—or six teeth. I talked about teeth at four months to give you an idea of what his dental development will be like.

The diet I have discussed each month under "Eating" supplies good nutrition as a background for good teeth. Sweets have not been included. In this way you can help to avoid dental cares and promote good dental health in your baby. Although his bite and type of jawline is determined largely by his heredity, you can try to guarantee good teeth by what you feed him. Tooth-brushing is in the future. The fluoride in his vitamin drops or water supply help give good tooth enamel and health.

EATING

Now you have arrived at another point of change. If you have been coarsening his foods as recommended, he has gone from a smooth, homogenized mixture to separate foods at four months, to mashed at six months, and coarser foods between six-eight months so that he may be ready for diced table foods this month. Babies are quite different about this, so your baby may not be ready. Perhaps you aren't quite ready yourself to have him grow up this way. As I have said so many times, try to look at your baby to find out what he is ready for and can do, then move with him.

SCHEDULE. Continue his three-meal schedule with meals 5½ to 6 hours apart, adjusted to the family requirements.

CEREAL (BREAD). Continue infant cereal for the morning meal but in addition, he may be able to use part of a slice of toast or zwieback for practice. At one meal the cereal substitute group, described last month, may be a replacement. Continue two portions a day of the cereal. Don't count on much toast being eaten. The cold or prepared fortified cereals that come in small pieces are good finger food as his pincher control comes into use. Avoid crackers or crumbly food.

MEAT—EGG. As before, try to present the meat—egg foods first at meals. If any seconds are needed, use the foods from this group. Include them in each meal and make every effort to choose a variety. Your choices will broaden now and in these months ahead as he is able to take and handle coarser food.

FRUIT. This month you will be able to give banana or any of his cooked fruits chopped, diced, or cubed. They are well-liked foods and good finger-feeding items. If your baby is an early self-feeder, he may do well with almost any fruit, cooked or raw. (See *The Ninth Month* for new fruit additions.)

MILK–MILK SOLIDS–CHEESE. Keep up your efforts to use milk solids in abundance in his foods so that he gets his portions without filling up on liquids. Cheese is a particularly good snack food as he begins to handle his food.

VEGETABLE (DARK-GREEN, DEEP-YELLOW). Just to remind you how wide a choice you have in this group, have you offered your baby greens other than spinach? Has he been exposed to the taste of vegetables other than the standard carrots, peas, and green beans? If you haven't done so yet, think now about bringing in new ones like broccoli, cabbage, green pepper, onions, and other kinds of greens. Don't forget that in the vegetable group are some Vitamin C-containing foods like broccoli, dark-green leafy vegetables, cabbage, green pepper, asparagus, and peas. For the most part, use the foods cooked. You may prepare your vegetables by quick boiling or baking. They keep their flavor and nutrients better if peeling or cutting is done just before cooking. Cook all vegetables for as short a time as possible. Drop into boiling water and cover. Small pieces will cook quickly. The vegetable is done when the fork goes through the pieces easily, but before they have lost shape or firmness.

Some of the vegetables may be offered raw now if your baby is handling pieces nicely and doing some chewing. If not, wait a little longer. Use a portion of one of the other vegetables as a substitute for the dark-green, deep-yellow group now and then to give your baby more taste-texture experience.

FAT–OIL. No great variation is possible at this age in this group. Continue one portion of the fats–oils in each meal, using it wherever it fits in best for mixing.

DESSERT. Perhaps a combination fruit-dessert portion is best. A solid custard with a high proportion of egg–milk, eggnog, or milk pudding are far better than a high-sugar type like iced cake or a piece of candy. But always treat dessert as dessert, something offered at the end of the meal. If he hasn't taken his main course, don't serve dessert.

BETWEEN MEALS. Between-meal snacks at this time should

consist of juice, at least one portion of the Vitamin-C type, not crackers or bread. If he is eating well, you can give a high-protein snack like cheese.

VITAMINS. Continue his regular vitamin supplement in his feeding.

Cup-Feeding

His performance with the cup is improving, but don't trust him. When he is finished, he will drop the cup or push it away. The remainder goes on the floor or walls. You have to watch that he doesn't sit there blowing bubbles in his milk.

Blowing food or squirting it back out may be a maneuver you laughed at when he was younger. You won't laugh now! He can spray everything within a four- to six-foot radius. Don't go along with this. Stop his feeding immediately and let him go until his next meal. Let him know by your tone of voice that he is misbehaving. Mean, you say? Not at all! He needs to know limits, even at this age. You don't spank him for this. You do use his hunger to show him what results his action produces.

Finger-Feeding

If he shows much desire to pick up food pieces, try some of the dry cereals that he can use his fingers on. You can also give him zwieback, soft finger-foods, or a bone to chew on. He may even make a good effort to get his fingers into his meal and up to his mouth on his own. Encourage this as you can. It can be very messy, so be prepared. Don't just turn him loose with his full plate and expect anything like eating to happen. The whole thing goes on the floor. Put just a few pieces down on his high-chair tray. As they disappear, add more. If they don't go down, move in and finish up the feeding.

Even if your baby is feeding himself nicely with his fingers your presence is still needed, and not just as catcher for your young pitcher. You don't need to hover. Be busy nearby, ready to add more food or make a shift in foods.

Talking pleasantly and responding to his jabbering are valuable reassurances to him.

But this may all be in the future, since you may have a young man who makes no effort to help himself yet except to open his mouth like a bird when the spoon approaches. Or you may have to spend what seems like an endless time slipping spoonfuls in while he concentrates on the mess he has made on his high-chair tray. Don't let this last too long. Stop and let him get hungry for the next meal. But do keep it pleasant. He has done no wrong except to be not very hungry and eight months old.

CONSISTENCY OF FOODS

If you have been gradually coarsening your baby's foods as recommended, he should be ready for cubed, diced, or chopped table foods. If you are using junior foods (chopped) you won't have to mash them any longer. You can give him any of the foods from your adult meals. You will find that the longer you delay introducing coarser foods the harder it is for your baby to accept the change, especially if you wait until he is a year or more. If you give him coarser food too late, he will take it in his mouth, roll it around, and finally, after an unreasonably long time of chewing it and getting the juice out, shove out several mouthfuls with his tongue. The adult who has trouble swallowing a pill can sympathize with this kind of late starter. A mother who feels sorry for her baby when he has to take that coarser stuff . . . and puts off making the gradual shift . . . does her child no service and creates problems for herself and her child.

You will see a great deal more chewing or gumming or jaw-motion in his eating now. He controls food in his mouth quite specifically and accurately. Now you have prepared the stage for his finger-feeding, which he may start this month or not for a time yet.

APPETITE

You are heading into another period of lessened or more erratic appetite. You saw one such period at the third or fourth month. Be ready to approach this new appetite change in the same fashion. Broaden his diet in all food groups. If there are to be second helpings, protein is first choice. If there is refusal, don't argue. Stop the meal there, and offer a cup of juice. Wait until his next meal to feed him. Don't give milk to substitute for his meal.

HIGH CHAIR

If you have not put him there earlier, he must be in his own high chair now. Although he is more impatient now when he has to wait, his impatience can be eased by a toy or distraction of some kind. Try to have his food ready when you put him in his chair.

When it does not interfere with his sleeping schedule, you may want to bring him to the table for dessert, but keep him elsewhere for the rest of your adult meal-time. Don't make problems for yourself and him by feeding him from your plate or with tidbits from the table. Keep his meal-time a definite event with clear limits for his behavior. Don't let him become a table-beggar or a dining-room bandit. You will be sorry later to have started this now.

BOWEL AND BLADDER FUNCTIONS

Your baby may be having a single daily bowel movement more consistently by the end of this month. But many babies may have several loose movements a day.

In spite of my advice against regularly using waterproof pants, you have probably done so. This may produce an irritated diaper area, which often results in an unhappy baby, particularly during the night hours. Check whether this may be the cause of a restless night's sleep.

SLEEPING

The patterns of last month are much the same for this one. If you have followed my suggestions thus far, the bottle as a source of food is a thing of the past, and so is the night bottle used as a pacifier. If you are in this pocket of trouble, offer only a bottle of water for a few nights—then an empty bottle for a few more nights—then let the bottle disappear altogether.

He may be trying to cut out his afternoon nap now because he is so busy doing things. But he still needs the two-nap routine. Try to keep it going.

EXERCISE AND PLAY

In his play he continues to enlarge his interest and activity. If you keep in mind how much more he wants to practice with his hands now, you will furnish him with toys he can grasp and get a grip on. (Look back to "Exercise and Play" in *The Third Month, The Fourth Month,* and *The Seventh Month* for suggestions on toys.)

His playing at simple games like peek-a-boo and bye-bye continues to help in his later understanding of coming and going. He may sometimes wave, pat, or hide on request. He also may show more signs of the dramatic. He knows how to act when he is center stage and has an audience. And can he laugh! Not only a show-off laugh but a good chuckling belly laugh.

But he still needs the chance to play on his own, both indoors and outdoors. You need to appear at intervals for short play times with him, but don't try to entertain him or keep him busy all the time. If you have been doing this, you will find your young man demanding your constant presence now. In fact, he can get to be quite a whiner or nagger. Also, he will depend on you to set the play pattern rather than discovering his own.

AWARENESS AND SOCIAL RESPONSE

He is coming into a period when he really gets himself somewhat out of step. You have probably noticed how much more unhappiness your baby seems to show now. He is trying so hard to find out so much that he gets ahead of his abilities. He has a need to succeed at any task he sets for himself. If he can't do it immediately, he is frustrated. This gets worse until he is able to get up on his two legs and walk. You can't help him much. The more you try to help or pacify him the more fussing you get back. His tears and his laughter are very close together—and he may drive you to the point where yours are, too. You may have a youngster who gets himself into a real rage, almost to the point of losing all control.

You may have noticed before this that your baby is showing some signs of rhythmic activity, which he uses to relax with. Thumb-sucking has been the commonest, but now that he is getting more able in his body control you may see ear-pulling, hair-twisting, head-rolling, or thumb-sucking while holding onto a favorite blanket or toy. During the day he is usually too busy to do much of this until he gets tired or bored. (Look back to the section on "Rhythmic Patterns.")

If he has had adequate social stimulation with sufficient —not excessive—physical handling, he will be moving along into an increasing awareness of people and things. He continues to develop the ability to distinguish the familiar from the unfamiliar. He pulls away from strange faces, strange voices, strange situations or places. If he has to pull away to avoid such a contact, he will often cry as well. Although such awareness of and reaction to differences has been called eight-month anxiety, your baby may have been recognizing such differences for several months.

He shows more reaching out to people even if he turns around and pushes them away in protest. This is all part of the business of learning to get along with people.

ORAL COMMUNICATION

He cries longer at one time and with greater emotion. His crying sounds give you more of an idea of how he really feels. He selects some special sounds that he uses to express his feelings. The violence of his movements is no longer a safe indicator to the violence or meaning of his crying. He can cry now while lying still.

His speech develops gradually from months of listening and months of voice play. He will have an easier time sorting out his brothers' and sisters' words, since children's speech is quite repetitious. They just use fewer words than adults. So try to talk to him in simple words and repeat some of them often, trying to associate the word to an object. But don't try to get him to repeat it after you at this point in his life. He doesn't have to understand what is said yet. He does need to find out that talking is something that people do. Each child handles this matter of speech a little differently. Your baby may not try to repeat a word until he knows its meaning and associates it with something he knows or understands. Or he may repeat sounds in a parrot-like fashion, without having any idea of their meaning. The latter child is the one who learns well by hearing, while the former may have what is called visual memory—he learns by seeing.

His early sounds were mainly vowels to which he has recently added consonant sounds which he practices. They appear in his babbling as single-consonant sounds like "da," "ba," "ka," "ma," "ga." When he puts together consonant and vowel combinations he may repeat one over and over. His sound-making moves outward from his mid-mouth with increased tongue-tip activity to the use of his lips so that he can make the "mmm" sounds. This is the reason "da-da" (tongue and palate) is said before "ma-ma" (lip control). Sometimes his word sounds resemble words. He won't know what he has said, though. He may put two syllables together like "mama," "dada," or "baba," but they don't mean any specific person. He doesn't do it in response to the adults around him. His babbling shows pitch and inflection change. He sometimes combines sounds with gestures. He seems to simulate a variety of animal sounds. Each of these can become imaginative play if mother picks up and makes the sound. He imitates it. This give-and-take simulation is another method by which he learns speech. He imitates clucking or "raspberry" noises.

He may understand some words or word sounds, especially the ones you use most often and use with gestures, like "no-no." He also knows when you are displeased by the tone of your voice.

This leads into the matter of discipline. Did you ever stop to think how the word "no" gets so ingrained in your youngster's vocabulary? You don't see it yet, but you are now starting this pattern. You say "no" so often to everything he wants to do. Why don't you try substituting something else—or distracting him to some other area of action? Your training is ahead as far as strict restrictions are concerned. But begin to think about your approach and method. In fact, why don't you be the one to set the pattern for your child? Give him a chance to feel secure and happy because he is firmly, consistently, and cheerfully led and kept out of trouble in a mutually respectful, courteous, helpful relationship with you. How much happier he will be than if you try to play a series of games with him in which you let him be the leader. You let him do the things that get him into difficulty, never stepping in to direct him until he *is* in difficulty. Then you blame or scold him, feeling that you are a very abused, long-suffering mother who has a problem child on your hands. (Look ahead to the section on *Discipline* for more on ways to direct your baby.)

IMMUNIZATIONS

As I have stressed, your baby should have had the series for diphtheria, tetanus, whooping cough, and polio. If not, get them completed as soon as possible! Your baby is important enough to need them.

BABY-CARE ROUTINES

BATH TIME

You should have him in the big tub by now. He is too active for the small tub. Make certain the hot-water faucet can't be accidentally turned on. Put in some water toys for play time—and scrub as you can.

He may be too lively by now for his bath table. You may have to shift to a bed or larger table for dressing and diaper changing.

CLOTHING

Be sure that his indoor clothes are suitable for crawling. His T-shirt, diaper, and overall combination is still good, but he scrapes and pushes with his feet so much that you may definitely have to use some form of food covering. You may find you need a somewhat thicker heavy-duty overall or coverall suit to protect his legs, especially his knees. Long-sleeved shirts or sweaters may be a help too. Unless your floors are cleaner than most, be prepared to launder a lot.

20.

The
Ninth Month

Your baby is becoming angry and difficult to please. He is reacting to the pressure of his development by being completely frustrated—which he takes out on you or anyone in the vicinity. A little simple encouragement with some patience is all you can really give him. Don't go overboard trying to keep him amused. You won't be able to do it.

WEIGHT

Ranges: Boys 16.6–24.4 lbs. Average 20.0 lbs.
    Girls 15.1–24.2 lbs. Average 19.2 lbs.

HEIGHT

Ranges: Boys 26.6–29.9 in. Average 28.0 in.
    Girls 25.7–29.2 in. Average 27.6 in.

This is a gain of two inches for boys in three months and 1½ to 2 inches for girls.

MOTOR DEVELOPMENT

At nine months your baby shows a definite urge to get
from all fours to two feet. He wants this so intensely that he
may be most annoying to his family. He doesn't always
have sense enough to know when to quit and sit. You should
watch this and set limits for him. If you have an efficient
mover on all-fours he may not bother you with a continual
demand to be on his feet, although he can be just as much
in your hair in other ways.

REFLEXES

The primitive reflexes of the early months are covered
now by his increasing control of his own body actions.

LYING, SITTING, STANDING, AND GETTING ABOUT

It's getting increasingly difficult to keep him on his back,
even for the short time it takes to change his diaper. Even
on his abdomen you won't have much better luck. He wants
to get perpendicular—none of this lying-down stuff for him.

His rolling is now often a very smooth performance.
When he rolls over he is more aware of what he is trying to
accomplish. He can still roll right off something, though.

By now, most babies get to a sitting position on their own
and are able to sit alone very easily, securely, and steadily
on a hard surface for ten minutes or more. (See plate 19J.)
Instead of leaning forward when you sit him down he comes
straight up on his own. He can lean forward to reach something and pull himself easily back to an upright position. He
can't lean sideways and come back up as yet. He can flop
down from sitting to his front or to an all-fours position.

Most babies will shift from crawling, that is, propelling
themselves on their stomachs, to do some creeping on all
fours at this time. (See plate 17J.) There are almost as
many ways to move about as there are babies doing it. The
baby's arms may carry most of his weight, or he may push
about on his fat stomach with his legs while he uses his
hands to hold or reach for something. A more active fellow
will be up on his hands and knees with his stomach well off

the floor—he creeps. He may be up on hands and feet with his bottom high in the air—he crab walks. You may find that he can do the same job of getting about by sitting on his bottom and pushing with his feet. Creeping gives him splendid practice for the development of his shoulder girdle, trunk, arm, leg, and neck muscles. Encourage the ordinary methods of creeping. Discourage any activity that uses one foot or arm more than the other.

Your baby may have pulled himself up at six months, but most babies can do it by the end of this month. The slow performer won't pull himself up alone for another month or more. Some of this depends upon his sitting ability and his desire to move to the upright. Like most babies at this age your baby is able to stand with help. (See plate 20J). His pulling up to standing helps you to see this. He may be quite good at it if he has practiced over this past month. Some won't do this for another month. During this month some babies already will let go and stand alone briefly quite well. Most babies are able to stand hanging on. The baby's first efforts are usually a struggle from a sitting position to all fours when he pulls himself up to his knees. He clings to the bars of his playpen and tries and tries—until he finally struggles up on his feet. He needs both hands to hang on with as he holds up his whole weight. He leans forward to manage it. Some babies stand on tiptoe. He has to have something firm to hang onto, and his crib side bars or playpen bars are fine for this. When he finally does it he gives you that big grin of triumph. "I made it!" He's a success. This may not come for another month, but you will see his struggles now as he learns how to do it. If you help him—as he asks repeatedly—he will stand where you put him. This is all right as a beginning, but don't keep it up, or he won't learn too much, except to expect help from you.

Your nine-month-old baby steps along pretty well with your help. He may have been doing this for the past two or three months—or maybe he won't be ready to until he is a year old. When he hangs on or stands, he does a stepping or stamping that he will later convert into walking. Sometimes, a baby will step right out on his own after a few steps into his first real walking. Usually, as he hangs on he will put one foot in front of the other. Each step is an individual effort.

Your baby may be one who is climbing before he can do much more than stand. Just make certain this is done under supervision.

HANDS

Last month you saw some thumb-and-forefinger grasping. Most babies will be doing this quite well by another month. This period seems to be a hang-on-to stage for him that limits to some extent what he can do with his hands. He is able to pick up small toys or objects at the end of his fingers and thumb quite efficiently. There is a space between the object and his palm as he holds it with his thumb and second and third fingertips. He uses his index finger as a poker or pointer finger. He uses it to touch something, poke it, push it, and explore it. This shows his use of different fingers for different things. His hand work is done with less whole-arm movement.

He continues to perfect his ability to handle two or more separate objects. He may try to put one object inside another, like dropping a block into a cup—then he tries to poke with his finger and fish it out. He will hit a toy in front of him with some object he holds in his hand. If you give him two objects at once he will grasp one, hold it, and then grab the other one. If you offer him a toy when he has both hands filled, he will drop one toy in order to get the third one. He is recognizing some relationship between things. When he drops a toy he will search for it. He is getting the idea of the near and far of things around him. (See plate 210.) He may hang onto a crayon or pencil, but he manages nothing but a mess with it. He may be quite interested in a scribbling demonstration on your part.

EYES AND OTHER SENSE ORGANS

Going along with his increasing finger ability is his coordination wih his eyes. By this age your baby is starting to get a useful perception of depth—three-dimensional—for the placing of things. You see this in his hand placement when he reaches for something. He doesn't grope for a toy —he places his hand on it. This is also due to better muscle control, but his eyes direct the action. This depth perception will become more acute in these weeks ahead. His macula matured last month. Now his depth perception has started. His control of his eyes is good in all directions.

His hearing is acute. He locates voices and sounds quite quickly and accurately. He may move rhythmically to music, sometimes with his whole body, sometimes with his head and arms. This may divert him when he is unhappy.

All of his senses show his general nervous-system development. You see this every day in what he does and how he responds to you and others.

TEETH

Most babies will have at least two teeth by now or by next month. Some will already have six.

EATING

By now your baby may be quite well along into finger-feeding, or his eating may be quite restricted, so that he demands your participation to shovel it in. Whichever way, check yourself to see that you are standing by to aid, not standing in the way.

MENU COMMENTS

Keep some regularity to his meal schedule, which must be related to the family schedule. Five-and-a-half to 6-hour intervals are advisable.

CEREAL–BREAD. His morning cereal is still the prepared infant cereal. For most babies, adult-type cold dry cereals are still finger practice foods. Cereal substitute foods may be used at one meal. He will do better with his other foods if you give the toast at the end of the meal as a taper-off event, like a dessert. Toast will become a more important substitute in these next months. Look back to p. 329 for the list of portions in this group.

MEAT–EGG. As your baby gains finger-feeding skill, I want to emphasize again that you should offer this group first.

You may find that he wants the more easily chewed and swallowed items. Textures and tastes should be varied to give an experience with the whole spectrum of meats. You may have to increase your own use of different meats. Don't neglect the high-value organ-tissue meats like liver, heart, tongue, which are often less expensive. With his finger-feeding, frankfurters, luncheon meat, pre-cooked meats, poultry, ground meat, are all helpful items. Look back to p. 331 for the list of portions in this group.

FRUIT. This month you will be giving more attention to the fruit group. Much will depend upon your baby and his ability to take food chopped, diced, or cubed. With the baby who has good hand skill you can start to use a wide variety of fruits, some uncooked. If he doesn't show this readiness you will have to wait. As you can, offer at least one portion of fruit during each day from the Vitamin C-containing group such as citrus fruit, tomato, or melon. In these next months add berries, cantaloupe, melon, dates, figs, grapes, raisins, grapefruit, mango, orange, papaya and nectarine, tangerine, and tomato to his previous list of prepared fruits. If there is a definite history of food allergy in the family, check with your pediatrician before giving the fruit group uncooked or fresh.

MILK—MILK SOLIDS—CHEESE. Cottage cheese, evaporated milk, and dry skim milk mixed in his foods take care of this milk group. Don't flavor his drinking milk to bribe him to drink it. This just says to him that it isn't very good stuff as it is, so you have to disguise it. He isn't fooled. You won't get any more milk down but you will have developed a taste for a sweet and flavored preparation. Just offer him one to two ounces in his cup after his solids if he has eaten well.

VEGETABLE. Your baby's increasing skills enable you to use more raw vegetables and more diced or chopped table-food-type cooked vegetables. Check back to last month on cooking suggestions. A green salad may be a little ahead of him.

BETWEEN MEALS. Snack time can be another time to encourage finger-feeding with cheese, soft meat, or fruit. However, his snack should be fruit juice if he isn't eating his meals well.

VITAMINS. Continue multiple-vitamins supplement in his food as part of his diet.

FINGER-FEEDING

His finger-feeding continues to improve if you give him a chance and aren't too squeamish about messes. How can you expect him to be neat and tidy when half the experience of feeding himself is in the feeling and tasting? He wants to test everything with his hands and mouth as well as look at it. He is going to chew on everything anyhow, so take advantage of it. Give him food to chew on. Give him cubed, diced, or chopped items you have available from your table. There should be enough firmness to the food so that he is encouraged to chew. After a trial period give him his regular foods in small pieces.

Notice that I talked only about fingers for food. A spoon may be a fascinating instrument to him, but this doesn't mean he is ready to use it for feeding himself. Let him learn to get good finger control and cup control first. Let him have a spoon to play with at some other time.

For some babies, this month may see the beginnings of the first real success in their efforts to feed themselves. Your goal from now on is to help your baby as comfortably as possible into feeding independence. It won't be a smooth progression. After all, none of his progress has been. Each fellow does it in his own fashion. Because of this, it may be another month or more before your baby really shows any enthusiasm for so much responsibility.

CUP-FEEDING

He is growing more daring with his cup. He is probably hanging onto it himself. Don't put very much in it at a time. Then you won't have so much to mop up. Don't trust him though. When he is done, he lets go.

APPETITE

His first six months was a period of very rapid growth with a large ever-increasing appetite. Now in this second six months his growth will be slower. He may want less food and become more finicky about it. When he isn't hungry try to be agreeable about it. Just let him go with juice to fill up on, not milk. He may fool you into letting him drink milk and refuse food. It is still not an adequate substitute, and not to be encouraged.

There is a notion that a child is able to select his own foods instinctively and wisely. This is based on a study done forty years ago when nutritional guidelines were very much different from what they are today. You are allowing a certain amount of choice but you are the parent. You must be the wise one to set up the pattern of his meal so that he has a choice among the basic protein foods. Don't give him the responsibility of choosing his own diet. He lacks the knowledge, instinctive or otherwise. He does have the opportunity of choice within the food groups. Don't give him an area of choice beyond this.

BOWEL AND BLADDER FUNCTIONS

You may find your youngster producing more stools daily now than he has been. This may tie in with his greater general activity or with changes in eating pattern.

SLEEPING

His total sleep time has been lessening. He is more interested in doing than in sleeping. Try to keep two nap—or rest—periods going. He—and you—need them.

Night waking is very common now. (Look back to "Sleeping" in *The Sixth Month* for suggestions on how to handle this.)

EXERCISE AND PLAY

As your youngster becomes more coordinated in his muscular control you will find yourself participating in more active play with him. But a little of this goes a long way with some babies. Watch for signs of fatigue or fearfulness. Be careful about lifting and holding him at this age. When you lift him, don't pull him up by his arms. You will protect him best by grasping his trunk under his arms and then lifting. Don't hold him by his hands and swing him about unless he is ready for it. This puts too much strain on the joints of his wrists, elbows, and shoulders. He has to support his full weight. A sudden twisting pull on a wrist or elbow may cause a common injury at this age. This is a dislocation of one of the bones—the radius—at the elbow.

Don't let him persuade you to give up his playpen. You will have to accept some of his complaints about almost anything you do at this age, so don't be bothered. Put his playpen where he can watch what goes on outside or in some area of the house where he can see what goes on there. Don't take him too seriously when he insists on your constant presence.

You can let him roam about on the floor with you part of the time when you are doing your housework if you're prepared to keep one eye on him while you carry out your chores. Once your child starts to move about, it is just more difficult for you to keep up with him. He is able to quickly and efficiently get into (and hopefully out of) all sorts of inconvenient and annoying places.

He will pull up on furniture, tip over wastebaskets, pull magazines off the rack and books out of the bookcases, mess up the shoes in the closet—but you must remember the old medicine you threw in the wastebasket, the sharp corner on the coffee table, the cigarette butts you tossed in the fireplace, the light cord with the loose wires.

As discussed earlier, try to avoid the "no-no" routine. By far the best approach is to distract him. Substitute something else—or pick him up and give him something else to play with in a safe spot. You can play this game of substitution for some time without once saying, "Don't," looking crossly at him, or scolding him with your voice and words. When you get tired of it, put him in his playpen or his room. Don't wait until you have to blow up at him.

AWARENESS AND SOCIAL RESPONSE

Your baby's social development has been so gradual that now you may suddenly realize he has become a person in his own right. He is placid or active, friendly or shy, fearful or fearless. Some babies seek lots of social contacts, but your baby may be a loner who is happier without too many people around. Watch for this in order to help him in either direction. Whatever type he is, he is there and he lets you know he is there. He is a busy, striving, adjusting, learning, fun-loving individual—and he is himself.

He has learned some things about other people. He knows the different signs you show in either your approval or disapproval—how you speak, how you move, how you hold him. You have to be careful here that he doesn't misinterpret your actions when they are the result of something not connected with him. Your strident voice after a recent quarrel may give him the wrong cue, just as your accepting behavior of a forbidden act when you are sleepy and tired will confuse him. You can see his hurt feelings when you scold, or his pouting when you forbid something he wants to do. You are in a continual process of socializing—teaching him lessons all persons living together must learn. This kind of lesson is never easy for either the pupil or the teacher. Your problem is to do it and still keep him relatively happy and unspoiled—which just means that he needs to get a feeling of his value while recognizing the rights of others.

He is more aware, too, of small variations in sight and sound in his surroundings. He is sensitive to what goes on around him. He is more ready to imitate what he sees, so that he is more responsive to your efforts to teach. This extends to people outside of his family, too, after his initial period of getting acquainted. He shows off and reaches out to people with a very appealing playfulness and expressiveness. He laughs and cavorts whether there is anything funny or not. He reflects the family expressions, which shows how sensitive he is to the feelings of those about him. He likes to be the center of attention.

ORAL COMMUNICATION

He has developed even more variety in his crying and babbling. His voice has a higher pitch to it—if you can believe it—and he changes the pitch up and down even more. He is using double syllables like "da-da" and "mama," but he isn't yet aware of their meaning. A few babies may recognize the association. He can give you some sounds you never heard of.

He may respond to his name. He can imitate a cough or tongue click.

As far as trying to imitate your words, if he is like most he isn't really doing too much of this yet. He may act as if he knows what "Where is the——?" and "bye-bye" signify. He strings a series of sounds together. They sound good, but you won't really be able to identify any words. As he listens to words and phrases he begins to put together words, sounds, eye recognition, and hand use. This is quite a complicated performance when you look at it. But he must know many words before he really speaks any of them.

BABY-CARE ROUTINES

BATH TIME

Your young sprout may very well recognize your whole pre-bath routine now. He may try to help you or do just the opposite. Either way it can be a noisy time for everyone involved. Give him a floating toy, a sponge, or a washcloth to keep him busy. He may even try to make rubbing motions with his washcloth or towel. He may put his hands up when he sees you coming with the washcloth.

CLOTHING

You will have continual trouble in changing his clothes. He just doesn't want to slow down or be put on his back. This may cause some friction between you. Use a voice tone and a firm grip that say you mean business.

21.

This month you are aware of your baby's developing independence—and his dependence. You may like the clinging he is doing, or it may bother you to have him drape himself about your neck and hang on for dear life the moment a strange face appears. You may enjoy his pushing you away to proudly prance about his playpen. Try to appreciate his push to explore as well as his need for reassurance.

WEIGHT

Ranges: Boys 17.2–25.4 lbs. Average 20.7 lbs.
              Girls 15.7–25.0 lbs. Average 20.0 lbs.

HEIGHT

Ranges: Boys 27.1–30.5 in. Average 28.6 in.
              Girls 26.2–29.8 in. Average 27.2 in.

MOTOR DEVELOPMENT

This period is another leap forward for your baby. Even pokey babies are moving and doing now. Your baby will show some interesting new patterns of behavior and control. If you think back, he spent his first three months getting the knack of making his eyes and mouth get together so that he had some kind of control. In his next three months he worked and worked to get the big muscles of his arms, legs, and trunk stronger and under his control. Recently he has been spending time getting his eyes and mouth and fingers to perform together under his direction. During these last three months of his first year he is going to apply all of this, so that with the help of his eyes he will improve the strength and control of his arms, legs, feet, and trunk.

LYING, SITTING, STANDING, AND GETTING ABOUT

No self-respecting ten-month-old baby takes kindly to a back position. He may give up long enough to accept lying down if he dozes off while he is on his back. But once awake—he rolls over, sits up, and stands up. He may deliberately roll over on his back to do some task, but this is just part of a step-by-step maneuver he is carrying out.

He sits alone very well for an indefinite period. He can also flip from almost any position to sitting without too much effort and with quite good control. He goes to his abdomen or all fours from sitting with definite purpose. There is no side-to-side wiggle first. His sitting is often just a temporary position before going on to something else.

At the end of this month his crawling has developed into creeping. His creeping is a rhythmical, coordinated movement of his hands and feet and arms and legs. He carries his body high off the floor, his weight suspended on his arms and legs or hands and knees. (See plate 17K.) A slow mover may be quite happy with crawling and continue to drag himself about the room on his stomach.

Your baby may like a stand-up position for as long as you and he can take it. He may continue to use his all-fours position most of the time—he has practiced enough to know that he gets places faster when he gets down on his hands and knees, even if he would prefer to move about standing up. He creeps, hitches, scoots, cruises, or uses any combination of movements to get where he wants—then he tries to pull up to stand. You may see more climbing efforts.

Last month you still may have had to help him to get up

into a standing position. Now he can pull himself up on his crib bars or playpen sides to stand on his own. At first, as he is learning this, he gets his feet twisted when he plants them down. After he finds out how to avoid the mix-up he pulls up to stand hanging on. This gives him confidence to go on to more things. He may feel so solidly planted on his two feet that he will let go with one hand briefly to manipulate something in his other hand. He may be so confident that he lets go with both hands. When he discovers he is on his own, he grabs hold again. He may let himself plop down on his bottom in a sitting position after a short time. He may stand on his tiptoes as a regular position.

He may get himself into difficulties when he tries to get down from standing. He stands there crying because he doesn't know how to let go, or is afraid to try. You unhitch him from the playpen rail to ease him down to sit. But you are scarcely out of the room when up he goes again, repeating the same cycle. Perhaps after a few times of this you will have to break into the pattern by putting him somewhere else, giving him a different toy, or playing some game with him. If you feel he has gone through this enough times and really could sit down if he had the courage, you'd better leave him alone to find his own way to get down. He may plop down or fall down, but sooner or later you will see him carefully lower himself to ease his well-padded bottom down to the floor.

Your baby may have already done definite walking with your help, or he may be trying it now when you give him your fingers to hold at his shoulder height. If he doesn't do this until a year he isn't unusual. The average fellow cruises or walks about his playpen now. He can sidestep along from one piece of furniture to another, never letting go. He can fancy it up a little and get along with just a fingertip contact to give him confidence. But this is a definite controlled effort on his part to put his feet where he wants them.

The very adventuresome baby can walk alone at this time. This usually starts as a few unsteady steps while he is hanging onto your finger. He has to combine moving forward with holding himself erect. He may be the fellow who steps right out on his tiptoes when you hold him under his arms, to put one foot in front of the other to do a type of walking. All of this may still be ahead of him since the average child walks alone sometime between eleven and fourteen months.

Hands

He has his thumb-to-finger pincher movement going well. He is now able to pick up crumb- or raisin-sized objects with his thumb and forefinger, with some help from his third finger. He plucks or grasps between the palm side of his thumb and his index finger. (See plate 21P.) When he picks up a large object it is held between his thumb and the ends of his index and third fingers, with a space between it and his palm. This is now only a hand movement. He no longer has to use his arm and shoulder to aid in it.

It is now that his index finger will come fully into its own. He uses his index-finger approach for everything. It allows him to explore ins and outs as he begins to understand that there is in-and-out depth as well as up and down.

He is able to do many things with an object. He not only can reach out and grasp it, but he shifts it about, hits the table with it, takes it in or out of a place, combines it with another object, or uses it as a social object by offering it to an adult. It is hard for him to let go. He resists any effort to take it away from him. This is the middle of his "hang on" stage. In the next few weeks he develops some ability to let go or release. His nervous system is just not mature enough to that extent yet.

He starts to use his hands in imitation. He puts his hands together to play patty-cake, waves bye-bye, imitates patting. He uncovers a hidden toy or tries to go after a dropped toy.

He will still grasp objects and bring them to his mouth as he did earlier, but you don't get the feeling that he is using his mouth as a sensing organ as he did in these past months. He uses his eyes more in handling and looking. He doesn't have to mouth an object to test it.

Eyes and Other Sense Organs

His depth perception is increasing. His universe is less flat and less simple. He watches an object that drops. He can realize what it is and may try to get to it. He is conscious of "2" as well as "1." He puts two things together. He needs two things instead of one to satisfy his impulse to combine, to bring things together when they are apart from each other. Although it's still rather vague, this awareness of two things is increasingly seen in his experimenting with play objects. He is more discriminating. He shows a very

keen interest in a small object and can very accurately get
to it with his hands, even when he has to look at it off to
one side.

TEETH

By this time your youngster has probably acquired several teeth. He may have two central incisors in his lower
jaw by now and one or two in his upper jaw.

EATING

Your baby's eating behavior now is quite astonishing. If
you compare it to his first two months you can scarcely believe it is possible for him to eat so much. Be aware of what
you have been and are trying to do. Furnish him with the
good basic building materials he needs, then leave him to
use them. But you can't force him into good nutrition any
more than you can force him in any other area. Your job is
to offer, his to grow. You can't eat for your child, although
many times parents continually try to do so. He must eat
and grow at his own speed.

MENU COMMENTS

By this time use table foods, or chopped junior foods, or
both, entirely. No more strained stuff! If your baby can
swallow the pieces, they are digested efficiently. You may
see vegetable or fruit pieces come through with his bowel
movements. This is not harmful.

CEREAL–BREAD. His morning cereal may be the prepared infant cereal or the cold dry cereal to which you add milk,
but no sugar. And note that you should never offer him the
sugar-coated varieties of dry cereal. He may enjoy feeding

himself pieces of dry cereal, but he probably won't get enough down to make an adequate portion. He isn't quite ready to do the feeding job for himself. You may give bread in place of one cereal offering now. Use enriched whole wheat or fortified white bread with margarine at the end of the lunch or dinner meal.

If your baby is doing very well in his self-feeding of his foods, this allows you to think about breads other than the whole wheat toast or prepared cereals. You can use a small muffin, a quarter of a waffle, or a pancake as cereal substitutes at lunch or dinner. Look back to *The Sixth Month* for the list of cereal substitutes you can use at one meal. Most of these are suitable substitutes now.

MEAT–EGG. Continue to give an egg at one or two meals daily. If he wants more than one egg, don't skimp. Let him have as much as he wants. Scrambled or hard-boiled may give him a better chance to use his fingers. In the meat group anything your family has as a meat course can be used. Pay some attention to the softness and size of the pieces. With his increased use of his jaws and fingers he may surprise you with what he can do when he is hungry.

FRUIT. Try some of the raw fresh fruits diced or cubed. Don't forget the dried fruits, like raisins, when you think of this fruit group. There are so many he will like as he is better able to feed himself. The Vitamin-C containing group of fresh fruits and melons are very appealing to many children.

MEAT SUBSTITUTES. Keep these in mind as replacements for one portion of the meat–egg at one meal a day. Except for peanut butter, they are more easily used mixed with other foods. Meat substitutes will be useful when he is older in making up lunch meals or stew combinations to which they can be easily added along with dry powdered skim milk. Some of them have been listed in the cereal substitute groups earlier.

> One portion = 1 ounce dried beans or peas
> = 2 tablespoons peanut butter
> = 1 ounce lentils
> = 3 ounces soybean flour

MILK–MILK SOLIDS–CHEESE. Your important milk–milk solids–cheese group must be watched now. You know your baby can't drink eight ounces of liquid milk and eat anything else. Try to include the equivalent of this (2 portions) of the milk–milk solids–cheese group in each meal. He takes this either as skim powdered milk, cottage cheese, or cheese. The cheeses are good finger foods. Continue to use evaporated milk whenever you need milk for mixing or drinking.

VEGETABLE. This group by now is often a favorite at the expense of the meat or perhaps milk–milk solids. Continue to offer new vegetables he hasn't tried. Try to keep to your dark-green–deep-yellow group as much as possible. Variety is what you are trying for. Don't be insistent if he doesn't manage more than a taste or two of something new in color and texture. Consider them fillers and not the primary items in his diet. Continue to introduce the stronger-tasting vegetables into his diet. As his finger and mouth control have improved the raw vegetables are now more than possibilities.

FAT–OIL. Continue one portion in each feeding.

DESSERT. If he eats well on his basics, offer a high-protein dessert after his night meal. Stay away from the highly sweetened foods. He doesn't need to develop a taste for them now, if ever. When you realize that a slice of chocolate layer cake is the equivalent of 450 calories, why give your small baby half of his daily calories in one inadequate food? This should explain to you my continual insistence on playing down sweets.

BETWEEN MEALS. Protein snacks like egg, meat, or cheese are the rule if he is taking his food well. If not, only juices. Your baby may prefer some juices over others but keep offering a variety. Don't encourage him to narrow down to just one or two. Let him have as much as he wants between meals, unless it is within the hour before his next meal. Give water during this interval.

VITAMINS. Continue his multiple-vitamin preparation in the drop form. He isn't quite ready for the chewable type.

FINGER-FEEDING

Your baby may be getting skillful enough so that he can really control his fingers to pick up pieces of food and carry them to his mouth. He does quite a good job. Continue to encourage him to do it when he is hungry, at the start of his meal, not at the end. Then he is only ready to play with his food. Continue to put a few bite-size pieces on his high-chair tray and to add more as he eats them.

As you watch him he gets a piece of food from his tray to his mouth. He mouths it around after feeling it well with his fingers. Then he takes it out again to put it back with the other foods to smear it around a little. Then back into his mouth it goes. This is part of his need to investigate and try everything for himself. Sometimes it is more important for him to mess and splash than to eat. Food seems to exist to be felt, to be tasted, to be tested, smeared on the face, smashed on the high-chair tray, and eventually put into the mouth, or dropped on the floor for the dog. He doesn't mind the mess, he likes it. He can't be neat. He isn't that well controlled yet. The only thing more powerful than his curiosity now is his hunger. So make use of it.

SELF-FEEDING

I hope that you haven't put off this gradual shift to chopped or diced foods and finger-feeding. If you have, you may have missed his cue. Now he may turn against coarse foods even though you decide he is ready for them. Earlier your fastidiousness or desire to keep the surroundings clean may have acted to deny him the experience he wants and needs. Now how do you suddenly untrain him to eat with his fingers? Let him practice. If messiness still upsets you, you can try to control it by letting him get good and hungry before meal time. Then he may eat more and mess less. When he starts to lag, lose interest, and play more than eat, help him to finish up.

CUP-FEEDING

His cup-feeding is quite messy because he is so determined to take over for himself. Continue to put a small amount of liquid in his cup and let him take that. Add more as long as he drinks. Stop when the fooling around starts to be all that he does. He either drinks or parts company with the cup.

SPOON-FEEDING

He's not ready yet to take this over by himself. With a full plate and a little help he may manage to load the spoon. But getting it to his mouth is a much more difficult process. On his own, he heads the spoon for his mouth but he turns it upside down on the way. It arrives at his mouth empty, which can puzzle or anger him.

APPETITE

Your baby may be showing some appetite drop now if he didn't last month or the month before. There is a good deal of difference in what a baby does about his needs now. For a while he may eat a large breakfast, practically no lunch, and a fair-sized dinner. Or perhaps lunch will be his big meal, with little eating at the other meals. This makes no difference. If he is healthy, active, and reasonably happy he will eat all the food his body needs. Many feeding problems start here when mother makes an issue of getting additional food into her baby after she feels he has had enough. If he eats lightly, say at breakfast, she anxiously gives him milk and crackers or cookies later because he has to "have something in his stomach." This is a mistake, as you will readily see if you think about it. Babies stuffed on crackers will not be hungry at lunch time. If you give him a mid-afternoon feeding of crackers and milk you will spoil his appetite for his evening meal. Before you know it, your well-trained baby has back-tracked to a six-meal-a-day schedule. And he will be eating far too much in the way of starches and milk in relation to the basic foods of meats, fruits, and vegetables he needs.

I have mentioned regularly that he should be fed in his

own dining area. Very few adult dining rooms are designed to withstand the young person learning to feed himself. If you have a tiled or hard-surfaced floor area with easily washable wall coverings you are ideally set up. Spread out a plastic sheet or newspaper if you don't have an invulnerable area. After what I have been saying about his eating habits, you can answer for yourself whether your young person should be at the adult dining table.

You can also see from what I have said that you are going to be intimately involved in his feeding process, either as umpire, catcher, or fielder. You really can't walk off and leave him to his own devices and then punish him for misbehaving when you come back to find the place a shambles. You have to be there and in the act! But this doesn't in any way suggest that you have to be a patsy to his shenanigans. Make this a reasonable affair for both of you. You know that if he is throwing food around and not eating, he isn't hungry. Take his word for it and take him out of his high chair. The meal is over until his next scheduled feeding.

SLEEPING

You may be concerned because you think he needs more sleep, since he is so active. If he has a regular sleep time and he is left alone, he will sleep as much as he needs. In the morning, if he is changed, given a drink of water, and left alone, he may play happily for some time.

Nap time is now about two and a half hours. Naps continue to be a long morning one with a short afternoon sleep period. There is a good deal more play involved during his nap periods than there has been before. This playing is usually happily carried out on his own. Afternoon nap times can be an off-and-on affair. Wakeful periods may occur at his regular nap times or in the middle of the night.

EXERCISE AND PLAY

Your baby may play contentedly with one toy for some time at this age. He is also quite determined to get at a toy

he wants. He doesn't give up easily. He may start the dropping game. He drops a toy for you to pick up. This can go
on as long as your patience holds out.

The toys that he uses now are about the same as before.
They are primarily soft, washable toys like rubber, plastic,
or wooly bright-colored balls, and knitted or cloth dolls.
He may also like spools, large beads, rattles, pots and pans,
blocks. He likes to pile things together. (Look back to "Exercise and Play" in earlier months for more about toys.)

His play with other children in the family will depend on
several things. If your baby has been regularly played with
by his older brothers and sisters it is a natural sequence of
his growing up. You have to be sure that they play with
him safely and in a safe place. They cannot be expected to
watch him as carefully as you do. They do need to know
the rules of safety. If they are old enough they can pick him
up, help him pull himself up, and take over some simple
baby-care chores. Don't let them put anything in his mouth.
If your oldest child is under three years, companionship
leads to play as a natural result. You must be available to
supervise such play. You can't expect so young a child to
have any judgment. Stay within hearing distance all the
time. You may have to stay right in the room.

Your baby can be played with and he may make some
effort to respond, but he really can't play with another
child. He shows some interest in what another youngster is
doing and may imitate some of his movements. He is upset
if he is ignored and the other child gets the attention.

A dog is fine as a companion for your baby if it is trained
and good around children. Your baby won't understand
how to be careful with the animal, so protect it from him.
He must learn to be gentle.

AWARENESS AND SOCIAL RESPONSE

He is both dependent and independent. You are not always certain at a given moment which he is. Since he wants
to move under his own steam he won't want to be held or
cuddled—until he gets tired, bored, or hurt. Then you have
a cuddle bug who wants your entire attention to get him
back into independent shape.

He shows definite emotional responses. In addition to

smiling at and patting his own image in the mirror he looks at and pats pictures or a doll. His crying is for either physical hurt or hurt feelings. Although he can express joy as well as anger, you may be more surprised by the anger part. He scolds, he shakes his head, even throws himself in his anger.

His interest increases in playing peek-a-boo, waving bye-bye, playing pat-a-cake, and clapping his hands. He will go in a big way for imitations. This tendency to imitate is an important factor in helping your baby's future personality. Every word, every gesture, each tone he receives in his observations he records in his sensitive mind so that you see it reappear later. He repeats, but not always with proper meaning. He repeats a performance that was appreciated and laughed at, like putting milk on his tray and mixing it with the food. He likes nursery rhymes with repetition. He can anticipate the action with body movements if you have done this with him before.

Although he will play by himself for relatively long periods, he is very quick to voice his desire for shifts of activity or company. He is anxious for social contact. He is still quite shy with strangers, and seems particularly afraid of a strange voice. Mother is still more in demand than the other members of the family. He usually manages better when he is alone with one person than with several.

ORAL COMMUNICATION

He is more able and more pushy with his voice. He makes his repetitive consonant sounds. He understands many words. He can imitate if adults use the same sounds as his in his vocal play. More babies definitely comprehend "no-no" and "Dada" by now, and will respond to words such as "pat-a-cake" or "bye-bye" with gestures. "Where is Daddy?" brings a response.

Voice use is difficult to predict at this age. He has given up the growling sounds he formerly used. He may not try many sounds on his own but may get the meaning of what is said. He may be attempting to use words meaningfully. He may know names that are frequently heard in the home, such as the names of his brothers and sisters or pets.

Don't use baby talk with him. Even if his baby words

sound cute, don't repeat them. He thinks he is talking the way you talk. Don't mix him up by giving him back his inadequate word sounds.

BABY-CARE ROUTINES

BATH TIME

Your baby may be active in his cooperation when he hears the water running and sees the preparations for his bath. He may like to get up on all fours, often creeping in the water. He often creeps in the water better than he does on the floor. He may rock back and forth. He may object to face-washing. The whole bath affair often has the elements of a friendly combat. He may increasingly try to use the washcloth or to rub himself with a towel. He may demand his bath toys with loud sounds. Bath toys are fine—but never let him play with the faucets.

CLOTHING

He associates certain clothes with certain activities. His sweater or snowsuit means going outside. He acts as if he anticipates this. He may hold his arm out for a sweater, put his foot up for a sock or shoe.

22.

The
Eleventh Month

You and your baby are getting closer and closer to that first birthday. You are nearing the end of his first year—maybe the end of your patience! By this time you know him pretty well—his personality, how he behaves, what he likes, what he doesn't like, what he can do, what he can't do, how bold or shy he is, and many other little details. You know by now that he can't be forced—at least, I hope you know that by now. You won't be successful in any such effort now or later, so don't try. If he gets out of line in his behavior, try to see what he is up to. Most often he is trying to do something that answers his need to investigate or just to be in motion. You can't expect him to sit still just because you want him to. You will, however, be able to interest him in something long enough to produce some more desirable activity—more desirable to you, at least!

WEIGHT

Ranges: Boys 17.8–26.4 lbs.   Average 21.4 lbs.
            Girls 16.3–26.0 lbs.   Average 20.8 lbs.

HEIGHT

Ranges: Boys   27.6–31.0 in.   Average 29.1 in.
            Girls 26.7–30.4 in.   Average 27.7 in.

MOTOR DEVELOPMENT

He increases his progress toward his goal—two-legged walking. A few babies have already achieved this, but your young fellow may be just average. Practice sessions are still ahead for him.

His motor development at this age is a very obvious testimony to the presence of individual differences.

Perhaps you have a young fellow who is slower than cold molasses as far as his locomotion goes. He isn't even about to creep. His self-limitation doesn't bother him. He could move if he wanted to, but he doesn't want to.

Then there is the middle-of-the-road fellow, who expertly and enthusiastically gets about on all fours, although he has walked hanging on to furniture for the past two months. His motor ambitions are a bit above his immediate abilities, so that he is restless and frustrated.

Then there is the baby who is a going concern. He already has such good balance that he boldly and nimbly gets all over the house. He is a self-confident one. This kind of baby has been performing ahead of average in the motor area since the very first. He rolled over at three months, sat at five months, was creeping at six months, walked with support at seven months, stood alone at nine months, and now walks alone at eleven months.

Lying, Sitting, Standing, and Getting About

He stays less and less on his back and abdomen. By and large, he uses both front and back positions primarily for resting, sleeping, or as the starting points for many of his actions. Sitting is often just a position of rest now too.

Rolling over is now more often part of a sequence of movements to accomplish some specific goal. Some babies still roll just for the sheer pleasure of it.

Your baby pulls himself up alone now even if he is a later performer. In fact he may do very little else all day but go up and down, up and down—and he may want you to do it for him, too. A little of this is fine, but as noted earlier, you may do better to let him get the knack of doing such things himself without too much help.

Crawling is now an accomplished fact, but the way in which the baby does his creeping is still his very own. He doesn't do it just for exercise. Now he is trying to get everywhere to satisfy his curiosity. (See plate 17L.) As mentioned before, his crawling soon becomes climbing, so you must be there to protect him if he tries the stairs or anything high. If you give him a little help, he may surprise you with how well he does. This is also preparation for walking.

He has learned how to place his feet better when he stands hanging onto something. Your early performer already may have stood alone in the middle of the floor. Your average fellow is just now starting to do it, although a slow performer may put if off for another couple of months. When he stands alone, he does a balancing act with his hands out and his bottom acting as a counterbalance. He may be so good that he can come up from the floor or lower himself down without hanging onto anything.

This may be a good point to talk about walking. Your early performer may have started stepping out on his own already. Some babies are trying a few steps on their own just about now.

If you give your baby a little support he will walk with his arms up, hanging tightly to your fingers. Just a little balance may be all that he needs, so that he uses very little actual support. He has reached the point of walking.

What decides when your baby will walk? His body make-up, weight, muscle strength, eye-hand-body coordination, general rate of development, his temperament. His temperament is a definite factor. If he is timid he waits—if he is a pusher he is off and gone. You probably know his temperament by now, since he has shown it in his behavior in so many other areas as he has progressed in his development during these months.

Learning to get up on two legs and take off on your own requires many steps of learning along the way—and courage or daring. After all, it is one thing to move your feet around the room while you hang onto the furniture, and another thing to take off across that big wide floor with nothing to grab, but finally he does it.

There he stands, feet wide apart for balance, knees bent slightly, stomach stuck out to balance his stuck-out bottom, arms raised shoulder height, head in line with his back. He shifts a foot forward and lets his weight follow it so that he can free the other foot to move. He teeters along, using his arms and upper body for balance. If he falls he may be discouraged briefly. If he is really ready he is back up again shortly, while his family sits there with held breath. Will he make it? Sooner or later he does, and you can't feel any prouder than he does. You would think that no one had ever done this before—and as far as he is concerned, no one ever has.

Don't act too concerned when he does his lurching walk and falls. Too much fussing and sympathy will give him the wrong idea. He may even look at you to see if he should cry or not. Save your sympathy for the really bad falls. Don't make him fearful. Bumps and spills are all part of his learning.

An upsetting event may temporarily slow him down. Don't try to push him back into action. Let him go back to crawling or walking around chairs if he wants to. Quite soon his urge to walk makes him forget whatever bothered him.

With the start of his walking it is perhaps time again to remind you about having him play in his playpen or room unless you are with him. You will find yourself at constant cross-purposes with him otherwise. His whole urge is to be independent and explore everything on his own—and you will just have to set limits on him for his safety and your peace of mind. As you get more and more exasperated he gets more and more confused. He doesn't know why you are angry, but he hears the angry voice and knows that you are. Put him where you don't have to be continually after him for something.

SHOES

Walking brings up the question of shoes. He won't need shoes until he is getting around on his feet most of the time. If he walked entirely on carpeted floors, you could use the soft moccasin type. But since he will have to walk on hard surfaces also, get a high shoe with a fairly stiff but flexible (not semi-soft) sole, wide at the toes and straight along the inside line of the shoes. This gives protection and shock absorption. It also directs the foot. Support for the ankle and arch is not as important in a normal foot as is the protection. A shoe is also a help since it is harder for the baby to take off—a favorite occupation at this time. Shoes do not help your baby walk sooner. If the soles are slippery, the shoes may actually make it harder for him to balance on polished or slick floors. Scratch the soles or put adhesive-tape strips on the soles to prevent his slipping.

His rapid foot growth makes it necessary for you to pay close attention to shoe fit. He can outgrow a pair of shoes before you think he has even broken them in. Check him weekly for size. When you buy shoes, don't get too big a pair in order to avoid buying shoes more frequently. And don't forget that his socks can get too small, too. Avoid curling or cramping his toes with too-tight socks. They should extend ¼ to ½ inch beyond his toes. Stretch socks avoid this problem to some extent.

The thickness of sole and heel in his walking shoes gives protection and support to help him balance on a broad base but still gives him foot freedom. The best shoes have flexible leather soles (foot motion), soft leather uppers (toe pressure), firm counter (heel position), and good shank (mid-foot support). Proper fitting allows his toes to lie straight without crowding, with room for movement, circulation of blood, and ventilation of his feet. This avoids pressure, friction, angulation, corns, calluses, and bunions. The length should be ½ to ¾ inch from his longest toe to the tip of the shoe. The width of the shoe should be ½ inch wider than his foot without wrinkling over his toes or causing pressure. As soon as his toes come to within ¼ inch or less of the end of his shoe, longer shoes should be bought. Blisters, calluses, or reddened pressure areas on the feet mean a recheck on the shoes is necessary.

The top of his shoe should be high enough to prevent pressure on his toes and instep. The ball of his shoe should fit the ball of his foot. The base of his big toe (first metatarsal head) comes at the point of rounding-in on the inner edge of the sole. The counter should be firm and fit the back of the foot snugly to provide stability for his foot. It need not be tight. It should not allow motion or irritation of his ankle.

To check the fit of his shoe, stand him with his weight evenly distributed on both feet. A properly fitted shoe should be trimly snug about his foot. There should be no large wrinkles running from one point to another. The bases of the toes (heads of the first metatarsal bones) should be felt to see if there is too much tension of the leather at these points. Try to determine if the base of his big toe is at the point of rounding-in at the inside edge of the sole. When his foot is bent, the "break" of his shoe shows by the lines running straight across the shoe. The position of the ends of his first and second toes is determined by pressure. Making sure that his heel is against the back of his shoe, press the toe to see where his toes end. The shoe should be examined at the heel to see that it clings properly. The outer margin of his shoe should show no gaping. Check the inside of the shoe to see that it is smooth with no rough seams. You may find one foot is larger than the other, either longer, broader, or both. His shoes are fitted to the larger foot.

Poorly built shoes that fit him are less apt to do harm than well-built shoes that do not fit.

Soft shoes, sneakers, or sandals may be used when he is in the yard or beach on soft surfaces and where he may get his feet wet. Avoid using them regularly when he is on hard surfaces. A child running about barefoot is not protected from hard surfaces, glass, or sharp objects.

When you look at your infant's foot, you may wonder if there isn't something wrong. It looks wrong. It is fatter and wider than an adult's, and doesn't seem to have an arch in either direction. A fat pad on the inner side of his heel makes it look flat. The infant foot is quite flexible because of the pliable muscle structure. When he stands, the line of the leg tendon in back is not quite straight. There are feet that look flat, pigeon toes, legs that look bowed and knees that look knocked. Many of these are entirely normal foot and leg conditions. Many of them change as development occurs. Some of them need simple shoe corrections. If you have any question, check with your pediatrician.

Walking on tiptoes is common. It causes concern in parents, but it requires no treatment if the child can walk with his feet flat on the floor. Time takes care of it.

Toes twisted or turned under each other are usually a hereditary condition, as noted earlier. In later years some of these conditions may require treatment. Nothing needs to be done at this time.

HANDS

By now your baby is so good at pincher grasping that he may put a toy in a box and take it out, sometimes cooperating long enough so that he will imitate you when you do it. His ability to use his hands makes everything more fun for him. His artistic ability with the crayon is still questionable, but his intentions are good since he scribbles with the crayon after you have demonstrated the technique for him.

EYES AND OTHER SENSE ORGANS

His eye-hand coordination has now become an intricate and integral part of his general behavior. This is important for walking and finger-feeding.

You continue to see signs of his hearing appreciation and his taste and smell use.

TEETH

He may have six teeth by now.

EATING

More than anything else, his eating now involves your patience and support as he goes about learning his new self-feeding skill. His diet continues the same but your effort is directed at feeding new foods, new combinations, new chances to discover. Not all of your efforts will make you feel wanted or needed, but you are.

MENU COMMENTS

You may have some concern that your baby won't get enough to eat as he takes over his own feeding. Have enough confidence in his hunger and appetite to permit him to eat as he needs. If your baby is hungry, he will eat. If he isn't, you will only make trouble if you try to feed him.

His growth rate is slowing down now so that his appetite and need for food lessen. It is well for you to keep this changing appetite in mind when you try to judge whether your baby is underfed or not. Your eyes will usually be bigger than his stomach. Some little people continue as large eaters.

CEREAL—BREAD. His increasing ability to feed himself makes it possible for you to expand the variety in this group, including the foods in the cereal substitute group. But be careful about relying too much on bread, especially as a snack.

MEAT—EGG. Egg in a variety of ways, and meat in almost any way your family has it, is and will be the basic part of his diet. Include adequate portions at each meal.

At luncheon you may have already been trying to make his meal simple. You can do this by using canned soup, undiluted, with added meat, powdered skim milk, cheese, dried beans or peas, to make it like stew. Another change to introduce will be the sandwich lunch with thick meat, cheese, egg, peanut butter on a slice of bread.

Another short-cut item is eggnog. This can be made with 2 eggs, 4 tablespoons of dry skim milk, and 2–4 ounces of water blended together. Vanilla and sugar can be added to taste. This can be used on cereal or used as a drink.

FRUIT. Be careful that his liking for and easy feeding of the fruit don't get you into difficulty with his diet. Keep the balance between your food group proportions even if it means some protest on his part about not enough fruit. Keep at least one portion a day for the Vitamin C-containing group.

MILK—MILK SOLIDS—CHEESE. This group should continue to be represented in each meal. Make full use of yogurt and cheeses. Cottage cheese goes well with fruit. If he self-feeds well on his solids, offer 2 ounces of diluted evaporated milk or pasteurized whole milk after his meal. Don't offer any if he eats poorly.

VEGETABLE. Keep a good variety of vegetables going in his diet, preferably the dark-green or deep-yellow type. Since he is getting many foods from the family table, you may have to look at your own adult diet to make certain it has sufficient variety.

DESSERT. Stick to the high protein desserts, making them higher in protein, if necessary, by adding more of the milk solids. Desserts of the sweet pastry type are definitely unnecessary extras. The end of the evening meal is the more satisfactory time to offer desserts.

BETWEEN MEALS. Snacks will be bite-size cheese, meat, egg, vegetables, fruit, or fruit juice determined by his eating behavior at mealtime. Your young fellow, now no longer such a baby, may like his juices better than anything else. Try to avoid giving him anything from this group within an hour before his mealtime.

VITAMINS. Continue the regular vitamin supplement in his diet.

SELF-FEEDING

Your baby may anticipate his mealtime with a happy smile as you slip on his bib. He "talks" to you and even goes to the high chair himself to be put in place. It is his good friend. He knows what it is used for.

Your fast performer has been at self-feeding for several months. Your average baby is just now coming fully into this stage. If he is like most babies at this age, he will be able to do a quite good finger-feeding job, starting out well and carrying through most of it. Don't expect a more finished performance than he is able to give. Before he gets tired and discouraged with this exciting but different system of eating, ease yourself into the picture to help him finish the last of it. Often he will object strenuously if you get into the feeding at all. He wants to do it for himself. Perfection does come, not at the start, but as a result of repeated attempts which gradually improve in quality. A new self-feeder is certain to make a mess. He may be less messy than last month but you may be hard put to agree. Be patient. You will soon discover that a messy face, smeared bib, and untidy kitchen are quickly repaid by his developing skills.

As an aware mother you will avoid telling him to "Hurry up!" Any request for speed from the self-feeder is discouraging to him. Your little precious will slow-down instead. Too much being done for him dampens his enthusiasm for doing. Too many "don'ts," anxious moves, or impatient admonitions discourage his drive to help himself.

SPOON-FEEDING

The gradual shift of the spoon-feeding process over to him will require still more teaching and patience on your part. Although your baby may be one who likes a spoon or fork from the first, usually he must become proficient with his fingers first. He may do very well with his fingers by 9 to 12 months, with a little help. Fingers are often used until 15 to 18 months, then a spoon becomes a necessity. Too early use of a spoon or fork may be frustrating. Your baby may be able to load the spoon but as he brings it to his mouth he turns it upside down. This leaves him angry and frustrated by an empty spoon. So ease along with him. He can do it eventually, but it will take much practice, years of it in fact. How many of you in your adult years never make a mistake in handling your eating tools? Before you answer look at the food spot on the front of your dress.

CUP-FEEDING

He may have started to hang on to his cup months ago. By now, he may be able to drink all alone. (See plate 22C.) (You still have to be nearby to watch him for that sudden move.) But he may seem more interested in picking food up from his tray or taking a gob of food out of his mouth to put into his cup. This is all part of his experimenting. He has to do it this way to learn how to be neat later. If he doesn't practice, how will he learn? So try to encourage his desire to feed himself. Finicky eaters are made, not born. Unfortunately, all too often they are made by over-supervising, interfering, too-neat mothers.

GOOD TOOLS FOR SELF-FEEDING

Now and in the months ahead he needs the right tools to work with. Nonbreakable plastic is a good material, but be sure it will stand washing in the dishwasher. Give him a spoon with a short, straight, broad handle about the length of his hand and with a shovel-shaped bowl so that he can slide it into his mouth sideways. A fork shaped like the spoon with short blunt points is a help. His cup needs a wide handle he can get his whole hand into, but not too heavy. A nonbreakable type of glass is a must. When he is ready for it, a straight-sided bowl or dish makes it easier for him to push food against the side and into his spoon.

SLEEPING

With some babies, reluctance to go to sleep and waking during the night may appear for the first time. Causes are both developmental and environmental. The baby's recognition of his parents as the most important people in his life increases his dependency on them. He does not want to be separated from them. Sleep then becomes a separation experience. He does not want to be left alone in bed. In addition, his motor abilities have developed considerably. His newly discovered methods of locomotion, his creeping or even walking, have opened a bright new world for him. Why give all this up for bed? This new ability may include attempts to climb out of his crib. Check this and make any necessary crib adjustments before he falls.

His nap patterns continue to change. Very often he absolutely refuses to take an afternoon nap. He sleeps eleven or twelve hours at night and has a long morning nap, but no afternoon nap. He may get a little tired and fussy, but you'll just have to put him to bed a little earlier. Let him sleep as long as he can in the morning. Get in a late-morning nap with a brief rest period in the afternoon. Keep the shades pulled down in his room and your housework quiet during his afternoon rest. Just about the time you have yourself adjusted to this new schedule, he may go into reverse and stay awake all morning and start taking nice long afternoon naps after his midday meal!

EXERCISE AND PLAY

He continues to delight in game playing, especially the peek-a-boo type. He covers his own face with a diaper or towel to start off the peeking. He likes the dropping game, too—he drops, you pick up. He likes the chasing games where he gallops off on all fours to get around the corner before you get him. He will hold out a toy for you, but he won't always let go without a little urging. He plays well on his own for some time. He explores all the possibilities of his toys. He looks for one he wants until he finds it, then settles down to work on it. If you show him how a new toy works he gets the idea, but he may not be able to make it work right away. He unwraps a toy you offer him —not neatly, you understand.

When you ask him "Where is ——?" about one of his toys or a household object, you may very well see a happy smile as he crawls off to look for it. But you may produce tears if he finds he can't move it to you.

He is developing a liking for massive color and picture books, especially if he gets a running description from you as you go through the book together. He can't quite turn the pages, but he gets the idea and tries.

His liking for imitations continues. If you make faces and put on a little show for him, you have an appreciative audience. He may learn to kiss you on request.

AWARENESS AND SOCIAL RESPONSE

At eleven months, your infant continues to grow more independent in some areas while he develops more dependency in others. He still carries his concern about strangers. You will also see the beginning of another type of concern, called separation anxiety. This may have manifested itself before now, but it is usually quite evident at eleven months. He is concerned when his mother leaves the room. This is why the peek-a-boo game should be encouraged earlier, so that he comes to understand going and coming. But this separation concern goes on for the next year or so. The degree of concern your baby shows has nothing to do with your way of doing things. You can't prevent it, so don't feel you have failed or have been neglectful. You may be annoyed by some of this, but try to treat it as a normal concern of his age. Go and come as you ordinarily would. Carry out your household tasks and let him continue his regular play schedule. If you overreact in either direction to his behavior, you don't help him at all. And you will have it to contend with off and on until he is about two and a half years of age. He can be quite pestiferous with his whimpering, clinging, and prolonged crying—or he may just come to you at intervals as if he has to touch home base once in a while. Just don't try to force independence on him. This can involve father, too. He may demand father just as he demands you—or he may refuse to have anything to do with him. If you can, create opportunities for father to take care of him—and be certain you are not around. Let them work this out themselves.

Baby-sitting can be a problem for your baby and the sitter. Try to get a sitter who is familiar. Expect some complaint from your child when you leave. Don't prolong your good-byes. Have your sitter briefed before you are at the door. Let the sitter contend.

He may show a violent anger response when something doesn't go well. He can be so frustrated and angry that he holds his breath, turns blue, and scares his family out of their wits. And they usually do the very thing that they shouldn't do—they get excited and try to get him to breathe. If he holds his breath long enough he will lose consciousness. Then he will breathe again. If he learns that he can frighten you and in this way control your actions, he will repeat the performance. He may anyway.

ORAL COMMUNICATION

At this point his language development may lag because he is spending so much energy in learning to walk. His emphasis is on navigation and not communication.

He says one word with meaning, perhaps "Dada" when he sees his father. He may say "Dada" and "Mama," and he does seem to connect them. He may understand simple commands such as "Give it to me," even though he does not obey them specifically. His behavior may clearly begin to show that he is learning what "no" means.

He can now imitate the correct number of syllables and sounds he hears when you give them to him. He imitates some new sounds he has not previously used. He shows interest in isolated words associated with objects or activities important to him, like "foot" or "sock." He can't say them yet. He will imitate two tones if you sing them for him. He continues to carry on quite a conversation in jargon. You know he is trying to say something by the tone of his voice.

Good manners are not for your baby at this time. They are a must for you. You should say "Please" and "Thank you" to help him make such words part of his vocabulary when he is old enough to do so.

IMMUNIZATIONS

This is an in-between stage if your baby has received all of the immunizations I have recommended up to this point.

BABY-CARE ROUTINES

CLOTHING

He may be so active by now that what was formerly a normal amount of clothing for him may be too much.

Look back to this month's "Motor Development" for suggestions on selecting shoes.

23.

The
Twelfth Month

Well, you've made it this far—and hasn't it really been quite an experience? I have talked about your baby's month-by-month progress, but do you realize that you too have been growing? You have moved from the helplessness of your first experience of motherhood to acquire a good many skills. It is rather a remarkable growth process, which has given you knowledge and understanding of your baby, which your husband shares to some extent also—hopefully, equally. Just as you encourage your child to learn, he in turn teaches you how to use your abilities and feelings. Certainly you are a far more confident person today than you were twelve months ago.

You have lived with your baby for a year. You are somewhat of an expert on children by now. You have found that your child doesn't break easily—bruise and bend, yes—break, not often. This is true physically, mentally, and emotionally. You have discovered, too, that you can make mistakes and that your baby will still continue to grow. Hopefully, you have discovered that what seem to be bad habits can be temporary situations of growth and development, and that some rebellion is necessary, even healthy—even if it is annoying to you. You have all kinds of signs that the sweetness and helplessness of the early months are being replaced by husky, even belligerent independence. It is difficult to be wholehearted in your welcome of this development, but this is part of your growing up too. He may convince you as you struggle to hold him on your lap while he grabs for the candle on his birthday cake to make it his own.

At the end of this first year he is in the middle of a period of development that began several months ago and will go on until fifteen months or later. He is still busy trying to master actions that he hasn't mastered as yet. His walking, talking, and self-feeding are all at an in-between stage as he enters his second year. So you don't see much change in his daily behavior from what I have described. Perhaps he isn't so frustrated now. He tries to get along socially even when his tasks challenge him. He has made his beginnings, but he still has a distance to cover before he will be successful.

WEIGHT

Ranges: Boys 18.5–27.3 lbs.   Average 22.2 lbs.
                Girls 16.8–27.1 lbs.   Average 21.5 lbs.

If you have the lean type of baby, he will weigh less than 3 times his birth weight. The stocky baby will often have gained more than this.

Your baby may be losing his chubbiness and lengthening out into the slender type of child seen so commonly in the second year on, or may continue heavy without growing tall—or grow tall without much weight gain.

If your baby is really obese—meaning too much flabby fat with poor muscle tone so that he doesn't move about much—you have probably not been following the menu suggestions I have made in previous months. A baby can be heavy, but this is all right if his muscle substance and tone are good.

HEIGHT

Ranges: Boys 28.1–31.6 in.   Average 29.6 in.
                Girls 27.1–31.0 in.   Average 29.2 in.

By the end of the first year, most babies have increased about ten inches over birth length. As soon as your child stands alone well, he should be measured standing rather than lying down. This may not be possible until later than one year. Measure him without shoes.

MOTOR DEVELOPMENT

As I have described your infant's progress through this first year I hope that I have made apparent to you the tremendous growth changes that have occurred. You started with a dependent little animal almost entirely governed by reflexes. In this twelve-month period he has replaced these reflexes to a great extent with voluntary activity, activity that is under his own conscious control. He has gone from a bunched-up four-footed creature to an upright human being.

LYING, SITTING, STANDING, AND GETTING ABOUT

Lying, sitting, and rolling continue to be means to an end —and that end is locomotion.

His efforts at getting about are still mostly in the creeping category. Even if he moves about on hands and feet rather than on hands and knees, he is still in a four-footed position. He may continue creeping long after this month, or at any time now he may give up creeping for walking.

Most one-year-olds are pulling up to a standing position, standing alone, and taking some steps with support or even alone. (See plate 20K.) Your baby walks off quite confidently now with his hand held. There is still a little of the balancing act about it, but he certainly is moving in the direction of two-footed locomotion. His backbone still has the curve of the four-footed little person he still is. He will get the S-shaped curve of the adult posture months after he actually walks alone. The full upright holding up of his body in a kneeling position doesn't come for several more months. It will be three to six months before he is able to back himself down to sit on a chair.

A baby is said to be in the toddler stage if he walks unsteadily with his feet wide apart. This is the broad-based gait where his steps are of different lengths. He steps off in different directions, holding himself balanced with his shoulders out and his elbows bent. He sways from side to side with each step, shifting his center of balance forward on the pivot. He starts the next step to avoid falling forward. He may fall backward or sit down with a thump. He practices and practices as he tries to get going alone.

HANDS

His thumb-finger use continues to improve. His grasp is still rather crude and not too well organized or smoothed out. When he handles a ball he can roll it or fling it. This is with a push-away type of thrusting motion which in no sense can be called a true throwing motion. His release ability is also still rather crude. It is more a total letting go all at once than a well-coordinated, smoothly carried-out sequence.

This is the age at which he begins to develop a better perception of face and form. It is now that he really begins to understand that there is an above and a below. This is the first space relationship that he discovers. There is some rudimentary investigation of in and out when he puts a block in a box and takes it out, but he doesn't understand this too well until he is older.

He is a single-minded fellow. You see this in his handling of objects in a group, such as blocks. He handles them one by one, not as a group. You may see some attempt on his part to put one toy on top of another by pressing it down on the other, but he still doesn't see things actually separate from each other.

You may be seeing some signs of hand preference. (See plate 21Q.) Some children don't show you which hand is their favorite until at least two years, others not until four years or older. Handedness may be inherited or environmental. How much is the result of the way the brain is constructed and how much is the result of imitation and instruction has been much debated. Early indications of a preferred side suggest that the baby is born with this tendency. Left-handedness is not the opposite of right-handedness. Right-handers stay quite consistently right-handed. Left-handers often show shifting use of either right or left hand. At this time you don't know what his real preference will be. Just try as much as possible to keep things presented at his middle, not off to one side or the other. If he seems to use his left hand more, let him. You may be loading him with a real handicap by trying to make him change. If you are right-handed now, how well would you do if you were forced to use your left hand? Answer this before you act to interfere with your child.

EYES AND OTHER SENSE ORGANS

By one year his pupils have enlarged to about their middle point, but their size will continue to increase. His central vision has reached 20/100 now. He has gained mature adult function of his eye muscles before this. He still doesn't coordinate very accurately into one the separate images he sees with each eye. You can break his focus easily by distracting him. The size of his cornea has reached adult size now.

TEETH

The average one-year-old has six teeth, all incisors, four in his upper jaw, two in his lower. Some babies have eight teeth at a year; others are just getting their first two. Don't be in any great hurry with that toothbrush routine. More important is what you are doing in his diet to prevent fermentable products in his mouth. After each meal give him a drink of water to rinse his mouth. Plan for a visit to the dentist when he has twenty teeth.

EATING

His eating patterns remain about as I have described them for the last couple of months. You are really in a waiting period. You are waiting for your young fellow to learn how to handle his fingers and cup well enough on his own to go on to spoon-feeding in the months ahead. But he isn't ready to make this next jump quite yet.

Continue a schedule with 5½-6 hour intervals or longer, particularly in this period of his erratic eating. Too frequent meals just bring him to his high chair not hungry. Adjust the times to your family schedule—although you may have a fellow who won't let you forget that 6 hours have gone by.

CEREAL–BREAD. You will have to watch your use of the bread–cereal group. Your year-old fellow may either ignore it completely or try to over-use it to the exclusion of other foods. This depends a little on how enthusiastic he is about self-feeding and chewing and how enthusiastic you are about pushing bread and cookies at him between meals.

FRUIT. Over these past several months you have introduced your baby to an increasing number of raw, dried, and cooked fruits, diced or cubed. Fruits are usually well accepted by your baby. He probably does most of his fruit feeding on his own without much help or interference from you. He may try to narrow the choices down to a few favorites, but offer a varied group. You want to give him a taste-color-texture food experience. In the fruits with large seeds or pits, always remove them before you offer the fruit to your baby. And at least one fruit portion a day must be Vitamin C-containing.

MEAT–EGG. In the months ahead this group continues to be the basic food group around which you arrange your meal plan. In any day's meals ⅔ of his protein should come from animal sources and ⅓ from the vegetable (cereal–bread) group.

MILK–MILK SOLIDS–CHEESE. Continue two portions of the milk–milk solids–cheese group. Add the milk solids to any of his foods that you can. Continue to avoid an effort on his part to substitute drinking large amounts of liquid milk for eating a balanced diet.

VEGETABLE. His vegetable group is now about the same as in an adult diet except for some extra care about raw foods and size of pieces. Although he can be an excellent chewer at this time, he may not always be patient enough. He gags on too large a food piece if you aren't careful. Raw vegetables will still have to be watched since carrot sticks, celery sticks, and the like may be a little bit too much at this time for him to handle. The vegetable group is sometimes a difficult one at this time. You are trying to increase his experience in colors, textures, and tastes. Your emphasis is on the dark-green, deep-yellow group. Try to keep introducing variety in both this group and the other vegetables. Don't expect enthusiasm for all of them. This is a highly individual matter. Just be content to introduce them. Let him have time to get to know them. Offer each one at intervals. Don't forget that in addition to the green tops there are bottoms which can be used.

DESSERT. Continue to keep his desserts simple and offer them only at the end of the meal. Plain cakes and cookies are probably part of his experience now. Don't get into pastries, heavily-iced cakes, or pies. Sweets are in this same problem area. Don't start the candy bar habit. Discourage such offerings from friends and relatives. If you must offer candy, use a plain sugar type after a meal, then have him drink water to rinse his mouth. Chocolate is the real offender in this group. It satisfies hunger so completely and for so long that he eats poorly at his next mealtime. Don't let him have sweets between meals.

BETWEEN MEALS. Avoid sweets or carbonated drinks now and later. If he isn't eating well, give him just juices between meals. Don't get in the habit of giving a cracker to quiet down your fussy young man. Fruit juice or a protein snack is better.

SPOON

A spoon will continue to be a problem, for him and for you. If he will tolerate your help, you can help him load it and guide it to his mouth. If he refuses your help, it will be better to hold off on the spoon-feeding for a time. Let him get more proficient with his fingers.

Babies are so different in their ability to use fingers, spoon, or cup that it is hard to be specific at this time. Your baby already may be handling a spoon with some skill or be so unready that he just bangs and waves it around. His finger-feeding and cup-feeding techniques are usually good by this age.

His growing independence shows up in his approach to feeding. It seems far more important for him to splash than eat. Food seems to exist not only to be eaten but also to be felt with his hands, smeared on his face, and dropped on the floor.

Just because he is messy now, don't worry about his later spilling or messy playing with food. And don't expect to give him any training in table manners at this point. But for your own later peace of mind, don't laugh at any of his antics or you will be in for a repeat performance.

APPETITE

But what about his appetite? It is often very good, but different now. He is much more choosy about his food as well as less hungry. As a result he can afford to skip a meal now and then.

Breakfast is usually a pretty good meal. You need to keep it a heavy protein meal with eggs, meat, cheese, eggnog, or similar proteins so that he is prepared for a heavy morning's work. His lunch is often an off-and-on meal, but don't ignore it. Your own attitude about lunch time can set up a pattern here. Dinner is usually a good meal, provided he is on his own without the social demands of the family dinner table.

MOVING TOWARD INDEPENDENCE

The increasing independence of your one-year-old may be causing you some concern in the eating area. Not only has his appetite decreased, but he doesn't have much patience either with you or with himself. He wants more attention in one way but less in another. He can be eating along perfectly well when suddenly he decides he would rather dump the dish upside down on his high-chair tray to mess with it better. He may drink beautifully with his cup, even holding it one-handed. Then suddenly he is done and what's left goes over high chair, baby, floor, and wall. He needs you there for the quick hand, the quiet voice, the companionship. But don't just sit there and look at him. This is just asking him to put on his little act after the edge is off his hunger.

Some of this you can avoid or cut down on by putting only bites or single spoonfuls of each food down on his tray at a time. You do better to give him small amounts so that he wants more. A big pile of food invites playing. Use his basic high protein diet and let him eat as much as he will. If he doesn't eat this meal, he will the next, or the next. Remember again, he isn't continuing to grow at the rate he did earlier. He just doesn't need as much food. You must have confidence in your child's appetite. It is difficult for you to avoid insisting that he take the food you have just spent time and effort preparing. But don't do it! You only start feeding problems where none exist. By ignoring his right to privacy and independent choice, you make him resist. End his meal with a casual "All done?" when he shows signs of ending it. Certainly don't follow him around the house trying to get another spoonful down. Game-playing, coaxing, forcing, bribing, are all invitations to further difficulty as he goes along. This is particularly true if he recognizes that he is able to control you in this fashion. It may be of some help for you to remember that this is a developmental change he is in the midst of.

Your baby may just now be coming to some of the things I have talked about. He may go backward for a time and want you to feed him. After all he isn't so settled in his independence that he doesn't get tired and bored with his attempts to feed himself. But watch his cues and get out of the way when he indicates his readiness. Just don't insist about it.

BOWEL AND BLADDER FUNCTIONS

Now that your youngster is showing so many abilities in so many directions you may feel that he should be ready to learn bowel control, if not bladder control. You know that you have changed his diapers at least a thousand times

—and it may have been much more than that. But stop and look at what you are asking of him. He is just now getting enough control of his legs to stand and walk. These are less complicated actions than the intricate systems of hold and release that exist in his rectum and bladder. And he has just learned how to release his grip on a toy. Although hand skill and walking are complicated skills, this doesn't mean that bowel control comes at the same level of development. Give him time to develop. If you have an insatiable urge to put your child on the toilet seat, limit this to the one time of day at which he seems to produce a bowel movement most regularly. Make certain he is secure on the toilet seat, feet supported, or put him on a potty close to the floor, where he doesn't get frightened. Don't flush the toilet when he is on it. You may scare him. Don't go out of the bathroom and leave him to his own devices. He plays with everything he can reach, from his own bowel movement to the toilet paper and his booties or socks. Save yourself a call to the plumber to clear a plugged toilet. The toilet paper unravels so quickly—his sock is right there to take off— what better place to put it than down the toilet? How can you punish him when you invited it?

If your baby is a quiet, placid one who doesn't mind sitting still and who has a regular daily bowel movement at the same time of day, probably you can accustom him to using the toilet to some extent. He comes to expect this, although he doesn't understand it. But the average active, on-the-go fellow doesn't like to sit still this long. He doesn't understand that this is toilet training. He understands it as a restraint and reacts accordingly. It becomes a battle, which develops later into a struggle over toilet training. If in addition he is also irregular in his bowel habits or has loose stools, why not forget about it? Wait until he knows what toilets are for. Ordinarily eighteen months or later is a much better time to start toilet training—in spite of your neighbor who claims that all of her children were trained at six months.

SLEEPING

The average one-year-old still totals about fourteen and a half hours of sleep in twenty-four hours, about two and a half hours of it in naps. The longest interval at night is almost twelve hours in length. Night sleeping at this time usually presents no great problem. He may go straight to sleep after his supper, or he may walk about his crib or play, going to sleep on top of his covers later. He tends to sleep quite soundly.

He may have given up his afternoon nap for good by now, or he may have a two-hour mid-morning nap and a short afternoon nap, or no morning nap and a two-hour afternoon nap. Even if he doesn't do much sleeping, a rest time when he plays quietly by himself is sufficient.

EXERCISE AND PLAY

Your baby makes his own play in his need to exercise. He is driven to pull up, sit down, crawl, stand up, walk about holding onto something, or do anything that uses his muscles. He likes to climb and cruise. A walker, "Tailor Tot," or "Kiddy Kar" can be good helping arms in his attempts at walking, but don't let him depend on them too much. He needs to practice on his own.

He likes to watch other children playing, but he won't be able to play with another child for at least another year. Even then he will have to be supervised in such play. At this time biting may be his only method of establishing some sort of social contact. This isn't because he is mean or angry or full of ill-will. It may be the only way he knows to find out about something in his surroundings. It may be a habit that you have allowed to develop from his need to mouth and appreciate everything. Always stop your baby from biting you—don't make a game of it. Anticipate it—don't wait for it.

He enjoys games that repeat the same simple motions. Rhythms continue to be attractive. He enjoys trying to get a toy hidden under a box, cup, or cloth. If he can hide behind a chair while you try to "find baby," he is tickled. He has developed to the point where he will hand you a toy when you ask for it—though he may want it right back. He may offer it to you to start a give-and-take game. He takes it from you with a pleased look—looks up at you happily—then places it back in your hand with a definite

"There it is" push. He may point to his eyes, nose, etc., at your request, show you how big baby is, and play other games mentioned previously.

His hand release and thumb-finger control gives him a new game with ball rolling. About half the time he can roll it in your direction. He does this most often in a sitting, crouched-down, or all-fours position. If he tries it standing he may throw himself off-balance and plop down on his bottom.

He may entertain himself for some minutes putting blocks in and out of a box. He puts small objects into a cup or can or box, then takes them out again. He can play with spools or large buttons.

He continues the dropping game described before. You may have to anchor his toys to his playpen. Just don't make the strings too long.

AWARENESS AND SOCIAL RESPONSE

Perhaps independence and negativism would be two good descriptive words for what his behavior represents now. His memory and association ability are growing. He has little sense of personal identity and no sense of personal possessions. "Mine and thine" is not in his mind yet. He is still very self-centered. He doesn't distinguish too clearly the difference between himself and others in his mind. But actions indicate that he has some rather definite feelings about his own individuality. He has his own feelings, his own anger, his own anxiety, his own affection. These may not be too separate and clear-cut yet, but he does try to transmit them to others—and he recognizes them in others.

He continues to approach his own mirror image socially. He talks to it. He may bring a toy along to get into the picture. He may offer the toy to the boy in the mirror, pat the toy or the boy, and talk to either or both.

As he moves out into his world he begins to act and think as an individual independent of other human beings. This is just another part of his drive to grow.

He is also a true Daniel Boone—he wants to pioneer, to

explore. He pokes himself into everything and everywhere. He digs, he shakes, he pulls, he climbs. He is a horrible nuisance many times, but you will be more lenient when you think of his drive and his needs. He has to find for himself the size, the shape, the mobility of everything. He has to discover, test, and retest each new skill before he is able to move on to the next.

Your "no-no" may not affect him at all. You can use his easy distractibility as a help in controlling him. He is so eager to find out about everything in this world that he isn't the least particular where he begins or where he stops. If he is deep in some work with his blocks, a spoon and a pan can make him drop that work at once.

His activity and practicing also extend to his social activities. He is better able now to deal with strangers. He will boldly make contact one minute—then break off to run back to you for protection and reassurance—then venture out on his own again. As he does this repeatedly his dependency is replaced with his confidence in himself. He needs the security he gets from you to gain his independence.

A year ago your baby wasn't even dimly aware of your existence. Everything was himself. He only knew when he was comfortable or uncomfortable. You had to give affection without receiving any for a time. As he has developed and matured he has come to recognize people as separate individuals—and his mother is the one most important to him. You are the best of all people as far as he knows. Your day-to-day care and affection now begin to pay off in the affection you see coming back to you.

He loves to have an audience. Since he is often the center of his family group, this comes about easily. He may squeal or show off to get the social ball rolling. He tries to do again what brought smiles or a laugh before from his family. His pat-a-cake, combing his hair, or powdering his nose may be crude imitations of ordinary events, but they draw his adults into his circle of charm. This helps him to distinguish himself as a person. He can imitate some simple social act.

If he is a baby who uses rhythmical patterns as part of his pre-sleep routine, he may be showing them strongly at one year.

If he hasn't before now, your baby may start to develop some fears. Sudden noises in themselves do not cause too much upset, but a loud noise may. People or objects that move suddenly into his range of vision may startle him. He is not immediately aware of what they are.

Your baby has no real sense of right or wrong yet. He doesn't know that he is being bad or doing a bad thing. He does know when you are angry or upset. He doesn't have any way of knowing why. Keep in mind that you don't stop him from doing anything by remote control. Go to him and either take him out of the difficult situation or supervise what he is doing.

Breath-holding may have started last month as a sign of frustration, anger, physical hurt, or temper. Temper tantrums may also be starting about this age. All children try them to some degree during the second year. If a temper tantrum works, the baby will try it again. A tantrum means that he has lost control of himself. Frustration is the usual reason, but anger for other reasons can also produce it. Either he can't have something, he can't do something because he isn't skillful enough, he can't make himself understood, or he doesn't understand pain. If these situations occur, a temper tantrum can result. You can try to help him avoid these situations, but you cannot avoid the temper tantrum. There are very few ways in which you can help him to meet his problems other than to ease them, if possible. He needs to know how to grow up. He needs to know how to get along with others around him. You do have to refuse unreasonable demands of his. You do have to ask for acceptable behavior. You do have to reject poor behavior. If you grant or give in to unrealistic behavior or each request, you teach him that he can control people by tantrums. You need to help him control himself. Put him alone until he is quiet. This gets results most rapidly. Spanking is definitely out—it usually just increases his anger and gives him more cause for it.

Let him understand that his tantrum is not the way to behave to get results. Don't have one yourself in trying to handle him. Don't give in just because he is frightening in the violence of his tantrum. Don't bribe to stop a tantrum. In public, it is hard not to give in to a tantrum. Actually, it is better to remove him from the scene kicking and screaming, as long as you yourself stay calm. Deal with the situation immediately and with confidence. Don't worry if someone criticizes the way you handle your child. You are the one responsible for him.

ORAL COMMUNICATION

At one year his vocabulary may consist of "Mama" and "Dada," and one to three other meaningfully said words. The rest of his word sounds are still gibberish. He may launch out into a lengthy conversation with you or his toy. His jargon may closely imitate the flow and rhythm of the language he hears, whether it is English, Spanish, Chinese, etc. His intonation is so similar to understandable speech that you are intrigued until you discover you don't know a word of what he is saying. His word sounds may be an attempt to imitate your adult words, using the initial sounds like "p" or "pu" for "pup." He often tries for two-syllable words. He may imitate a dog, cow, clock, or your adult exclamation. Some of his talking may be accompanied by gestures. By and large his speech is not a put-together process yet. He uses all vowel sounds and consonants m, b, k, p, g, w, h, n, t, d. He omits final consonants and some initial consonants. He substitutes the consonants just mentioned for the more difficult ones.

Your baby may be the quiet type who doesn't make much effort at word sounds, although he understands quite well what you are saying. When he is ready, he will start. Then you may wish for a little silence again. Or your baby may be in the more language-minded group and have half a dozen words or more by now.

You will be aware that his understanding of words and nonverbal talking comes before his spoken words, as when he responds to "Where is the shoe?" by looking for it. He may recognize some words by their sound. He indulges in a great deal of nonverbal communication. The most evident is his pantomime language, which he uses most often to ask for things he wants. Games like "show me" help him to learn to imitate word sounds. When he follows simple directions, he shows you that he understands a great deal. He more definitely associates the words with objects and people now. He also knows from your voice whether he is "good" or "bad."

He may use some of his sounds as attention-getters, too. A cough or a Bronx cheer or blowing bubbles can all be used as social demands for attention and the beginning of some type of interchange with people.

Keep on with your talking. Use gestures and demonstrations of objects to show what your words mean.

IMMUNIZATIONS

During your visit to the pediatrician this month, your baby should receive immunization against measles (rubeola). He will be given a protective dose of an inactivated measles-virus vaccine. Measles can be a serious disease in childhood, not only because your child can be quite ill with the primary infection, but also because secondary complications can be so devastating. Since this highly successful protection is available, take advantage of it for your baby. This single dose gives a long-lasting immunity. Reactions have been quite infrequent and mild; if they occur, they are usually about a week after the injection. If your child has shown a severe allergic reaction to egg, be sure to advise your pediatrician prior to administration of the vaccine.

Immunization against German measles (rubella) and mumps may also be given at this time, frequently in combination with the above measles vaccine.

BABY-CARE ROUTINES

BATH TIME

He prefers to sit in his bath now. He is less interested in splashy play and more interested in washcloth, soap, or float toys. He grabs at them and lets them fall over the edge of the tub. Then he pulls up to lean over to try to get them. If you want the washcloth, he may put it in a container for you.

He is learning how to get up on his hands and knees and then lunge down with a great splash. Discourage him from standing in the tub. He can slip and fall just as readily and disastrously as an older person.

CLOTHING

He is getting more know-how about dressing and undressing. He doesn't resist as much as he did. He cooperates more. But he is still more interested in taking off his clothes than putting them on. He may very easily pull his pants off by himself, especially if his diapers are soiled or wet, usually when he is alone in his crib. This may lead to some stool smearing on his crib and walls. You will just have to be alert to catch him sooner.

He may enjoy playing with his shoes and their laces as well as taking them off. He tries to put his shoes on, but he won't help you by pushing his foot into the shoe.

He fights diaper changes, probably because when he is flat on his back he isn't in control. Putting him in a partly sitting position or on all fours may be an answer, but it is difficult to put on the diaper in these positions.

Clothing designed for a child of one year should embody the principles of "self help." Garments should have front openings and only a few buttons, preferably large ones, which slip easily in and out of buttonholes. Shoulder straps should not fall over the tip of his shoulder and limit his arm actions.

24.

Discipline

The word "discipline" may mean punishment to you. This is often the way you hear it used. Punishment means a penalty imposed for a fault or crime, while discipline means training or development by instruction in self-control. So, in this sense, discipline means to guide, to educate, to teach, to lead. This is a far cry from the idea of punishment.

If your discipline then is to be teaching, what do you want to teach your child? Don't you want to help him to learn how to behave so he can get along well with other people, be comfortable and happy with them? Discipline then is a positive learning experience—how to learn the rules of behavior for living with other people in a way that is best for him and his own individuality. He has to learn self-control so that he can live in harmony with other human beings. You are teaching him socially acceptable behavior—the ability to do the right thing at the right time in the right way. He can grow into a happy, loving, giving person who feels secure and comfortable. What things are important to accomplish this?

In this first year, your discipline has been made up of many little things. Discipline is an everyday affair. Each month I have mentioned a variety of procedures and suggestions that contribute to this teaching process that is going on. You feed him, bathe him, talk to him, clothe him, handle him, and put him in a comfortable bed—so that he is not hungry, not too tired, and is treated as an individual with courtesy and affection. When you try to understand and answer his needs, you teach. When he demands attention at inappropriate times and you leave him alone, you teach. These are the little things that add up to a series of little lessons.

There are some general principles that are guideposts for your daily coping with your child's learning. Perhaps I can give you a little different approach, at least present a modified way to look at your infant. You can use this to give your baby the help he needs to learn the rules of the road of living ahead of him. This is really a compromise between the children-are-to-be-seen-and-not-heard method and the method where children must be allowed complete freedom of expression. Perhaps in talking about some of the factors that go into your discipline, I may be able to help you see what a balance between the too-strict and too-lenient approaches might give you. This middle-of-the-road way is a little hard to follow, since you have to pay attention to the child, to his individuality, to his stage of development and his readiness. No parent ever always works at his best level. So you can't expect yourself to do this perfectly or all the time. After all, mothers get tired, fathers get overworked, so that no one method can be used consistently or exclusively. Perhaps some of the considerations as to what goes into helping your child learn will be pertinent now.

Too many parents today have difficulty deciding just what their role is in discipline. They are afraid of frustrating their child. But there is no proof that all frustration is an unhealthy thing. In fact, it may be a needed part to all learning. I've been telling you about the frustrations your baby has as he tries to get up on his two feet. This same kind of frustration comes at all stages of learning in these years ahead. You don't regard this as either avoidable or unnecessary. You have no hesitancy in stopping your baby from burning his hand in a fire, sticking his finger in the light socket, running in front of a car—you know just what to do. You expect him to be frustrated and upset with you, but you want him to listen to your prohibition. You don't worry about any permanent injury to his psyche or any conflict over your invasion of his privacy. You put it down to a learning experience. Why should you treat learning to obey as anything other than this kind of learning experience? You cannot set limits without producing some frustration. The response to it can vary all the way from a momentary pause before a new activity is picked up to a full-blown caterwauling, maybe with a physical demonstration. He has a right to make his protest. He doesn't have a right to be too annoying to the persons around him. If he is too disturbing, his room is available for isolation until he gains control. You can't avoid these conflicts and confrontations if you want him to grow up with respect and consideration for others, especially his parents. You may be anxious about such conflicts, but you won't cause harm either to your child or to your relationship if your action has been taken with the long-range result in mind.

Parents do need to agree on methods of discipline and to back each other up in the carrying out of the various parts. This doesn't mean you have to agree on every little point before you act. This is an unlikely situation, since no two people always agree on everything. Your child can learn to fit into and around these differences within your family if they're not too opposed.

By this time, you recognize the type of baby you have and realize why it is so necessary to individualize your discipline. You may use the same principles of teaching, but you take into consideration his capacity to learn the basic principles and follow them. If you watch the manner in which he goes at walking or talking, enthusiastically or impatiently, you have a good indicator of how he will accept training rules for living with other people. After you see the nature of his inborn disposition, you adjust your teaching.*

Another way to look at this individual approach to teaching is to keep in mind at what level of development your child is. You can use this as a guide to tell you when he is or isn't ready for any certain experience. If he can't manage it, then don't let him. You fit your teaching to his abilities, his interests, and his weaknesses at that point. You won't be successful if he isn't ready. You didn't expect your newborn baby to hear your "no-no," but you do expect a response now when you say it. (I didn't say obedience to it. I said response to it.) Your lessons in discipline are like any learning experience you have seen—a little at a time—and not always successful for a time.

I have suggested the readiness concept many times in discussing your baby's developmental process. He needs to try and fail. With your encouragement and his own will to do, he will try again and finally succeed. This doesn't mean you can't help him, but you may have to help by distracting him to something else. He may be trying something just beyond his readiness level. Readiness applies particularly in the area of discipline. Are you asking more from him than he is able to do at his stage of maturing? Is he ready for doing what you demand? Your common sense tells you the answers if

---

* For a much fuller description of this important aspect of temperament refer to *Your Child Is a Person* by Drs. Chess, Thomas, and Birch (Viking Press, New York, 1965).

you are aware of what he is and has been doing in other areas of his development.

But here are some suggestions for your teaching.

Make certain your baby understands what you expect of him. Make it simple, exact, and clear. A simple "no" with a restraining hand will get the message to him. He learns faster with clear direction.

Be consistent with him. Consistent behavior on your part is the basic building block of your discipline. Set up intelligent rules of behavior. Then stick to them. Be clear in your own mind what you want and expect so you don't go around changing your mind or forget you made a rule. This way he knows what to expect, then he can go ahead and do it without confusion. This does not mean an inflexible rigidity. This kind of consistency is out except for safety rules. Common sense can tell you when to make exceptions.

Be patient with him. You may get impatient with yourself and your own failures, but he needs time to learn. Obedience is really cooperation, which is what you are always working to gain from him. You have to insist at times on what you regard as acceptable behavior and to set limits for unacceptable behavior. The big question always is how firm should you be in setting and enforcing limits. If you are the rather permissive, oversoft type of parent, you may have to be a little more strict and demanding about your own rights in order to teach your child about the rights of others. If you are too rigid or overstrict, you may have to learn how to bend a little in order to help your child realize that he has rights.

Keep your rules few and simple. It's easier to be consistent and firm about a few than too many. If you make too many rules, you and your child will both get confused and forget. The more rules, the less performance.

If your demands are always negative and prohibitive, you are not disciplining. You are repressing. Your "No, don't do that" is never balanced by anything positive, helpful, or comfortable. Your rigid forcing methods can only produce trouble, never obedience or cooperation. You pose a choice for your child. He can submit timidly, dawdle, and refuse in every subtle way to cooperate with your efforts. Or he can rebel, be negative, have temper tantrums, or cause unending trouble.

Your baby may need your guidance in a new experience or situation. This is leading, not taking over for him. You help him to learn to do the right things at the right time and for the right reason.

Correction is best done by one parent at a time and not for every trivial little thing. When there are other adults in the home, you will have to watch that each of them is not picking at the child separately or all at once.

Your examples of courtesy and manners are powerful in getting him to adopt habits of courtesy, consideration, and manners. Obedience or discipline is not so much a matter of making your child mind as it is the process of making it easier for your baby to learn to do the right thing by imitation or example. As he grows in his love and trust he wants to please you and to imitate you.

A sense of humor is an invaluable asset for any parent. This is an excellent way to keep your perspective. Every baby has this immense store of built-in pleasure. He wants to learn, to grow, to love, to act like the grown-ups around him. He is driven by it to learn their ways in every manner he can. When he finds that what he does pleases people, he tries to remember to behave that way.

Your baby enjoys attention. He will do whatever gets attention. He wants center stage, but he doesn't always know—or care—whether this is scolding or a praising response. If you pay attention to his less satisfactory acts, he repeats. If you pay attention to the less satisfactory ones, he again repeats. This should give you a lead. Make a pleasant fuss over his acceptable accomplishments. If he repeats this often enough, it becomes habit. So you do have some influence as to what he learns.

This very urge to do and learn at this time gets him into difficulty. He practices and practices how to drop things as well as pick them up—how to get up and down and around. You praise him when he puts his doll in the toy box. He can't understand why you are upset when his teddy bear is dropped in the toilet. When he has mastered one skill he is enthusiastically off to the next to give you a new set of problems to deal with. But you can't very well punish him for accidents as a result of his efforts to control his body.

You can take the first step in discipline. Prepare his surroundings so that he is protected from doing anything for which he is not yet ready. Don't ask too much of him. You make it easy for him to be good by preventing the difficulties. You think ahead to anticipate what his needs will be as well as what his abilities are.

In this first year, you won't find much cause for punishment. There isn't much a developing child does that deserves anything but the simplest measures. If you don't want your baby to misbehave, remove him from the situation in which he will misbehave.

In general you're teaching your baby how to behave all through the day. It isn't just when you say "no" and scold him for his mischief. You're teaching him good behavior when you simply accept the behavior that you recognize as part of his babyhood. You give him simple, interesting toys and safe places to play. You allow him as much freedom as you safely can. You cheerfully accept his offered attempts to do things. You don't punish him for accidents, but you do stop him promptly from getting into danger. You give patient and gentle understanding about the many things he needs to learn, but you keep showing him what you expect.

Never spank a baby under a year of age. He simply does not understand what you mean. He learns nothing, or worse yet, he learns to fear you instead. The impulse to strike a baby often comes from anger within the adult. He may be very exasperating to you. Or you may be reacting to things that have nothing to do with any act of the baby. Although the impulse to strike a baby may be strong, especially when you are tired or worried, you'll find that it is deeply upsetting to him. It doesn't improve his behavior.

Discipline—education for living—is much simplified when you recognize that it is a natural process of teaching, necessary and a help to your child and to your family. Children are very durable. They are also very human humans. Parents are the same. Humans make mistakes. A parent can ignore all that I've been talking about. A tired, worried, angry, frustrated parent can easily forget all about the suggestions for teaching at times. But his child mirrors the prevailing family attitudes and actions of his father and mother. And a child forgives and forgets much better than his parent does.

During this first year then, your discipline can be suggested by these guide words: consistently, patiently, firmly, lovingly, gradually, gently—and you will be on the road to good discipline.

25.

Baby-Sitters

The baby-sitter is a very prominent figure in American homes. She would be sadly missed if she suddenly vanished. Millions of couples would prowl their apartments and suburban homes like so many caged animals. Many amusement businesses would feel the pinch. The teen-age group would have less money to spend. Baby-sitting is big business in terms of the number of people involved and the amount of money spent.

Money for a baby-sitter can be money well spent. You need time to do shopping, to go to the beauty salon, to attend to errands. Above all, you need to get yourself out of the house—out of the baby-care routine. You also need to get out with your husband. This provides both a physical and emotional break in the pattern of your daily living. You get far enough away to get a little perspective and balance as to what you are doing and aiming for in your home affairs and tasks.

FINDING A SITTER

You may be faced with a real problem in finding a sitter. There is no one way that works for everyone. You will usually have to search.

Perhaps you are fortunate to have a built-in baby-sitter in the shape of an older child. Older children can be a real help if they are sufficiently mature. If you ask your older child to baby-sit, make it a formal request to perform a responsible job—and pay for it! It is neither fair nor forward-looking to make it a duty or to demand it in return for the weekly allowance. The teen-ager can make an excellent baby-sitter. The ten- or eleven-year-old can be quite a mature little person, but don't push this too soon. If you have any question about your eleven-year-old's adequacy, wait.

If your relationship with her is a good one, perhaps the best all-around baby-sitter is a real, live, honest-to-goodness loving grandmother. (Look back to the section on *Grandparents* for possible problems about this.)

Other relatives are often available for baby-sitting. You may be able to work out a trade-children policy if they are relatives with families.

If no relatives are available, what about the people in the neighborhood or in your apartment building? If they aren't available to come to you, you can perhaps take your child to them. The neighbor does the same.

Exchange baby-sitting is sometimes shared among several families with similar-aged children. This saves you money and gives you reliable and capable sitters. You must be a little cautious about the choice of families involved in this. Too wide a difference in child-care policy is going to lead to friction. Be tolerant of minor differences as long as your child is not in danger. A few hours of a different kind of handling won't change your child's life.

When there is a teen-age high-school girl in your neighborhood you may have found your sitter. They are generally responsible, full of energy, adore babies, and enjoy taking care of them. You won't go far wrong with a well-recommended, conscientious teen-ager. A young high-school person is willing to learn and will obey your rules. You can have several paid and supervised practice sessions with her so that you know that the job will be done right when you aren't there. With your help and instruction, she can do a good, responsible job.

A younger teen-ager may be very willing, but you will have to estimate her judgment and experience when you talk to her. Get to know her. Check on her references from the people who know her or have hired her in the past. Know about her family. If she has younger brothers and sisters, her experience may be quite adequate. A telephone acquaintance with her family is advisable, as she may use her mother for advice when she runs into a problem. Her family needs to know something about you, too.

If your friends can't recommend such a person, you can look up professional baby-sitting services in the phone book. Their applicants are drawn from college-age people and older persons like grandmothers, mothers, teachers, retired nurses, and governesses. Many of them have been bonded, medically checked, and trained in baby or child care. Expect to pay more for this type of service. You will also be expected to pay extra for late hours and to supply cab fare.

The nursing school of your nearby hospital may be a source. Student nurses may be interested in child-care experience as well as the extra income. Expect to pay a higher fee, for these girls are professional people.

You may find a young person who wants a live-in arrangement. Whether you pay her a wage in addition to supplying room and board depends on how much work you are asking for. Students and unwed mothers are usually the ones interested in this kind of arrangement. But look into it carefully first. Make certain you have sufficient room for a nonfamily adult. Also check out her background.

Sometimes community organizations like the Red Cross, the Y, a church group, or a residence club will be good sources for baby-sitters. But with all of these except for the professional baby-sitter service, you will have to spend some time beforehand checking on your future sitter.

Unless a new baby-sitter is personally recommended to you by a friend who has used her herself, you will do well not to hire a sitter sight unseen. A face-to-face interview in advance is an absolute minimum precaution with any baby-sitter about whom there is the slightest question. Meet her in advance so you and your husband are satisfied she meets your qualifications.

WHAT TO EXPECT OF YOUR SITTER— AND VICE VERSA

The safety of your baby is your first concern. When you choose a sitter, you want a person who can be trusted, who is competent and reliable, who has had some experience in handling children, who is watchful but not rigid, who is gentle in her manner and has a real liking for them, who is in good health, and who can be depended upon in any emergency that is likely to come up. Your baby-sitter will be able to do a better job of caring for your child if she understands what is expected of her.

Your sitter should remain awake while you are away. A

sleeping sitter offers no protection for your baby. If you plan to get home very late, you may agree to her napping, but in most cases you should make it clear she is to stay awake.

But you have responsibilities also. Call your sitter sufficiently ahead of time so that she can plan accordingly. Be definite about the time she is to arrive, how long she is to stay, what her duties are to be, what the pay rate will be, and what arrangements in transportation there are.

The sitter has the right to expect you to return when you said you would. If you are delayed or late, use the telephone to make new arrangements. Your sitter may be agreeable to your change in plans. If she isn't, return home as soon as you can.

Make certain that you deal with some of the questions about your sitter's safety. During nighttime sitting, have her keep doors and windows locked. She should deny admission to anyone unknown during your absence. Always be sure that she arrives home safely.

While it is important to impress on your sitter your ideas about safety and accident prevention, you have the primary responsibility of making your home safe for your child and giving your sitter specific information she needs. (Look ahead to the section on *Accident Prevention* for safety reminders.)

Keep a list of emergency phone numbers on the telephone base or near the telephone. It should be something like the following:

TELEPHONE NUMBERS

> Fire Department
> Disaster Unit
> Police
> Pediatrician's Office
> Father's Office
> Mother's Office
> Neighbor
> Relative

It's also wise to prepare an information sheet for your sitter. Keep it simple. You don't want her to spend the evening deciphering detailed instructions that she won't need anyway if she is a competent and experienced person.

If she has not been in your house before, you should not just hand your sitter the list and leave. You need to show her around, point out where necessary items are to be found, familiarize her with the household routine, be sure she understands all her duties.

You must be definite in advance about what privileges your baby-sitter is to have. Most problems center about food, phone calls, boyfriends, TV, and disorder.

Once you've gotten everything set up to your satisfaction, don't keep calling home to find out how things are going. If you plan to call once during the evening, let the sitter know beforehand that you will do so.

26.

Accident
Prevention

Accidents are the commonest cause of death and serious injuries in the early years. Poisons kill more children than illnesses do. Eighty percent of poisonings occur in a child under six years, 65 percent under three years.

The tragedy in all this is that most accidents are preventable. They occur as the result of carelessness, thoughtlessness, or lack of knowledge.

Listed below are some safety rules that you should follow zealously. Some apply more to the younger baby, some to the older one. All are important. Some have already been mentioned in the descriptions of your baby's development and your baby-care routines. Perhaps reading them all together will help you to keep them more clearly in mind.

SAFETY RULES

Never leave your baby alone in the house, or in the care of young children, even if it is only for a few minutes.

Never leave your baby unattended on a bed, table, or anyplace from which he can fall. Don't trust safety straps.

Never leave your baby unattended in the bath, or near water.

Never put your baby in the bath without first testing the water to make sure it is not too hot.

Never add hot water to the bath while your baby is in it.

Never let your baby play with the water faucets.

Keep safety pins, plastic sheets or bags, or any objects small enough to go into his mouth out of your baby's reach.

Make sure that anything your baby plays with has no sharp points or edges and no small removable parts.

Never carry anything else when you are carrying your baby. Watch your footing, especially on stairs.

Always have your baby sleep alone in his crib.

Never take your baby into your bed.

Check the crib before you leave your baby's room to make sure the crib sides are raised and locked into place.

Never use pillows.

Never tie your baby down in bed, or use a sleeping gear that can twist or tighten around his neck. Anchor the bedclothes firmly so they won't twist or wad about him.

Never prop your baby's bottle.

Never put your baby's high chair close to a table, stove, or anyplace where he can reach out and grab things.

Never use cellophane or adhesive tape anywhere near your baby. He may be a great picker.

Never use plastic bags anywhere near your baby.

Keep electrical outlets covered.

Keep your baby's medications separate from the rest of the family's.

Keep poisons and medicines out of your baby's reach.

Label medicines with name and date of purchase. Protect the labels with transparent tape so they won't become illegible.

Read the label and note the dose under a good light before you use the medicine.

Give only the dose indicated.

Always throw away prescription items when the illness for which they were prescribed has been relieved. Throw away prescription medicines that have gone beyond their expiration dates.

Never give a medicine prescribed for another person to your baby (or to anyone else in your family).

Dispose of medicines and household products by flushing the unused portions down the toilet and rinsing containers before discarding them.

Store household products like lye, ammonia, cleaning and polishing agents, detergents, kerosene, or insecticides in cabinets out of your baby's reach.

Always remember to return hazardous products to their proper storage places immediately after use.

Never store nonedible substances in food or beverage containers. In the event that your baby swallows something that you think may be toxic, call your pediatrician or poison-control center immediately. Don't wait for symptoms to appear.

Keep the following item in your medicine chest for emergency: Syrup of Ipecac U.S.P. In case of poisoning with materials other than petroleum products, give two teaspoons of this and follow with abundant water. Repeat in a half hour if no vomiting has resulted and you haven't been able to get your baby to a hospital or to get further instructions from a doctor or poison-control center.

Keep the phone numbers of your pediatrician's office and your druggist posted on your telephone or medicine chest. Keep a poison reference chart (you may be able to get one from your druggist) fastened to the back of your medicine-chest door. Keep a first-aid pamphlet handy (Red Cross and other agencies issue such pamphlets).

THE OLDER BABY

The safety rules given above apply to the older baby as well as to the younger one. However, once your baby begins to get around, the possibility of accident-producing situations increases enormously. It will be worth considering some of them.

Now that he is beginning to move around, your baby may discover trouble for himself. A good safety rule is to expect him to be able to do more than you think he can and to get into more places than you know he can. What he couldn't do yesterday he may demonstrate for you today.

Go over your house and yard for anything that can hurt him.

Keep doors closed, especially those leading to stairs or out-of-doors. If there is no door, you must put up an adequate gate or barrier. Keep stairs free of clutter.

Keep your baby out of areas that have furniture he can climb on or pull over on himself. Hanging cords and drooping tablecloths are an invitation to him—and can be dangerous.

Breakable objects can be a risk because at this age he doesn't know what breaks and what doesn't. If you don't get them out of his reach—or keep him where he can't reach them—you will be continually prying him loose from something. This is never a help because he doesn't understand this kind of prohibition, and your "no-no" soon loses its power to dissuade. You just have to use it too often.

Many common household preparations are dangerous: cosmetics, hair oils, coughdrops, dyes, household cleaners —the list is long. You may say this isn't a risk since your baby doesn't get into things. The next time he plays with your purse—which you gave him to keep him quiet—may change your mind quickly. Even a can of talcum he is given to play with can be a real catastrophe if he breathes in the contents.

Don't let him play in the kitchen while cooking is going on. Hot liquids or foods burn quickly and sometimes deeply. A cooking-pot handle, a turned-on stove burner, a hot coffeepot or cup of coffee—all these are hazards.

As your youngster gains better ability to get around he will increase his chances for falls. You will have to be alert to this, but you can't always anticipate his headlong dashes across the room on his unsteady legs to land flat on his face in the brick fireplace—or bang into the corner of the coffee table. As he propels himself with increasing skill, his fingers have increased their power of exploration, too. So watch out for the poisoning possibilities in your home. Child-proof any areas he will be in as far as possible. Take into consideration loose items on the floor, lamps and cords, bookcases, electrical gadgets, knives or scissors, heaters, cluttered table tops, windows and window coverings—and more.

You can let him have the freedom of some rooms when you or another adult is present, but if he is to do his exploring alone, he should be, as I have said many times, in his playpen, his play yard, or his own room. These will protect him as he tests and tastes his way out into the world.

Do a quick check on your own actions. Do you put things away and avoid clutter? Are you careful with breakables? Do you close drawers and doors so that they are out of the way? When you smoke, are you careful with the matches, the ashtray, and the lighted—or unlighted—cigarette?

Your baby may learn to climb in and out of his high

chair, using it as a sort of modified jungle gym. His high chair must be strongly made, with legs on a wide base, and should be fitted with a safety strap or harness. Bouncing chairs, swings, and strollers need to be well balanced so that tipping over isn't easy. Harnesses or safety straps are needed with these too.

Your baby must be carefully watched in any room that has a fireplace. A baby should never be left to roam in a room where a fire is burning. Even with a dead fire you have to avoid problems with the ashes and what they contain.

Playpens and cribs must have safety catches that don't pinch inquiring fingers. Spaces between the bars must not be wide enough to let a head through. Watch for the time when he can climb over the crib side—and then make some other arrangement. Guard rails can be attached to make the crib sides higher.

Make certain that his crib or playpen is far enough away from articles he can grab and get into trouble with, like drapes or blind cords.

By this time your baby has probably traveled a good many miles in your car. As I have mentioned before, he needs a securely anchored car seat to sit in with a strong harness. Many of the available harnesses are nowhere strong enough to stand a hard stop or accident, so choose carefully.

Never let anyone sitting in the front of the car hold the baby on his lap. It is a very dangerous spot. Never let your baby move about while you are driving. Never leave him alone in the car.

27.

Sick-Baby
Care

CALLING THE DOCTOR

Your baby—like most others—is probably going to have at least one illness during his first year. So you will need to be aware and recognize the cues and little signs he gives you that he isn't feeling well. You will be able to do this better than anyone else as you become acquainted with him. You become an expert about your own baby—but don't try to be an expert diagnostician on your own. Use the telephone so your doctor can help you interpret your findings—and try to be as specific as you can.

You may hesitate to call because you hate to bother the doctor or you think that it is just a little thing. Serious illness may have a mild beginning, just as a not-too-serious situation may start off with a frightening series of symptoms. You will be on the safe side to call. Your doctor would rather be bothered by calls about trivial illness than have you neglect to call him about the signs of a really serious one.

Following are questions your doctor may ask about the baby:

Does he have signs of a cold, such as a runny nose or cough?

Does he have a fever (101° or higher)?

Is he refusing to eat—not taking one or two feedings or taking nothing?

Is he vomiting? Is he losing an entire feeding? Is he bringing up both liquids and food?

442

Is he crying or wailing as though he were in pain?
Does he show any other signs of pain?
Is he unusually listless?
Has he a flushed or pale complexion?
Is his skin hot or dry?
Are his eyes red or sensitive?
Does he have loose stools, diarrhea, or show any sudden
    changes in his stools?
Is his urine output decreased? How long since he last
    urinated?
Is his breathing hoarse or labored?
Does he just act differently?

TEMPERATURE-TAKING

What about his temperature? Feeling his forehead is not
a method for temperature-taking. Use a thermometer. Take
your baby's temperature rectally. Use a blunt-bulb rectal
type for this. The mouth type can be used rectally if the
blunt type is not available. The mouth type has a slender
end.

Before you start, shake the thermometer down so that
the mercury column is below 97°F. To do this, hold the
upper end (not the bulb end) firmly in your fingers and
snap downward a couple of times. Smear Vaseline on the
bulb end. Place your baby on his abdomen on your lap or
on the table. Put the Vaseline-covered tip 1 to 1½ inches
up into his rectum. Slide it in easily. Don't push it in. Let
it follow the natural curve of his rectum. Keep it in place
for five minutes. Keep his buttocks squeezed together and
his legs anchored during the waiting period. Don't let go of
him or the thermometer. When you remove the thermometer, wipe it clean and rinse it in cold—not hot—water
after reading it. Wipe it with alcohol before you put it
away.

Use the rectal approach for your youngster until he is
old enough to hold an oral thermometer in his mouth under
his tongue for five minutes. This is usually from nine years
on.

Take his temperature in the morning, late afternoon, and
evening so that you can get a record of any variations from

the normal levels. Read his temperature exactly as it registers on the thermometer.

READING A THERMOMETER

The column to read is either in silver or in red. Hold the thermometer horizontally between your fingers until you spot the height of the red or silver column. The numbers

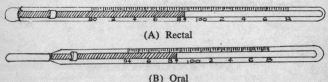

(A) Rectal

(B) Oral

Fig. 51. Reading a thermometer.

are in degrees F., usually 92 up to 106. The little markings between these are 0.2 degree divisions. The arrow indicates 98.6 degree F. Exaggerating the size a little, this is the way it looks. (See fig. 51.)

FEVER

Normally your baby's temperature taken by rectum will vary from 98.6° to 100.6°. His mouth temperature is usually less accurate—about one degree off his actual body temperature. His morning temperature is usually lower than his mid-to-later afternoon temperature. Any rectal temperature of 101° or more must be considered above normal— it indicates infection until proved otherwise. Often when he is sick his morning temperature may be normal, with a high rise in the afternoon or evening.

Your baby's temperature responds easily and quickly to illness, with much higher swings than in an adult. His temperature regulator is not well enough developed so that he can handle these changes without fluctuation. His flushed face and hot-to-the-touch skin should suggest fever to you. This is his body's way to handle illness. It is not good or bad in itself. Fever is not a disease, but a defense reaction on his part. It is a symptom—an alerting signal. It doesn't tell you what the disease is.

Fever isn't something to be feared in itself. A high temperature frightens most parents, but you can often let fever be. It indicates a disease process, but you don't have to knock yourself out in your efforts to bring it down. You may be interfering with a natural defense mechanism.

Don't imagine the worst. The greater the temperature rise doesn't mean the greater the illness. High fever alone does not cause brain problems. Certain diseases with fever may.

GIVING FLUIDS

With a fever you should give fluids, if he is not vomiting. Give water and diluted sweetened fruit juice, ginger ale, 7-Up, clear broth, weak sweetened tea. Any high-water-content sweetened fluid will do.

Give him small amounts frequently rather than letting him gulp it down in large amounts. They may go down since he may be quite thirsty—but they bounce back just as readily.

Don't give milk as a fluid at this time. He may be more easily upset by milk than anything else. He can often take clear liquids well.

DIET

He may eat his regular diet if he wishes, but don't insist that he do so. Most babies eat less when they don't feel well. He is better off to skip a meal or two and stay with clear liquids than to eat and start vomiting.

DRESSING

Dress him as you normally would. Don't overdress him just because he has a fever. His body is trying to combat his illness by raising his temperature. If you overheat him with too many clothes, you interfere with his protective body processes and his heat loss. The same thing holds true of bedclothes. Cover him more lightly when he has fever—add covers when his temperature drops and he is sweaty and easily chilled. Don't button your feverish child into warm pajamas, wrap him in a heavy blanket, and keep him in an overheated room. Room temperature should be between 68° and 70°F.

ACTIVITY

You do not need to try to keep your sick child in bed. Bed rest is not significant in his recovery. In general you should encourage him to rest. This doesn't mean that he has to be forced to lie down when he is actually well enough to be up. Putting a child to bed in the daytime doesn't mean he will rest. In fact, he may be more active in bed than if he is up and dressed. Let him decide how he feels and how much activity he wants. Watch his actions and put him to bed when he feels too sick to stay up. He may do better on the couch in the living room where he can see all that goes on. If he hurts, he will stay quiet in the position he finds most comfortable. Don't forcibly restrain any child in any particular position except under unusual circumstances. Try to give him activity that slows down his usual push.

Don't take him to bed with you or get into bed with him. You won't rest at all—and there are emotional considerations involved as well. Sit by his bed, hold him or rock him in a chair, sing to him, play quietly with him and tell him stories. Anything but an actual bed association.

BATHS

Give him his regular daily bath. He will feel more comfortable. A bath is often restful, too. If his temperature is above 104° and he seems very drowsy or excessively agitated, twitchy, or on the point of convulsive seizure, put him in a warm bath at once. Make the water comfortably warm—you don't need to shock him with cold water. You're trying to soothe him and relax him. Even a warm tub of water is cooler than his body temperature. He will gradually cool down. Keep him immersed for fifteen or twenty minutes and then get him out. Dry him quickly and put him in his regular night gear. If his temperature rises again later, and he seems uncomfortable, repeat the process as often as necessary.

Alcohol or tepid-water sponges or ice packs or wrapping in a wet sheet may be used, but they are often more upsetting than a warm bath. They may not be any more or as effective.

MEDICINES

You may give aspirin for fever or for pain if your youngster is not vomiting. The dose is one grain per year of age up to five years every four hours. Baby aspirin comes in 1¼ grain tablets. An adult aspirin tablet is 5 grains. This can be used by cutting it into quarters so that ¼ tablet equals one baby aspirin. Aspirin compound may be used, but other aspirin combinations are not needed. Stay with straight aspirin.

You can crush or dissolve the aspirin tablet and add it to some sweet food like jelly.

Vitamin C may also be of help in your child's defense against illness. It does not affect an infection directly.

Do not give medicines unless your doctor has given you specific instructions to do so. Self-medicating can produce some unhappy results.

CONVULSIONS

Fever may sometimes precipitate a convulsion. It may be your child's response to illness, just as a shaking chill is a response in an adult. Temperature doesn't have to be very high with some children to bring on a convulsion. A convulsion can be a frightening thing to you. It may be a more upsetting experience for you than it is for your child. It is not often dangerous in itself, but the average parent doesn't know this—or can't remember at the time. Permanent damage occurs not with the convulsion but because of the underlying condition.

As has been stressed before, *under no circumstances is teething ever a cause of convulsions.*

There may be some early signs of a coming convulsion. Your youngster looks a little out of touch, rather twitchy and overactive. Then he suddenly loses consciousness. His eyes roll back or become fixed and staring. He doesn't respond to you. His teeth clench and he holds himself rigid and tight. His breathing becomes noisier, heavier, and more difficult. He may show some blueness, or cyanosis, as he holds his breath. He may show spasm of his whole body, of one side, or of an arm or leg. This twitching can be with or without wetting or soiling his diaper. This spasm lasts a few minutes—it always seems much longer—and then he relaxes. More severe convulsions than the simple fever convulsion may accompany several serious diseases.

Delirium is another part of the same thing. There may be no convulsion or there may be a combination of both convulsion and delirium.

WHAT TO DO

No matter what its cause you may not shorten the convulsion. You do need to prevent your youngster from doing damage to himself—you must do nothing which will do damage to him either.

First—don't panic. Keep calm. Simple advice but hard to follow. A convulsion always seems to last longer than it actually does by the clock. Panic is contagious. Don't infect your child. Use your wits and not your anxiety in handling your child. Keep your voice quiet. Don't yell or shout. Touch him gently and confidently. Place him on a flat surface. Get objects away from him. Try to get him on his side or stomach to avoid breathing difficulties. Get a pad of cloth or handkerchief between his teeth to keep him from biting his tongue. Wrap him in a sheet or blanket to keep him from thrashing about.

When you call your doctor, keep your head. If he asks questions instead of springing into some kind of action, understand that he is seeking out the underlying cause.

Draw a tub of warm water and get him into it as quickly as you can, just as advised under "Fever." If he is con-

vulsing, you should have help to manage him. Don't forget
to check the temperature of the water before you dunk
him, in your excitement. Keep him in the tub until he relaxes and seems to respond somewhat. Fifteen to twenty
minutes is usual. *Don't leave him alone at any time,* of
course.

When he is ready to come out of the tub, lightly dress
and cover him. Let him sleep if he wants.

As noted under "Fever," alcohol or tepid-water rubs, ice
packs, or wrapping in a wet sheet can be used instead of the
bath, but they are more disturbing to the baby. After he is
thoroughly responsive, aspirin for sedation may be used.
Don't ever try to push anything down him when he is unconscious or not responding. Retub him if he seems about
to do the same thing again later. You will have to check
him frequently for a time and don't let him try to move
about on his own until you are certain of him.

If your baby has a generalized convulsion without a high
fever, prevent any injury to your child. Follow the previous
suggestions. Your doctor will have to determine the cause
behind this type of nonfever seizure.

FOOD REFUSAL

If your child suddenly refuses all his food, he may be
saying he is heading for trouble. A throat ache may be the
cause. He may have early feelings of nausea, which tell him
to be careful. If you insist on food at this point you may
start off a vomiting sequence. It is better for you to wait.
Let him skip a meal. Give fluids—and watch. Make certain
he gets nothing else to eat that you are not aware of.

VOMITING

If his nausea bubbles over into vomiting, or there is a
sudden attack of vomiting, you are alerted to the fact that
something is going on. It may or may not be serious. Un-

usual or sudden vomiting is another symptom by which your child tells you that he is ill. It doesn't tell you in what way he is ill, since vomiting can come not only with intestinal problems but with upper respiratory infection, beginning appendicitis, or as the aftermath of a head injury. It just says he isn't well. This type of vomiting is considerably greater in quantity than the baby's normal spitting back.

First, do not try to give anything by mouth for several hours. Let his intestinal apparatus rest and quiet down if it will.

Secondly, if he has vomited several times or is retching, get a special suppository to use to relieve his nausea and vomiting.

Call your doctor for directions.

Give some thought to what is causing his vomiting—food indiscretion, infection, intestinal problem, head injury. You need to observe, and report to your doctor so that he can arrive at a diagnosis. Again, vomiting is a symptom, not a disease.

GIVING A SUPPOSITORY

A suppository is a bullet-shaped object containing medication for special purposes. You insert the suppository into the rectum. Put your baby on his abdomen. Put Vaseline about the anal opening of the rectum. Slide the suppository into the opening about 1 to 1½ inches. You may gently push it in with your finger covered with a finger cot. It must go beyond the circular muscle at the opening of his rectum to remain in place. Keep your youngster quiet and gently squeeze his buttocks together for five minutes. Try to distract his attention to some other area.

After several hours have passed without further vomiting, start one-teaspoon amounts of water, weak sweet tea, 7-Up, or Coke. Repeat at ten-to-fifteen minute intervals for an hour—then start to increase each portion by a teaspoon, working up to six or eight teaspoons or more. The idea is to give small amounts frequently rather than large amounts less frequently. Don't let your baby take all he wants at first, or you may start the whole vomiting cycle over again.

If he doesn't want anything, leave him alone for several hours. Then try again. Don't start food until he has taken fairly large quantities of clear liquids without difficulty.

If he starts vomiting again, repeat the suppository and the sips-of-water routine—and be more cautious about increasing amounts the next time around.

As you increase fluids, you may use diluted sweet fruit juices, liquid gelatin, gelatin desserts, carbonated beverages, clear soups, broth, or bouillon.

After he has taken liquids comfortably and in adequate amounts, offer him any well-cooked food that is low in roughage and fat. You can offer a soft-cooked egg, bananas, ground lean meat, cooked vegetables or fruit, puddings or gelatins, custards, cereals, ice milk, toast, soda crackers. In the smaller baby start with cereal and banana or other fruit sauce.

Get back to his regular diet as he is able to take it. Let liquid milk or fatty foods be the last things added back to his diet.

Avoid a feeding problem at the end of his illness. If your child has had fever several days and wants little to eat, he naturally doesn't gain weight. He may even lose weight. This worries you the first time or two that it happens. When his fever is finally gone you can begin to work back to his regular diet. You may be impatient to feed him up again. Often he turns away from the foods which are first offered. If you urge meal after meal day after day, his appetite never picks up at all. He is not too weak to eat, but at the time his temperature went back to normal there was still enough infection in his body to bother his stomach and intestines. Just as soon as he looks at his first foods his digestive system warns him that he is not ready for them.

When you push or force food into your baby when he already feels nauseated because of illness, his disgust is built up more easily and rapidly than if he had a normal appetite to start with. He can acquire a long-lasting feeding problem in a few days' time if you persist in this.

Just as soon as his stomach and intestines have recovered from the effects of his illness and are in condition to digest most foods again, your child's hunger will come back with a bang—and not just to what it used to be. He usually is ravenous for a while in order to make up for lost time.

Your cue at the end of any illness is to offer your baby only the drinks and solids he wants without any urging. Wait patiently but confidently for signs that he is ready for more. If his appetite has not recovered in a week, your doctor should be consulted.

DIARRHEA

A change in your baby's bowel movements may be a symptom of trouble. This change may be anything from more frequent stools to a purging type of watery, fluid-losing bowel movements. This very messy, unpleasant symptom can be serious in a younger child because of possible heavy fluid loss leading to dehydration. Always pay attention to this symptom, since it may be a very uncomfortable affair for your child, and can indicate infection or intestinal disorder. This often goes with vomiting or abdominal cramping.

Give him only well-cooked, low-fat, low-roughage foods *without milk*. Urge clear liquids to compensate for the fluid loss he shows in his stools.

Your doctor may advise Kaopectate or a similar intestine-soother. The dose is usually one or two teaspoons every four hours or with each bowel movement. If this is not effective, he will order a special medication.

The cause of the diarrhea symptom needs to be found. This should be done as promptly as possible if the diarrhea is severe.

CONSTIPATION

Constipation is also a symptom—usually not of any serious illness but reflecting the amount of bulk coming down the intestine and the amount of water taken out. Some children have bowel movements only every few days—others have several a day.

When a child is ill, eats less, and has fever, he often shows fewer bowel movements. He not only dries uot the food residue in his bowel because he needs the fluid, but there is less food residue available.

As has been stressed before: Never give laxatives or drugs.

Your doctor may advise an enema. Enemas or suppositories are not to be used without his recommendation.

GIVING AN ENEMA

An enema is an injection of a liquid into the lower rectum, usually to produce a bowel movement. The fluid can be plain water, 1 pint of water with ½ teaspoon of salt, or whatever solution your doctor advises. An enema can be used also to administer fluid when a child is unable to take fluid by mouth. For your baby a bulb syringe is generally used.

Place your baby on his back or on his abdomen. Have a pad or towel under him to catch moisture. Try to get him to relax and remain quiet. Vaseline the tip of the syringe and gently insert into the anus to a depth of 1 to 1½ inches. Hold it in place. Slowly give three to four ounces of liquid for a young baby (up to eight ounces for a larger, older baby). When the liquid has been injected slowly, remove the tip, put him down on the towel or pad, and keep his buttocks squeezed together. Be prepared to catch the returning fluid.

If the enema is not expelled, you do not need to be concerned. It may mean he needed the fluid and absorbed it. You may have to repeat the enema.

BREATHING DIFFICULTIES

Irregularities in his breathing can be a distressing symptom for your youngster, and for you too. Hoarseness may be the first symptom you notice in your youngster when he is starting a throat infection. It is a symptom to be watched but not treated unless other symptoms occur with it. A croupy sound to his breathing means that you hear a noisy passage of air through his throat and vocal cords. If this goes along with increasing difficulty in getting air in and out, some blueness about his mouth, and pulling in of his lower chest with each breath, then you must contact your doctor at once. If his breathing is just noisy and he doesn't have any of the other symptoms, you can safely use steam vapor to give him relief.

Quick relief can sometimes be obtained by taking him into the bathroom and turning on the hot water to make a steam room. This is a great help when croup appears in the middle of the night, as it usually does.

You can use a vaporizer or cold steam machine if you

have one available. You can construct a vapor tent, but always be certain fire hazard is eliminated. A UDL-approved, cold steam unit is the best all-around type. Do not use a hot plate, boiling kettle, or any unprotected heat source.

Coughing can be of all varieties and degrees. It can be from an irritated throat, a discharge of material from the back of his nose, an allergic response, or the sign of a lower respiratory difficulty. Try the usual home remedies, such as honey and lemon juice. If a cough persists, check with your doctor for further measures to determine other treatment. Don't give any special cough mixtures oftener than the directions say.

Just because you hear a rattle in your child's chest when he coughs does not mean pneumonia. It means you are hearing or feeling the transmitted sound from the material rattling back and forth in the back of his throat.

SKIN RASHES

Any rash or sign of skin eruption should be considered as a possible sign of illness. If it appears with a fever or other symptoms, you should phone your doctor. He will usually have to see a rash to definitely diagnose its cause. But you can describe it as to location on the body. Does it vary from one spot to another? Does it itch? What does the rash look like: spotty, blotchy, little blisters, blush, scaling, dry, moist, crusts or scabs? Does it come and go?

Baking soda paste, calamine lotion, or any plain soothing ointment may help itching. Your doctor will have to examine the rash before any other measures can be taken. There is medication available to be taken internally to relieve itching.

(Check back to *The First Month,* "Baby-Care Routines," for more on skin rashes.)

BURNS

Do not put grease or oil of any kind on the damaged area. With small burns of the scalded-skin type, your doctor may prescribe a special cream to apply liberally to the area. With larger burns accompanied by blistering or loss of superficial skin, use the cream but avoid breaking the blister. Put the cream on liberally and cover the area with a dressing to protect the damaged skin. With serious burns do not put anything on the area except to cover it with a clean white cloth— and then get in touch with your doctor at once. He will tell you what to do next.

PIMPLES, BOILS, AND ABSCESSES

These are all skin infections. You must always treat them with respect. *Do not squeeze, pinch, or try to open them.* You will cause more damage and increase the risk of trouble if you do. Keep the skin well cleansed with soap and water. Your doctor may prescribe an antibiotic ointment. You may have to apply heat to the inflamed area with hot packs, hot soaks, a hot-water bottle or heating pad. Your doctor will decide when incision and drainage are indicated.

PAIN CRYING

If your baby is crying with pain, you may be frightened because you feel so helpless. He can't tell you where he hurts or how bad it is. Perhaps he will show you in other ways.

With a severe pain his crying may seem sharper, louder, and more persistent. There is a note of urgency and fright. If this comes at intervals with rests between, he tells you that it is an off-and-on pain or cramping. If he has a complaining, whimpering kind of continuous crying, it has a different meaning.

The way he holds himself and moves may give you another clue as to the source of his pain. He may claw at the side of his head or ear when he has a sore throat or earache. If his pain is in his abdomen, he lies quiet with his legs pulled up. Leg, neck, or back pains cause him to lie very still, since movement brings on pain. He may cry out and pull away if you touch the spot where he hurts. He may not have a local pain but may just feel miserable all over, so that he just cries, acts unhappy and uncomfortable.

You can check out the usual causes of discomfort discussed earlier in the section on *Crying*. If none of these seems likely, then look for further signs of illness and report to your pediatrician.

Appendix

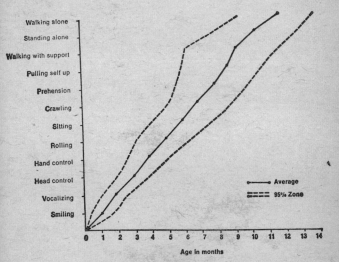

Fig. 52. First Year Development

This graph shows the average age for most infants to achieve each of the designated acts. (Modified from Aldrich, C.A., and Norval, M.A.: *J. Pediat.* 29:304, 1946)

RECORD OF WEIGHT AND GROWTH

Date	Age	Weight	Length

NOTES ON FORMULAS AND FEEDING

Date   *Notes*

IMMUNIZATION RECORD

POLIO—ORAL (SABIN)	Dates					
WHOOPING COUGH						
DIPHTHERIA						
TETANUS						
SMALLPOX						
RUBELLA						
MUMPS						
MEASLES						
TUBERCULIN TEST						

Bibliography

Ames, Louise Bates. *Child Care and Development.* Philadelphia: J. B. Lippincott, 1970.

Arety, Leslie Brainard. *Developmental Anatomy.* 7th ed. Philadelphia: W. B. Saunders, 1965.

Baldwin, Alfred L. *Theories of Child Development.* New York: John Wiley & Sons, 1968.

Breckenridge, Marian E. *Child Development.* 5th ed. Philadelphia: W. B. Saunders, 1965.

Bundeson, Herman N. *The Baby Manual.* New York: Simon & Schuster, 1944.

Chess, Stella, & Thomas, Alexander. *Your Child Is A Person.* New York: Viking Press, 1965.

Church, Charles F. *Food Values.* 11th ed. Philadelphia: J. B. Lippincott, 1970.

Erikson, Erik H. *Childhood & Society.* 2nd ed. New York: W. W. Norton, 1963.

Flanagan, Geraldine L. *First Nine Months of Life.* New York: Simon & Schuster, 1962.

Fomon, Samuel J. *Infant Nutrition.* Philadelphia: W. B. Saunders, 1967.

Fraiberg, Selma H. *The Magic Years.* New York: Charles Scribner Sons, 1959.

Gersh, Marvin J. *How to Raise Children at Home In Your Spare Time.* New York: Stein & Day, 1966.

Gesell, Arnold. *Infant and Child in Culture of Today.* New York: Harper & Brothers, 1943.

Gesell, Arnold. *First Five Years of Life.* New York: Harper & Brothers, 1940.

Goodrich, Frederick W., Jr. *Infant Care.* Englewood Cliffs, N. J.: Prentice Hall, 1968.

Heinz Co., H. J. *Nutritional Data.* 5th ed. Pittsburgh: H. J. Heinz Co., 1963.

Illingsworth, Ronald S. *The Normal Child.* 4th ed. Boston: Little Brown & Co., 1968.

461

Illingsworth, Ronald S. *Development of Infant & Young Child.* 3rd ed. Edinburgh: E. A. Livingston, 1966.

Jensen, Gordon D. *Well Child's Problems.* Chicago: Year Book Medical Publishers, 1962.

La Leche League. *Womanly Art of Breast Feeding.* Franklin Park, Ill.: La Leche League, 1963.

Langman, Jan. *Medical Embryology.* 2nd ed. Williams & Wilkins, 1969.

Lynch, Harold D. *Your Child Is What He Eats.* Chicago: Henry Regnery Co., 1958.

McGraw, Myrtle B. *Neuromuscular Maturation of Human Infant.* New York: Hafner Publishing Co., 1963.

Sachett, Walter W. *Bringing Up Babies.* Harper & Row, 1962.

Saltman, Jules. *Your New Baby & You.* New York: Grosset & Dunlap, 1966.

Schaffer, Alexander J. *Diseases of Newborn.* 2nd ed. Philadelphia: W. B. Saunders, 1965.

Shettles, Landrum B. *Ovum Humanum.* New York: Hafner Publishing Co., 1960.

Silver, Henry K. *Healthy Babies & Happy Parents.* New York: McGraw Hill, 1960.

Smith, Clement A. *Physiology of New Born Infant.* 3rd ed. Springfield, Ill.: Charles C Thomas, 1959.

Spock, Benjamin. *Baby & Child Care.* New York: Duell, Sloan & Pearce, 1946.

INDEX